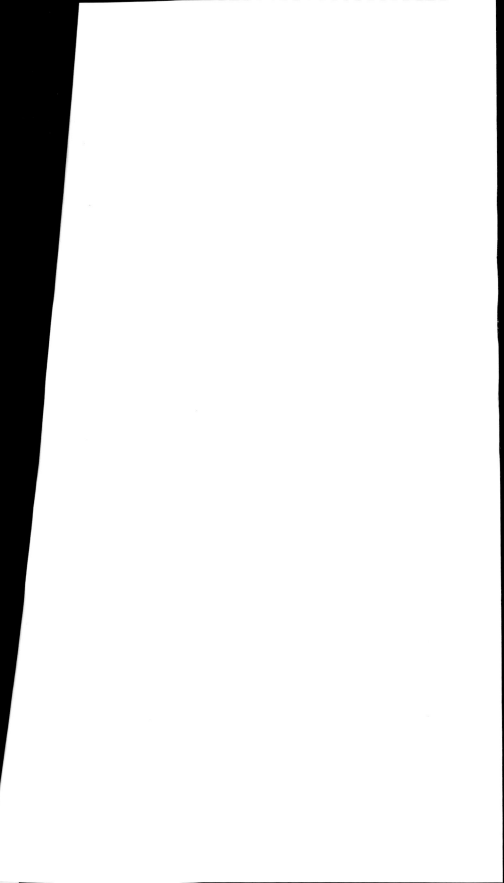

MOL
PATHOL
DRUG DISC
AND DEVELOP

MOLECULAR PATHOLOGY IN DRUG DISCOVERY AND DEVELOPMENT

Edited by

J. Suso Platero

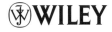

A JOHN WILEY & SONS, INC., PUBLICATION

Published by John Wiley & Sons, Inc., Hoboken, New Jersey
Published simultaneously in Canada

For general information on our other products and services or for technical support, please contact our Customer Care Department within the United States at (800) 762-2974, outside the United States at (317) 572-3993 or fax (317) 572-4002.

Wiley also publishes its books in a variety of electronic formats. Some content that appears in print may not be available in electronic formats. For more information about Wiley products, visit our web site at www.wiley.com.

Library of Congress Cataloging-in-Publication Data:

Molecular pathology in drug discovery and development / [edited by] J. Suso Platero.
      p. ; cm.
   Includes bibliographical Referencess and index.
   ISBN 978-0-470-14559-3 (cloth)
  1. Drug development.   2. Pathology, Molecular.   I. Platero, J. Suso.
   [DNLM: 1. Drug Design.   2. Molecular Biology–methods.   3. Pathology–methods.
4. Pharmacogenetics. QV 744 M7183 2009]
      RM301.25.M65 2009
      615'.19–dc22

                                                                          2008049906

Printed in the United States of America

10 9 8 7 6 5 4 3 2 1

To Begoña, Pablo, Santiago, Maria, Laura, Lucas, and Cecilia
the reason for my existence and to Joel C. Eissenberg, who taught me
how to do science

CONTENTS

9 MOLECULAR PATHOLOGY: IMMUNOHISTOCHEMISTRY ASSAYS IN DRUG DEVELOPMENT PERFORMED BY A CONTRACT RESEARCH LABORATORY **221**

Frank Lynch and Steve Bernstein

11 AQUA® TECHNOLOGY AND MOLECULAR PATHOLOGY 295

*Mark Gustavson, Marisa Dolled-Filhart, Jason Christiansen,
Robert Pinard, and David Rimm*

PREFACE

During the last few years there has been a great deal of public interest in the area of personalized medicine. News articles, scientific magazines, and entire books have been dedicated to the subject. While a lot has been said about the subject, there is little done in practice. Nowadays there are only a few examples of personalized medicine. One of them is the use of the HER2 diagnostic test, in breast cancer patients, in order to treat them with Herceptin, a drug that works well in that subpopulation. Other tests, like the estrogen receptor (ER) or the progesterone receptor (PR), are also used to put breast cancer patients in hormonal therapy. All these diagnostic tests could be characterized as molecular pathology tests.

My intent in putting this book together was to show others how one can develop new molecular pathology tests for use in personalized medicine. I have used the process of drug discovery and development as the outline of the book for a simple reason, the discovery of the molecular pathology test could be done at the same time that the drug is been discovered. In Chapter 1, Dr. Franz Fogt gives an overview and historical perspective of the field of molecular pathology, and I follow it with a simplified overview of the drug discovery and development process. Chapter 2 follows with a view of the drug discovery process and how molecular pathology could be used to identify and validate new drug candidates. Chapter 3 introduces the reader to the world of biomarkers, and how biomarkers could be found using transcriptional profiling. These biomarkers can then be used as surrogate endpoints, and molecular pathology could play a significant role in validating these biomarkers and developing tests for use in hospitals. This chapter is followed by examples of molecular pathology in safety assessment in the area of toxicology. It also gives an overview of toxicology and its methods to identify off-target liabilities of drugs in both small molecules and biological compounds. Chapter 5 looks at toxicogenomics, a new way of doing toxicology by looking at transcriptional profiling to identify genes that are relevant to the safety of compounds. This chapter is followed by the use of molecular pathology in clinical trials. Examples of how molecular pathology assays have helped identify the right dose for different drugs are shown. Not only is molecular pathology useful in finding the right dose but also in finding the right patients for treatment, which is discussed in Chapter 7. Here again is the area of personalized medicine that is directly affected by molecular pathology. Several examples are shown of how this is done today in the clinic. The following chapters deal more with direct applications of molecular pathology. Chapter 8 shows several examples of usage of molecular pathology in molecular therapy. Chapter 9 is a practical approach on how to do immunohistochemistry (IHC), one of the most important and useful techniques in molecular pathology. This chapter also indicates if you do not have the expertise in house how to use other companies, contract research organizations, to do this type of work. The last two chapters look more at the future of molecular pathology. Chapter 10 deals with the quantification of the colorimetric signal while Chapter 11 looks at fluorescence as a way to quantify and normalize the signal.

Color representations of selected figures in the book are available as pdf files at the following ftp site address:

ftp://ftp.wiley.com/public/sci_tech_med/molecular_pathology

I want to thank all the authors for their work. Each chapter has the contributions of people who are truly experts in their fields. Also, thanks to Jonathan Rose at John Wiley & Sons for his patience in guiding me through the whole process.

J. Suso Platero

Radnor, Pennsylvania
March 2009

CONTRIBUTORS

Dr. J. Albanell
Experimental Therapeutics Unit and Medical Oncology Department
IMIM-Hospital del Mar
Barcelona, Spain

Dr. Ricardo Attar
Ortho Biotech Oncology R&D
Centocor R&D
Radnor, Pennsylvania

Dr. David Berman
Global Clinical Research
Bristol-Myers Squibb
Princeton, New Jersey

Dr. Steve Bernstein
QualTek Molecular Laboratories
Goleta, California

Dr. Wayne R. Buck
Global Pharmaceutical Research and Development
Abbott Laboratories
Abbott Park, Illinois

Dr. Eric A. G. Blomme
Global Pharmaceutical Research and Development
Abbott Laboratories
Abbott Park, Illinois

Dr. Jason Christiansen
HistoRx, Inc.
New Haven, Connecticut

Dr. Marisa Dolled-Filhart
HistoRx, Inc.
New Haven, Connecticut

Dr. Franz Fogt
Chairman, Department of Pathology
Penn-Presbyterian Medical Center
University of Pennsylvania
Philadelphia, Pennsylvania

Dr. Mark Gustavson
HistoRx, Inc.
New Haven, Connecticut

Dr. Hewei Li
Discovery Medicine and Clinical Pharmacology
Bristol-Myers Squibb
Pennington, New Jersey

Dr. Cornelia Liedtke
Department of Breast Medical Oncology
University of Texas M. D. Anderson Cancer
Houston, Texas
 and
Department of Gynecology and Obstetrics
University of Münster
Münster, Germany

Dr. Matthew V. Lorenzi
Oncology Drug Discovery
Bristol-Myers Squibb
Princeton, New Jersey

Dr. Frank Lynch
QualTek Molecular Laboratories
Newtown, Pennsylvania

Dr. Raphael Marcelpoil
Senior Scientific Director
Becton Dickinson Biosciences
Le Pont de Claix, France

Dr. Robert Pinard
HistoRx, Inc.
New Haven, Connecticut

Dr. J. Suso Platero
Director Oncology Biomarkers
Centocor R&D
Radnor, Pennsylvania

Dr. Lajos Pusztai
Department of Breast Medical Oncology
University of Texas M. D. Anderson Cancer Center
Houston, Texas

Dr. Martha Quezado
Laboratory of Pathology, Surgical Pathology Section
National Cancer Institute
Bethesda, Maryland

Dr. David Rimm
Yale University School of Medicine
New Haven, Connecticut

Dr. F. Rojo
Pathology Department and Experimental Therapeutics Unit
IMIM-Hospital del Mar
Barcelona, Spain

Dr. A. Rovira
Experimental Therapeutics Unit
IMIM-Hospital del Mar
Barcelona, Spain

Dr. Brent A. Rupnow
Oncology Drug Discovery
Bristol-Myers Squibb
Princeton, New Jersey

Dr. Rolf-P. Ryseck
Oncology Drug Discovery
Bristol-Myers Squibb
Princeton, New Jersey

Dr. S. Serrano
Pathology Department
IMIM-Hospital del Mar
Barcelona, Spain

Dr. W. Fraser Symmans
Department of Pathology
University of Texas M. D. Anderson Cancer Center
Houston, Texas

Dr. Carlos A. Torres-Cabala
Assistant Professor, Department of Pathology
University of Texas M. D. Anderson Cancer Center
Houston, Texas

Dr. Richard A. Westhouse
Department of Discovery Toxicology
Bristol-Myers Squibb
Princeton, New Jersey

MOLECULAR PATHOLOGY AND DRUG DEVELOPMENT

Franz Fogt and J. Suso Platero

1.1. GENERAL PATHOLOGY

The histopathologic assessment of tissues and, for that matter, body fluids serves to diagnose alterations and disease state and helps to categorize and collect information about disease. The pathologic assessment of tissues and organs itself is a stepwise process of progressive analysis of the present disease, and the next possible finding one can describe with (relative) certainty. This is, naturally, only possible when a sufficient amount of tissue is submitted to pathology. If fluid material, only cells present in that specimen can be assessed and further evaluation can mostly not be done with certainty. For the diagnosis of a colon carcinoma, a microscope is rarely necessary. When opened, the colon will reveal the tumor, the size, and, at least semiquantitatively, the invasive depth. However, to assess the correct depth and the type of carcinoma, a section of the tissue must be reviewed with the microscope. The next necessary diagnostic step to categorize, grade, and stage the lesion is the review of the lymph nodes as to their involvement by metastatic disease. Traditional histopathology uses the morphologic aspects of tissue and cellular arrangement to provide diagnosis as to the cellular origin of malignant tumors.

Similarly, morphologic features can be used to predict behavior and outcome of malignant tumors and can influence the way certain tumors are treated. This is illustrated by the relative bland morphology of bronchioloalveolar carcinomas of the lung with a relatively benign outcome compared to the guarded outcome of poorly differentiated small-cell carcinomas of the same organ. In the case of colorectal carcinomas, the morphologic aspect of tumor transgressing through all layers of the bowel wall and its presence as metastatic tumor within lymph nodes indicates a higher stage of disease and predicts a guarded outcome. At the same time, based on such information, specific treatment, that is, chemotherapy, radiation, and surgery can be initiated.

1.2. GENERAL ASPECTS

Molecular pathology generally describes the aspect of pathology that is removed from the purely histologic aspect of diagnosis and uses information on the molecular level for diagnosis and prediction of outcome. Thus, the molecular aspect of pathology deals with identification of genes and the subsequent change in cellular architecture and expression of proteins in a given disease. Taken in such broad terms, molecular pathology is something pathologists have done for a long time, even before biochemical techniques were invented to analyze cellular DNA. Application of molecular pathology was used to imply the analysis of cellular structures at the electron microscope level or the analysis of proteins within the cell (Roizin, 1964). Staying with malignant tumors, identification of specific proteins within tumor cells can aid in the diagnosis of cellular origin, which may be important for both diagnostic and therapeutic purposes. The presence of tumor within the lung that expresses prostate-specific antigen (PSA) will undoubtedly define this tumor as a metastatic lesion and exclude a pulmonary primary tumor. These proteins may be visualized both by immunohistochemistry, that is, staining with immunohistochemical stains for PSA in case of prostate carcinoma, or by histochemical methods, that is, visualization of mucins with mucicarmin stain for other lesions. These examples use the expression of normal proteins in a tumor, which is, naturally, gene driven. Further assessment of tumors can identify expression of proteins that are not normally expressed in normal cells and, again, be of diagnostic use. The wild type of the p53 protein is a short-lived protein. The probability to have wild-type protein present in a given cell at a given time is quite low, and, thus, staining of tissues that contain wild-type p53 will result in a negative staining. Mutated p53, on the other hand, has a long half-life, will be present in tissues containing that protein, and will stain positive for p53, indicating its abnormal presence (Rom et al., 2000).

1.3. MOLECULAR PATHOLOGY, THE MOLECULAR WAY

The genetic code represents a specific code of four desoxynucleotides, which combine with complementary strands of DNA. When isolated from the nucleus, DNA usually breaks easily at random areas, resulting in DNA strands of various lengths making it difficult to impossible to analyze a specific area of a DNA strand. The invention of restriction endonucleases in the 1970s allowed for the first time to produce specific DNA fragments of defined areas and length. This allowed identification of specific DNA sequences when those DNA strands were, after detachment from their complemetary strands, hybridized with marked deoxy-nucleotide oligonuceotide complementary strands. Such strands with known sequence, usually radioactive marking, have been produced in the laboratory and could be performed with the enzyme DNA polymerase. The idea that DNA poly-merase was also able to multiply in an exponential fashion a specific strand of DNA flanked by oligonucleotide primers was first introduced by Mullis in the early 1980s (Mullis, 1990). The first methods to use polymerase chain reaction (PCR) for diagnostic purposes were applied to the diagnosis of hemoglobin diseases in the mid-1980s (Saiki et al., 1985). This technique allows one to analyze the genetic abnormalities that make up specific parts of the DNA and to analyze alterations that are represented within the genome. One such technique would be the analysis of loss of heterozygosity (LOH). Here, one assumes that all genetic alleles are present in duplicate within a given somatic cell. Those alleles may be identical, called homozygous, or slightly different, called heterozygous. In tissues with het-erozygous alleles comparisons can be made to malignant tissues within the same body by testing for LOH. Primers flanking the alleles of choice are produced and the DNA strand of interest is multiplied and analyzed. If the normal tissue con-tinues to show two distinct allele bands but the tumor has lost one of the two bands, the tumor is said to show LOH of the given gene tested. Other abnormali-ties may be analyzed with the same basic technique by sequencing the DNA strand of interest to assess whether the base pair sequence differs from the normal tissue.

1.3.1. Loss of Gene Expression

The previous example of p53 expression representing the assessment of cellular proteins is the result of genetic alterations, specifically the loss of genetic function of the *p53* gene. Typical examples for loss of function of genes are mutation, methylation, loss of heterozygosity, and so forth. Inappropriate silencing of genes through the mechanism of methylation has been described specifically in tumors of the gastrointestinal tract in patients with hereditary nonpolyposis colorectal cancers (HNPCC) (Chen et al., 2007). Methylation of genes or promoter regions of genes can inhibit the function of the genes or promoter regions and result in loss of genetic function without change in the sequence of the genetic code. In vertebrates a methyl group is bound to the 5-carbon of a cytosine base, which is located next to a guanine through the enzyme DNA methyltransferase, resulting in a CpG dinucleotide pair. The effect of methylated DNA on transcription is probably not related to its physical change but more by abnormal protein binding capacities (Wajed et al., 2001). Microsatellite instability (MSI), on the other hand, is a situation in which a microsatellite allele changed the number of repeat units resulting in a change of length. If this change is present in a given neoplasm, it can be concluded that this neoplasm is monoclonal. One of the first lesions in which MSI has been observed was HNPCC, where it was associated with defects in the DNA repair mechanism. Involved genes of MSI were *hMLH1*, *hMSH2*, and *hMSH6*. Normal DNA repair will correct the mutation, but in patients with deficient mismatch repair function, a high percentage of mutation risk is present, which can also affect coding of DNA regions. If regions involving proliferation or programmed cell death are affected, cancer can develop. This genomic expression of MSI can be tested in family members, and affected persons can undergo regular surveillance examinations (Baudhuin et al., 2005). Such testing involves the analysis of tumor and nontumor tissue and the comparison of dinucleotide repeats between the tissues. To evaluate for low microsatellite instable and high microsatellite instable patterns, five markers have to be tested. If at least two markers show mutational pattern, the tumor is said to be high microsatellite instabile (Fig. 1.1).

Other tumors may show loss of heterozygosity of specific tumor suppressor genes. Here, two alleles of the tumor suppressor gene are present with one of the alleles being genetically altered, that is, silenced. If the second allele, which must have been genetically stable, is damaged by a second hit, that allele may no longer be present but only the one previously nonfunctional. Those changes may be present as germ cell mutations, such as hereditary retinoblastoma or acquired as in cases of usual colorectal adenomatous polyps.

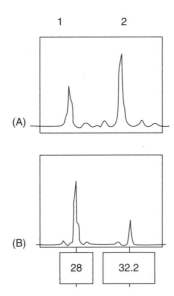

Figure 1.1. Microsatellite instability. Set (A) represents normal tissue. Lanes 1 and 2 show almost equal size of the two heterozygous alleles 28 and 32.2, respectively. Set (B), representing tumor, shows a >50% loss of height at marker 32.2 (lane 2). This loss represents LOH. (Courtesy of Zoran Budimlija, Department of Forensic Biology, Office of the Chief Medical Examiner, New York, New York.)

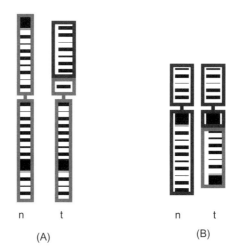

n   t   n   t
(A)   (B)

<u>Figure 1.2.</u> Translocation. Translocation defines the exchange of fragments of DNA between chromosomes. The figure shows normal chromosomes (A) and (B) (n) and the same chromosomes after translocation of fragments of DNA has been taking place (t).

1.3.2. Translocations

Molecular pathologic analysis of specific tumors is also of diagnostic use both in routine cases, such as malignant lymphomas, and in the diagnosis of soft tissue sarcomas, which may show signature genetic aberrations diagnostic for a specific disease entity and possibly predictive for specific tumor behavior. In lymphomas, genetic analysis may reveal specific translocations and predict the development of genetic alterations that make mucosa-associated lymphoid tissue (MALT) tumor of the stomach no longer susceptible for antibiotic therapy. Translocation is the rearrangement of fragments of chromosomes that are nonhomologous. They are usually denoted as t(A;B) indicating that the translocation is between chromosome A and B and $(q_x; p_x)$, indicating the location on gene A and B, respectively; p and q stand for short and long arm of chromosomes (Fig. 1.2).

In soft tissue sarcomas, histologic similarity between spindle cell sarcomas may make it difficult to diagnose with certainty the presence of synovial sarcoma. The tumor-specific translocation (tX;18) can aid in the diagnosis of synovial sarcoma and lead to specific therapeutic intervention (Fig. 1.3).

1.3.3. Detection of Pathogens

In nonmalignant aspects of disease, molecular pathologic techniques may be able to detect specific pathogens, that is, viruses and bacteria, associated with disease. The typical examples here are the genetic detection of specific viruses in patients with human papilloma virus infections. Here, the routine genetic testing for specific virus types has not only led to therapy and surveillance for specific patient

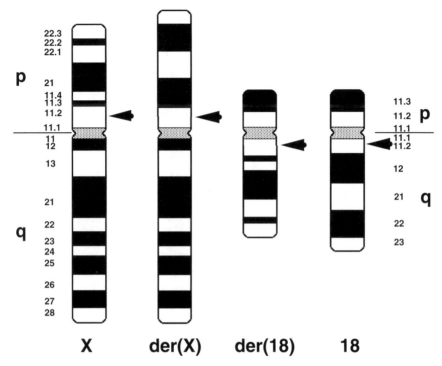

Figure 1.3. Synovial sarcoma x;18 Translocation. t(X;18)(p11.2;q11.2) in synovial sarcoma G-banding; substitution of the 8 last amino acids of SYT by 78 amino acids of SSX1 and SSx2. (Courtesy of Dr. Frederic Barr, University of Pennsylvania, Philadelphia.)

populations, but is, at least indirectly, involved in the recent successful development of vaccine for high-risk human papilloma virus infection. In addition, the molecular biologic techniques can be used to compare genetic information of current pathogens with historic pathogens, such as comparison of the current bird flu H5N1 and the virus that caused the 1918–1920 influenza pandemic (Wang et al., 2007).

1.3.4. Forensic Identification

At the same time, molecular pathologic techniques may be applied to assess for presence of specific normal genes when attempting to identify origin of tissues, that is, identification of unknown persons/victims. The theory is that, although the DNA between one human to the next is rather identical, short repetitive DNA areas exist, which are known as polymorphisms. Short tandem repeats (STR) are such short sequences of DNA, 2 to 5 base pairs in length, which are quite individual in different persons. By testing 9 to 15 such areas of STR, the probability that one person shares the exact STR with another person within a specific

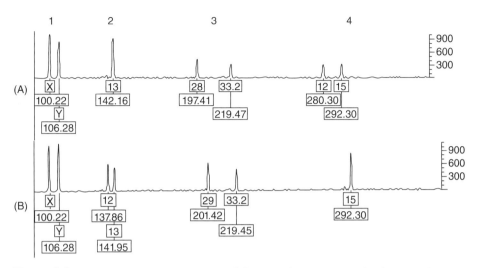

Figure 1.4. Forensic STR testing. Two runs of short tandem repeats. Individual A and B. STD 1 and 3 are shared by both individuals. For STD 2, individual A is homozygote (single peak at point 13), whereas individual B is heterozygote with two peaks at 12 and 13. Similarly at STD 4, individual A is heterozygote with two peaks and individual A homozygote with one peak. These features indicate probability that the individuals tested are not identical.

regional pool of persons decreases at least logarithmically and allows the determination of the origin of specific tissue samples (Fig. 1.4) (Tamaki et al., 1996).

1.3.5. Protein Changes

Assessment of specific DNA alterations, such as mutations, may indicate a specific tumorigenic pathway, but the changes in the DNA may not necessarily predict whether the altered DNA leads to altered protein expression downstream. Areas in which genetic alterations and specific protein expression patterns have been observed are specifically evident in the expression of c-Herb in carcinomas of the breast or in staining for *hMLH1* in colorectal carcinomas of patients with familial nonpolyposis colorectal cancer. Both have been used to specify further diagnosis of disease but also for therapeutic application. In patients with proven c-Herb expression, specific treatment options can be used, which are not applicable in tumors not expressing this protein. In patients with familial colorectal cancers that are microsatellite instable, the diagnosis of MSI will lead to more frequent surveillance and examination of other organ systems prone to develop tumors in this state of disease. Testing for epidermal growth factor receptor (EGFR) in patients with epithelial carcinomas has led to treatment options with antibodies to EGFR in expression-positive patient populations.

Testing for the presence of altered, that is, increased or mutated, messenger ribonucleic acid (RNA) may provide more insight into the effect of genetic

DNA-based alterations on the development of tumors. Messenger-RNA-dependent protein expression may again provide additional insight into the alterations that resulted from the original DNA damage. Thus, the circle to the analysis of cellular proteins is closed.

1.3.6. Other Methods of Detection

Beside the immunohistochemical analysis of cellular proteins, newer techniques allow for the analysis of vast amounts of proteins present in a given tissue substrate. Proteomic analysis uses two-dimensional gel electrophoresis to dissociate proteins that can subsequently be isolated and sequenced both for identification of the native protein and the presence of mutated forms of a specific protein. Newer proteomic techniques allow for dissociation and analysis with a one-step procedure. Protein signatures can be used to identify tumors or predict presence of tumors when found in surveillance specimens, for example, serum analysis. Historically, the time from the determination of the correct number of human chromosones in 1956 (Tjio and Levan, 1956) to the discovery of constant genetic alterations in malignant disease process such as chronic myelogenous leukemia (Nowell and Hungerford, 1960) was very short. To date most human genes have been deciphered and a vast number of disease processes has been linked to specific genetic alterations, and a much fewer number of those genetic alterations have been specifically used for pharmacologic application.

1.4. APPLICATION OF MOLECULAR PATHOLOGY

How molecular pathology has aided in the understanding of the development of the malignant phenotype may be underscored by the discovery of differences in colorectal carcinomas. It has been shown previously that colorectal carcinomas develop frequently from adenomas, which are adenomatous polyps found in the colon of patients. At the same time, there is a familial disease in which patients develop thousands of adenomas and have a 100% certainty to develop invasive tumor by age 50. Early molecular pathologic studies have shown that these tumors follow a specific stepwise progression with accumulation of chromosomal damage that leads to the invasive phenotype. The same stepwise progression was found in patients with single adenomatous polyps and is the base for the adenoma-carcinoma pathway of the majority of colorectal carcinomas (Fig. 1.5).

However, it was soon noted that not all carcinomas are associated with polypoid adenomatous precursors and that there are tumors that are histologically different from the typical adenoma-associated tumors. Following the histologic findings, analysis of chromosomal aberrations showed that many of those tumors are associated with a lack in the DNA repair mechanisms, such as *hMLH1*, *hMSH2*, and *hMSH6*. Those tumors with microsatellite instability are the result of methylation of the normal DNA repair mechanisms that lead to the clonal proliferation of DNA-damaged cell populations that would have otherwise

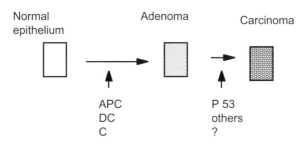

Normal epithelium   Adenoma   Carcinoma

APC
DC
C

P 53
others
?

<u>Figure 1.5.</u> Adenoma carcinoma pathway. Stepwise progression of genetic changes from normal colonic mucosa to the development of adenoma and finally invasive carcinoma. Cumulative genetic alterations lead to dysplastic features of cell populations and development of invasive phenotype.

undergone DNA repair. Analysis of these tumors resulted in the finding of other associated tumors in this syndrome, namely uterine and ovarian carcinomas. Analysis of family members can aid in the timely diagnosis of this disease and adequate prophylactic surveillance studies. Additionally, histologic observation that some hyperplastic colonic polyps, which are typically harmless proliferations, are associated with fast proliferationg tumors, lead to the genetic analysis of those lesions. The analysis of these tumors showed that there are in fact specific *BRAF* mutations followed by methylation defects leading to dysplasia and invasive phenotype (Higashidani et al., 2003). Similar lesions in yet another form of colonic carcinoma show hyperplastic-like polyps with histologic changes that are representative of dysplasia. Those serrated adenomas follow a genetic progression different from the above described ways in that those tumors have changes in the *Kras* gene and develop DNA repair defects through the MGMT (O6-methylguanine-DNA-methyltransferase methylation) pathway (Hiyama et al., 1998). It should be of note that in all of these lesions, specific histologic differences between these tumors had been described before implication of molecular pathology and that molecular pathologic data have supported the diagnostic differences and expanded the knowledge of these lesions.

In fact, many systematic molecular pathologic analyses of lesions follow histologic differences made by observant pathologists. Hyperplastic polyps have for the longest time been considered nonneoplastic lesions. Pathologists have described lesions that are very similar to hyperplastic polyps but that have a high malignant potential. Those sessile serrated adenomas show very little histologic difference to hyperplastic polyps, but subtle differences in the glandular structure and the extent of hyperplastic cells along the crypts were a constant feature with polyps associated with malignant tumors.

Molecular pathologic studies not only showed that these polyps are, in fact, different from hyperplastic polyps, they were able to define an entirely new pathway of malignant progression (Makinen, 2007). Whereas many molecular changes have been supporting morphologic observations, other molecular pathologic changes may precede histologic changes visible through the microscope. In ulcerative colitis, normal appearing colonic mucosa is apparently not affected by the disease process as the histologic features show no significant abnormalities. It has been shown, however, that early genetic alterations that are carried through the stages of low-grade dysplasia, high-grade dysplasia, and invasive carcinoma are already present in histologically normal tissues (Fogt, 1998). This has been shown to be the case in Barrett's esophagus as well, where metaplastic epithelium carries early genetic changes, that is, LOH of the *APC* gene, which are carried through the dysplasia carcinoma progress (Zhuang et al., 1996). Similarly, the observation of blood vessel and clear-cell proliferation in hemagioblastomas in patients with von Hippel Lindau syndrome were thought to represent the proliferation of all genetically altered tissues involved in this tumor (Vortmeyer et al., 1997). Molecular pathologic analysis of these lesions, however, demonstrated clearly that the blood vessels are benign proliferations, which follow the proliferation of the genetically altered clear cells.

1.5. MOLECULAR PATHOLOGY IN DRUG DEVELOPMENT

Application of molecular pathology to drug development has been specifically successful in treatment of chronic myelogenic leukemia (CML) and gastrointestinal stromal tumors. The *BCR-ABL* gene in cell-mediated lysis and the *c-kit*-associated fusion genes in gastrointestinal stromal tumor (GIST) result in an altered tyrosine kinase. Whereas the normal tyrosine kinase is inactivated by the binding of its own terminal phosphotyrosine (P) with the activation center, in *c-kit*-positive GIST tumors, this phosphotyrosine cannot bind and inactivate in the genetically altered tyrosine kinase. Here, molecular pathology has proven its place in the pharmaceutical arena with the development of a molecule that can fit into the activation center binding site. Imatinib mesylate (Gleevec) has been introduced as highly potent therapy to suppress the uninhibited activation of the genetically altered tyrosine kinase by binding as an alternative molecule into the inaccessible activation center of the *c-kit*-altered molecule. This treatment has been applied with a high rate of success in chromic myelogenic leukemia and in patients with gastrointestinal stromal tumors that demonstrate similar changes in the tyrosine kinase protein.

The obvious problem that divides the purely academic application of molecular pathology to the pharmaceutical aspect is the way research is performed and supported. The discovery of specific mutations in a given malignant tumor may indicated a pathway of disease development from its earliest beginnings toward the invasive phenotype. This has been shown in colorectal carcinomas, with the *APC* gene on chromosome 5q21 being the first step in the progression from the normal epithelium to dysplastic epithelium. Additional stepwise progression of genetic damage has been shown to lead to advanced malignant and invasive phenotype and, later on, to metastatic phenotype. This kind of progression has been shown to exist in other organ systems as well, such as development of melanomas from dysplastic nevi and the development of breast carcinomas from noninvasive precursor lesions. Unfortunately, there is rarely one single mutation or genetic loss, through whichever mechanism, that can be pinpointed as the truly first step toward tumorigenesis. The *c-kit* story is the famous exception here; the academic research approach in this field, as has been the case when immunohistochemistry was first discovered as a powerful tool to diagnose tumors, is, in many, but clearly not all cases, the categorizations of genetic alterations in given tumors. This may be reflected by the development of a cancer genome atlas that is to be developed to list all genetic alterations, mutations, loss of heterozygosity, and genetic loss found in specific tumors. This is likely not to be helpful in the development of pharmaceutics' progress in cancer treatment as the multitude of genetic alterations will not likely be reversed by acting on one genetic change. Additionally, the listing of genetic alterations is not likely to be followed in the foreseeable future to a cause and reaction analysis. Furthermore, analysis of the main tumor for genetic alterations may not catch the subtle alterations of some tumor clones that will acquire the possibility not only to invade surrounding tissues but the ability to cause metastatic disease, which is what kills the vast majority of cancer patients.

1.5.1. Most Important Molecular Pathologic Consideration

The most important aspect when dealing with molecular pathology research is the quality of the tissue in question. When specific tumors are reviewed for molecular pathologic differences or specificities, large numbers of tumors may be obtained from collaborative researchers or from tissue banks. Banked tissues represent small amounts of tumor tissue, usually cut at the working bench, for storage and later research. The labeling of the tumor will be the same as the final pathology diagnosis. Some tissue banks will include quality measures by sectioning at the borders of the tissue and at least review for presence of tumor and/or presence of viable tissue. Not in all cases will the original diagnosis be confirmed on the sections. The tissue blocks received from outside suppliers therefore may or may not contain significant amounts of true tumor and, if necessary, viable tumor, within the specimen. Often a tissue bank specimen will contain mostly necrotic tumor elements; in other cases much of the tissue may represent reactive tissue surrounding tumor material. Before implementing any kind of studies, it is necessary to have the material that is being worked on reviewed by a trained pathologist to ensure that both tumor material and the correct tumor diagnosis is being studied. Depending on the source of the tissues for research, lesions may be solely marked by diagnoses such as the "adenocarcinoma of stomach." It should be noted that such diagnoses will not suffice to characterize the tissue for research sufficiently. One should not combine in a gastric carcinoma study the usual intestinal-type adenocarcinomas with its signet ring cell counterpart, as the cell of origin and the biology of these tumors are quite different. The same is true for many other tumors in different organ systems. Blindly trusting that tumor material is present in the tissue obtained will lead to diluted results, wrong conclusions, and an increase in the cost of research. When reviewing the results of a study, it is again necessary to ensure that the data are read from malignant tissue and not from benign counterparts or reactive tissues. This may be done by having cases reviewed by pathologists after staining of tissues for immunohisto-chemical stains, fluorescence in situ hybridization (FISH), or other in situ stains on the slide. When tissues are removed from the slide for microdissection, again, this should be done after a pathologist has marked the tumor areas on the slide in question or a slide of a deeper section. Optimally, microdissection is performed with a trained pathologist reviewing the microdissection itself.

1.6. PHARMACEUTICAL DRUG DEVELOPMENT

1.6.1. Introduction

The drug development process is a long and arduous road. Nowadays, it takes a compound around 10 years from the time it is discovered to the time it is approved and able to be used by the general population. In addition, it is esti-mated that the costs associated with developing a new drug are from around $800 million to a billion dollars. And the costs are getting higher and higher each year. It is not our intention to give an exhaustive review of the drug development process in this chapter; rather we want to use this as a general overview of the process. There are a lot of good books published on the subject that can be used if a more thorough knowledge of the subject is wanted. An understanding of the overall process is necessary to better understand the role that molecular pathol-ogy can play during this process.

1.6.2. Drug Discovery and Development

The whole process of drug discovery and development is summarized in sche-matic form in Figure 1.6. Each step comprises multiple processes with variable amounts of experimentation associated with them. Several of the steps could be carried out one at a time or simultaneously in order to finish the process in the least amount of time possible. The faster the development of a compound the less cost and greater benefit will be achieved. The role that molecular pathology can play in each of the steps will be expanded in later chapters.

Target Discovery. In order to develop a drug candidate first the clinical condition is identified that needs to be address. Nowadays the question that most people ask themselves is what the unmet medical need is. This need could be in

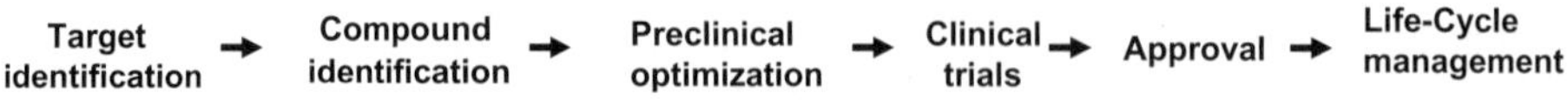

Target identification → Compound identification → Preclinical optimization → Clinical trials → Approval → Life-Cycle management

Figure 1.6. Simplified drug development process.

several fields, cardiovascular, metabolics, immunology, or cancer to name a few. Once the specific medical need is identified the druggability of the process is ascertained. This may require obtaining a better understanding of the disease. This part could be done by reviewing the existing literature in the field and additionally by carrying out experiments to focus in a particular molecule that may play a role in such disease.

Biology is the main driver in this step. Techniques associated with classical biology, like genetics, are employed to find new genes that may lead to new targets. One example of this is in finding drugs in the area of cancer. Cancer is a disease that has been proposed to arise due to mutations in certain genes. It is a stepwise process requiring several mutations to be present for a full-blown expression of the disease. One theory is the two-hit theory developed by Horowitz and colleagues. They postulate that one hit is needed for the cancerous condition to arise and the second hit arises in order for the disease to spread (Horowitz et al., 1990). One of the genes that have been shown to play a role in the cancer pathway is the retinoblastoma gene. This gene plays a major role in the development of a malignant tumor of the retina. The gene is a tumor suppressor, which means that its absence in the cells leads to the development of cancer in the retina. Therefore, this gene may be a target for making a drug. Once this gene has been identified as a key regulator of cancer progression, the biological pathway in which this gene is found could provide several additional targets. If the literature does not provide the pathway genes, then experimental approaches could be utilized. One way that has been used in the past is by identifying other proteins that interact with this gene. One method to do this type of work is by using the genetics of the fruit fly, *Drosophila melanogaster*. Using screens in these animals can lead to the identification of new genes that play a role in cancer. Such a type of screen led to the identification of a new gene, a novel peptidyl prolyl isomerase gene that could be a new target of anticancer agents (Edgar et al., 2005).

Another approach to identify new targets is by looking at proteins already known to be involved in the progression of cancer. An example of this could be the EGFR in colon cancer. This molecule plays a crucial role in the development of this cancer. The EGFR molecule was then chosen to become a target for the development of drugs. Today, there are several EGFR inhibitors on the market. These inhibitors can take several forms; they can be either small-molecules or antibodies. Iressa is an example of the small-molecule inhibitor, which are small molecules synthesized in the laboratory or isolated from nature. The antibodies can be divided into humanized antibodies (a chimeric mouse human antibody that has been modified to elicit no immunological response) and in human antibodies. They have the advantage of being more selective and they tend to have fewer side effects. Erbitux is an example of a humanized antibody, and panitumumab is an example of a fully human antibody. All three of them have been developed as therapeutic agents and are currently available to cancer patients (Mendelsohn and Baselga, 2000; Amado et al., 2008). A consequence of developing these drugs has been the declining mortality of colon cancer over the past few years, demonstrating that this approach to find targets is very useful.

With the advent of the genomics revolution, methodologies that explore the whole human genome are being currently used to find new targets in diseases. Some of those technologies are transcriptional profiling, which will identify all the messenger RNAs (mRNAs) present in a specific sample, proteomics, which will find out the proteins present in the sample of interests, or SNPs (single nucleotide polymorphism) used to find changes in the DNA sequence that may lead to mutant proteins or proteins that are overexpressed.

Identification of a Drug Candidate. Once the protein has been identified to target, we need to find out how to suppress its function. Chemistry, and recently biotechnology, plays the most important role in this arena. There are now two classes of molecules that can be developed to be used as drugs, one is the small inhibitors, chemical entities produced through synthetic chemical reactions or isolated from nature. The other is antibodies, large molecules that are produced in cells through new biotechnology techniques. These molecules are also called biologics to distinguish them from the chemical entities.

Pharmaceutical companies have used the products of chemistry synthesis to discover and refine the small molecules that target specific compounds. One such example is the development of a small molecular inhibitor named dasatinib (Sprycel is its commercial name). This molecule inhibits the *src-abl* oncogene, the main culprit in the disease associated with the Philadelphia chromosome. The presence of such chromosome leads to the development of chronic myeloid leukemia, a devastating type of cancer. The *src-abl* gene was identified as the culprit protein in the translocation whose aberrant function leads to leukemia. Therefore, pharmaceutical companies targeted the protein by making small molecules that were able to knock out the function of the chimeric protein. Chemical synthesis of a battery of related compounds was used to screen for the best candidate to inhibit the *src-abl* oncogene. Upon the production of these compounds, they were further screened for their ability to inhibit other tyrosine kinases and for their antiproliferative effect in human cells and xenographs (Lombardo et al., 2004). Xenographs are human cancerous cells grown in nude mice, mice lacking the immune system. They are a wonderful in vivo model for mimicking human cancers in mice. After the cancers are grown, they are tested for the activities of the compounds. Such models allow for the screening of numerous small-molecule inhibitors before they are even tried in human subjects.

A different way to reduce the function of a target protein is to use antibodies against the molecule that block its properties. This approach has been pioneered by biotech companies and is now widely used. The main advantage of this approach is the increase in specificity due to the use of antibodies. This specificity tends to lead to a decrease in toxicity because there is less off-target effects than using small-molecule inhibitors. While the difference in toxicity and specificity are important, a bigger difference is the manufacturing process required to produce such antibodies. Instead of using chemical synthesis, monoclonal antibodies are produced in cells. The cells are grown in incubators and the antibodies purified from them. The process is not as controlled as the chemical synthesis, and there are greater variations in lot to lot that need to be carefully monitored. One such example is Erbitux. This molecule is a humanized monoclonal antibody that specifically targets the EGF receptor. It binds to the receptor blocking the signaling from the receptor to its downstream targets (Mendelsohn and Baselga, 2000). This is an important process in colon cancer; blocking this pathway leads to the disappearance of certain types of colon cancers.

Obviously, this is an iterative process. Using either small molecules or antibodies as starting materials, new rounds of compounds or antibodies are tested until the desired characteristics are found. Once that is achieved the compound is now ready for further testing.

Preclinical Optimization. After the identification of a small molecule or an antibody, the next step is to test the compound for toxicities. This testing is administered in vitro and in vivo settings. In vitro refers to the testing conducted in cells in the laboratory, while in vivo refers to the testing carried out in animals. In vivo analysis is required before the drugs are applied to humans. Here the important point to consider is what are the potential side effects or toxicities associated with the compound. Testing is initialized with small animals such as rats and then moved to higher animals such as dogs and chimpanzees. Pathology plays a major role here. Compounds are dosed to find the maximum tolerated dose in each animal species, and pathology is often used as one of the methods to try to find the mechanism of toxicity. After the animals display physical symptoms of side effects, a full physical and pathological examination is carried out. Organs are taken from the animals and examined under the microscope for morphological changes in all the tissues. Here is where classical pathology is doing most of the work in the pharmaceutical development process. Here is also an opportunity to start using molecular pathology. The pathology could give us clues regarding the mechanism of action of the toxicity. This could point to a specific pathway, which can then be investigated using molecular pathology to specifically ask what proteins, mRNA, or DNA are doing in those tissues where the toxicity is observed, thus blurring the lines between classical histopathology and molecular pathology.

If a specific mechanism of action is found for the compound, or a particular side effect is identified, this is a great place to start developing assays that could point them out later during clinical trials. After examining all the experimental results of the in vivo and in vitro experiments and determining what an adequate toxicological profile is, the compound is now ready to start the next phase of human clinical trials.

Clinical Trials. This is the first time that compounds are used in human experimentation. There are four phases of clinical trials: phase I, phase II, phase III, and phase IV.

Phase I is carried out to determined the metabolism and pharmacologic actions of drugs in humans. (For a thorough review of the clinical process see http://clinicaltrials.gov.) These are medical trials that enroll a small number of patients and try to demonstrate that the drug does not have significant adverse events in humans. The way these trials are normally designed is to start dosing human subjects with the smallest amount of the drug possible and then raise the amount while carefully monitoring the patients. The starting dose is obtained by taken into consideration the preclinical results with animal experimentation. The equivalent starting dose is the dose that when extrapolated from animal results in the lowest dose at which no side effects are expected and efficacy is expected. If there are toxicities associated with the compound, an even smaller equivalent dose is used to start dosing human patients. This dose is progressively increased, keeping the patients under conditions in which the possible side effects can be monitored and brought under control. Obviously, the importance of safety cannot be underestimated in this process and priority has to be given to patients' well-being. The side effects could expand the whole rage of illnesses: from rash to vomiting, hepatocellular abnormalities, or even cardiovascular abnormalities. Some of these could be easily monitored, like checking for specific enzymes in the blood that are associated with tissue disease, such as elevated levels of lactate dehydrogenase, or LDH. The threshold for accepting side effects varies with each indication. Depending on the disease in question, the safety barrier associated with a drug may be put at different levels. For example, if the indication is for a population of terminally ill patients, like those associated with some types of metastatic cancer, higher tolerance for abnormal side effects, such as high-grade rash, loss of hair, or vomiting, may be allowed. While if on the other hand the drug is for an indication in which there is not immediate death, such as ulcerative colities or rehumatoid arthritis, then the safety barrier is higher.

Another goal of the phase I trials is to start gaining early data on the effectiveness of the compound. While these trials tend to be small in number, raging from 20 to 100 patients, and the results may not be statistically significant, they may provide some guidance for a subpopulation of patients to conduct the following phases of clinical research.

Phase II is started after concluding phase I. These are controlled clinical studies that start to look at the effectiveness of the drug. Part of the emphasis is in identifying the right population that the drug is going to target and to find the right dose for the patients. In this phase safety is still being evaluated, side effects are continually monitored, and the risks keep been assessed. A larger number of patients are used to try to get statistically significant numbers to answer questions of effectiveness. Lately, it is very common to include as a secondary goal in these trials some biomarkers. Biomarkers are surrogate measurements that may indicate that the drug is having an effect. There are several types of biomarkers. Those showing changes that correlate with drug dose are named pharmacodymanic markers, and others that may select which population of patients is more likely to respond to the treatment are called predictive biomarkers. Nowadays, there is a lot of emphasis and research in this area. Even the Food and Drug Administration (FDA) is getting in the act, and it is issuing new guidelines regarding the use of biomarkers in clinical trials. One nice effect of utilizing these markers is that it could find faster the patients most likely to improve with treatment, with lesser side effects, use a smaller number of patients and therefore lower the cost of developing the drug, which in turn will reduce the overall cost of drugs in the market. Thus, the use of biomarkers may benefit both the patients and the pharmaceutical companies. Further use of biomarkers is explained in several of the chapters in this book, and the demonstration of the use of biomarkers in the drug development process is shown in more detailed in Chapters 3 and 6, where the authors show several examples of biomarkers for both predictive and pharmacodymanic uses in early clinical trials.

Once a phase II is completed the process moves to phase III. Here, the trials are with an even greater number of patients with the goal of getting at the effectiveness of the drug. At the same time, additional information is gathered regarding the side effects, and an overall picture of the risks and benefits is obtained. These will serve as the bases for the product description that appears in the label of the drug. Each new drug carries a label. In it, the intended use of the drug, the population to which the drug is targeted for, and the known side effects are enumerated. This label will contain the basic information needed by physicians to prescribe it to their patients.

Approval of a Drug. After completion of the three first phases, the data is presented to the medical authorities for approval of the drug. In the United States, the FDA is the governmental body entrusted with deciding the safety and efficacy of all new drugs. In Europe, the European Agency for the Evaluation of Medical Products (EMEA) fulfills the same role for the European Union. For the rest of the world each country has its own rules and regulations. Some of those countries will first ask that a drug be approved by the EMEA or the FDA before they even look at the application. Other countries, like Japan, require that the clinical trials may be done in patients that are genetically similar to the population present in their respective countries. This is to prevent the appearance of new side effects in the native population that may be due to a different genetic background from the subjects that were used for the initial clinical trial. Interestingly, the agencies may approve, request additional information, or deny a drug application. Approval from one agency does not automatically mean the other agencies may conclude the same. Additional information may be required for each agency, such as the running of new clinical trials to specifically target an observed anomaly in a subpopulation of the patients' that was observed previously. An example could be to repeat a clinical trial with an expanded number of patients where a specific cardiovascular risk is examined.

Life-Cycle Management. After a drug has been approved for a specific disease, other clinical trials may be started to look for additional indications in the population. These clinical trials are referred to as phase IV. As before in the other phases of the process, information regarding safety and side effects is of vital importance. It is at this point of the process that doctors can start using the medication in other areas as appropriate. For example, in the case of Erbitux, it was first approved for use in colon cancer patients as a single agent, in EGFR-expressing metastatic colorectal cancer after failure of both irinotecan- and oxaliplatin-based regimens, or in patients who are intolerant of irinotecan-based regimens. Also, it can be used in combination with irinotecan, in EGFR-expressing metastatic colorectal carcinoma in patients who are refractory to irinotecan-based chemotherapy. Then, new clinical trials were carried out in patients with head and neck cancers (Burtness et al., 2005). This has led to approval of the drug in this new indication. In head and neck cancer, Erbitux can now be used in the treatment of locally or regionally advanced squamous cell carcinoma of the head and neck in combination with radiation therapy. It could also be used in recurrent or metastatic squamous cell carcinoma of the head and neck progressing after platinum-based therapy (Erbitux label).

Note that it is not only the drug companies that push for new applications of approved drugs; doctors also have perhaps the most important role. They can design and conduct their own clinical trials if they think the drug could be used for a particular indication. Then, they contact the pharmaceutical company that has designed the drug and ask it for the specific application that they want to test. A new clinical trial can then be designed for that indication.

While this process is long, complicated, and expensive, all the parties involved—the pharmaceutical companies, the doctors, the government agencies—all have one single purpose, the eradication of illnesses in the human race. With the advent of genomics and the marriage of old and new technologies, molecular pathology could play a significant role in the discovery and development of new drugs.

REFERENCES

Amado, R. G., Wolf, M., Peeters, M., Van Cutsem, E., Siena, S., Freeman, D. J., Juan, T., Sikorski, R., Suggs, S., Radinsky, R., Patterson, S. D., and Chang, D. D. (2008). Wild-type KRAS is required for panitumumab efficacy in patients with metastatic colorectal cancer. *J. Clin. Oncol.* 26:1626–1634.

Baudhuin, L. M., Burgart, L. J., Leontovich, O., and Thibodeau, S. N. (2005). Use of microsatellite instability and immunohistochemistry testing for the identification of individuals at risk for Lynch syndrome. *Familial Cancer* 4:255–265.

Burtness, B., Goldwasser, M. A., Flood, V., et al. (2005). Phase III randomized trials of cisplatin plus placebo compared with cisplatin plus cetuximab in metastatic/recurrent head and neck cancer: An eastern cooperative oncology group study. *J. Clin. Oncol.* 23:8646–8654.

Chen, H. Taylor, N. P., Sotamaa, K. M., Mutch, D. G., Powell, M. A., Schmidt, A. P., Feng, S., Hampel, H. L., de la Chapelle, A., and Goodfellow, P. J. (2007). Evidence for heritable predisposition to epigenetic silencing of MLH1. *Int. J. Cancer* 120:1684–1688.

Edgar, K. A., Belvin, M., Parks, A. L., Whittaker, K., Mahoney, M. B., Nicoll, M., Park, C. C., Winter, C. G., Chen, F., Lickteig, K., Ahmad, F., Esengil, H., Lorenzi, M. V., Norton, A., Rupnow, B. A., Shayesteh, L., Tabios, M., Young, L. M., Carroll, P. M., Kopczynski, C., Plowman, G. D., Friedman, L. S., Francis-Lang, H. L. (2005). Synthetic lethality of retinoblastoma mutant cells in the Drosophila eye by mutation of a novel peptidyl prolyl isomerase gene. *Genetics* 170:161–171.

Fogt, F., Vortmeyer, A. O., Goldman, H., Giordano, T. J., Merino, M. J., and Zhuang, Z. (1998). Comparison of genetic alterations in colonic adenoma and ulcerative colitis-associated dysplasia and carcinoma. *Hum. Pathol.* 29:131–136.

Higashidani, Y., Tamura, S., Morita, T., Tadokoro, T., Yokoyama, Y., Miyazaki, J., Yang, Y., Takeuchi, S., Taguchi, H., and Onishi, S. (2003). Analysis of K-ras codon 12 mutation in flat and nodular variants of serrated adenoma in the colon. *Diseases Colon Rectum* 46:327–332.

Hiyama, T., Yokozaki, H., Shimamoto, F., Haruma, K., Yasui, W., Kajiyama, G., and Tahara, E, (1998). Frequent p53 gene mutations in serrated adenomas of the colorectum. *J. Pathol.* 186:131–139.

Horowitz, J. M., Park, S. H., Bogenmann, E, Cheng, J. C., Yandell, D. W., Kaye, F. J., Minna, J. D., Dryja, T. P., and Weinberg, R. A. (1990). Frequent inactivation of the retinoblastoma anti-oncogene is restricted to a subset of human tumor cells. *Proc. Natl. Acad. Sci. U.S.A.* 87(7):2775–2779.

Lombardo, L. J., Lee, F. Y., Chen, P., Norris, D., Barrish, J. C., Behnia, K., Castaneda, S., Cornelius, L. A., Das, J., Doweyko, A. M., Fairchild, C., Hunt, J. T., Inigo, I., Johnston, K., Kamath, A., Kan, D., Klei, H., Marathe, P., Pang, S., Peterson, R., Pitt, S., Schieven, G. L., Schmidt, R. J., Tokarski, J., Wen, M. L., Wityak, J., Borzilleri, R. M. (2004). Discovery of N-(2-chloro-6-methyl-phenyl)-2-(6-(4-(2-hydroxyethyl)-piperazin-1-yl)-2-methylpyrimidin-4-ylamino)thiazole-5-carboxamide (BMS-354825), a dual Src/Ablkinase inhibitor with potent antitumor activityin preclinical assays. *J. Med. Chem.* 47:6658–6661.

Makinen, M. J. (2007). Colorectal serrated adenocarcinoma. *Histopathology* 50:131–150.

Mendelsohn, J., and Baselga, J. (2000). The EGF receptor family as targets for cancer therapy. *Oncogene* 19:6550–6565.

Mullis, K. B. (1990). The unusual origin of the polymerase chain reaction. *Scient. Am.* 262(4):56–61,64–65.

Nowell, P., and Hungerford, D. (1960). Chromosomes of normal and leukemic human leukocytes. *J. Natl. Cancer Inst.* 25:85–109.

Roizin L. (1964). Some basic principles of "molecular pathology." 3. Ultracellular organelles as structural—metabolic and pathogenetic gradients. *J. Neuropathol. Exp. Neurol.* 23:209–252.

Rom, W. N., Hay, J. G., Lee, T. C., Jiang, Y., and Tchou-Wong, K. M. (2000). Molecular and genetic aspects of lung cancer. *Am. J. Respirat. Crit. Care Med.* 161:1355–1367.

Saiki, R. K., Scharf, S., Faloona, F., Mullis, K. B., Horn, G. T., Erlich, H. A., and Arnheim, N. (1985). Enzymatic amplification of beta-globin genomic sequences and restriction site analysis for diagnosis of sickle cell anemia. *Science* 230:1350–1354.

Tamaki, K., Huang, X. L., Nozawa, H., Yamamoto, T., Uchihi, R., Katsumata, Y., and Armour, J. A. (1996). Evaluation of tetranucleotide repeat locus D7S809 (wg1g9) in the Japanese population. *Forensic Sci. Int.* 81:133–140.

Tjio, J. M., and Levan, A. (1956). The chromosome number of man. *Hereditas* 42:1–6.

Vortmeyer, A. O., Gnarra, J. R., Emmert-Buck, M. R., Katz, D., Linehan, W. M., Oldfield, E. H., and Zhuang, Z. (1997). von Hippel-Lindau gene deletion detected in the stromal cell component of a cerebellar hemangioblastoma associated with von Hippel-Lindau disease. *Hum. Pathol.* 28:540–543.

Wajed, S. A., Laird, P. W., and DeMeester, T. R. (2001). DNA methylation: An alternative pathway to cancer. *Ann. Surg.* 234:10–20.

Wang, M., Lamberth, K., Harndahl, M., Roder, G., Stryhn, A., Larsen, M. V., Nielsen, M., Lundegaard, C., Tang, S. T., Dziegiel, M. H., Rosenkvist, J., Pedersen, A. E., Buus, S., Claesson, M. H., and Lund, O. (2007). CTL epitopes for influenza A including the H5N1 bird flu; genome-, pathogen-, and HLA-wide screening. *Vaccine* 25:2823–2831.

Zhuang, Z., Vortmeyer, A. O., Mark, E. J., Odze, R., Emmert-Buck, M. R., Merino, M. J., Moon, H., Liotta, L. A., and Duray, P. H. (1996). Barrett's esophagus: Metaplastic cells with loss of heterozygosity at the APC gene locus are clonal precursors to invasive adenocarcinoma. *Cancer Res.* 56:1961–1964.

2

MOLECULAR PATHOLOGY IN ONCOLOGY TARGET AND DRUG DISCOVERY

Rolf-P. Ryseck, Ricardo Attar, Matthew V. Lorenzi, and Brent A. Rupnow

2.1. INTRODUCTION

Historically, drug discovery was a largely empirical process where pharmacologically active compounds were identified either by isolating them from traditional remedies or by chance observations that a specific compound had a biologic activity that might be useful in treating an illness. During this era of pharmaceutical research, little emphasis was placed on the molecular pathology underlying a drug's activity until after it was proven to be effective. Only then was the mechanism of action for a drug determined. Often, the mechanism by which a drug worked to reverse a disease process led to a better understanding of the pathophysiology of the disease.

Over recent decades, our understanding of the molecular and cellular biology fundamental to healthy and disease states has grown exponentially. This is, in large part, due to breakthroughs in genetic and genomic technology. The sequencing of the human genome as well as those of model organisms from flies to mice has revolutionized biology and in turn drug discovery. Today, pharmaceutical researchers have the capacity to manipulate the activity of specific genes in cells as well as whole organisms to understand whether a specific gene, or the activity of its protein product, might be relevant to progression of a particular disease.

Molecular Pathology in Drug Discovery and Development, Edited by J. Suso Platero
Copyright © 2009 John Wiley & Sons, Inc.

Using molecular pathology and genomics, we are also beginning to understand that conditions once described as a single disease entity can be categorized into several smaller disease types, each of which might respond better to different therapies. Given this wealth of information, today's pharmaceutical and biotechnology companies as well as academic and governmental institutions are approaching the hunt for new and better drugs starting with the molecular target(s) believed to be causative or required for the maintenance of a specific disease defined by its molecular characteristics. With a molecular target in hand that has been demonstrated to support the initiation, progression, or maintenance of the disease, biologists and chemists collaborate to identify small molecules or biologic modulators of the target usually by screening a large collection of synthetic chemical compounds, natural products, or antibodies. Once "hits" are identified, an iterative process of lead optimization continues until an agent is identified that acts as a potent modulator of the target protein, has little effects on other proteins, and demonstrates pharmaceutical properties (e.g., absorption, metabolism, stability, solubility, etc.), allowing it to be tested for activity in vivo and eventually be assessed in human clinical trials for safety and efficacy. The drug discovery work flow, from target identification through clinical testing, is illustrated in Figure 2.1. At each stage of the process, the level of validation for a specific cancer target increases. However, many targets fail along the way for various reasons. Therefore, one must experimentally test many potential cancer targets in order to find those few that eventually prove to be essential for cancer cell growth and/or survival and for which drugs can be developed. Molecular pathology plays a crucial role at each step on this ladder of target/drug progression.

In this chapter we will review modern, target-based, oncology drug discovery emphasizing the role that molecular pathology plays at each step of the process from target discovery to patient selection. Although the focus of this chapter is on drug discovery for cancer, the paradigm can, for the most part, be applied to any therapeutic area.

2.2. HISTORY OF CHEMOTHERAPY AND CANCER DRUG DISCOVERY

The first chemotherapeutic medicine originated from a chemical warfare agent used in World War I. It was observed that individuals exposed to mustard gas exhibited profound reductions in white blood cell counts. In the mid-1940s, physicians tested the first nitrogen mustard chemotherapeutics in lymphoma patients where they observed dramatic, albeit transient, reductions in tumor mass. These early studies demonstrated proof of principal that cancer could be treated with drugs [reviewed by Papac (2001) and Scott (1970)].

In subsequent decades, cancer drug discovery and development focused on identifying compounds that exploited the rapid proliferation rate of cancer cells relative to normal cells. It was rationalized that agents that targeted a cell's ability to divide either by blocking the cell division machinery or by starving the cells

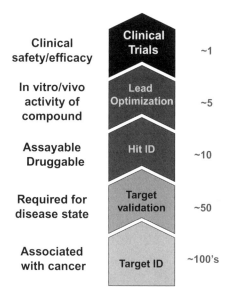

Figure 2.1. Progression of targets through drug discovery pipeline. Target-based drug discovery begins with the identification of genes and proteins associated with disease. Targets are subsequently validated to demonstrate that they are required for maintenance of the disease. Those whose activity can be measured and are amenable to small-molecule or biologic modulation are progressed into compound screening. Identified compounds that modulate the target are tested for desired effect in disease models with in vitro and in animal models. Drug candidates that can reverse disease in vivo with acceptable toxicology profiles progress into clinical trials to determine safety and efficacy in human patients with the disease. Most candidate targets/compounds fail at some step along the path to clinical proof of concept (see numbers at right for reference). Therefore many targets must be evaluated to ensure the success of a few.

of essential nutrients to make new DNA would preferentially kill rapidly dividing cancer cells but not quiescent normal cells. This marked the beginning of the era of rational drug discovery for cancer. The first example of a rationally designed chemotherapeutic is methotrexate, an analog of folic acid. This antifolate blocks the function of the enzymes that utilize folate to synthesize the nucleotides required for nascent DNA synthesis. By the late 1940s methotrexate was demonstrated to have antitumor effects in children suffering from acute lymphoblastic leukemia [for detailed review see Welch (1983)].

Further advances in chemotherapy for cancer came from the discovery of additional compounds that targeted DNA directly, including alkylating agents such as the nitrosoureas and platinum agents (Braña et al., 2001; Wheate et al., 2007) as well as agents that targeted enzymes required for DNA synthesis including topoisomerase I inhibitors such as camptothecin and the topoisomerase II inhibitors such as etoposide (Sriram et al., 2005; Meresse et al., 2004). Another major breakthrough was the discovery of antimitotic natural product compounds including the vinca alkyloids and taxanes both derived from plant toxins [for detailed reviews see Cragg (2007) and Noble (1990)]. These compounds were shown to bind to microtubules, the structural components of the mitotic spindle, and either stabilize (taxanes) or destabilize (vinca alkyloids) the structure. In both cases, the ability of cells treated with these agents to segregate their chromosomes to daughter nuclei is compromised resulting in death of cells attempting to divide.

Aside from the discovery of these individual compounds that have proven effective in treating cancer patients, the rational design of drug combinations provided another remarkable leap forward for cancer chemotherapy. The rational combination of chemotherapeutic drugs along with radiotherapy led eventually to curative regimens for diseases such as Hodgkin's lymphoma and testicular cancer [reviewed by Kardinal (1985), Zubrod (1979), Longo and DeVita (1992), and Hoppe (1992)].

For decades, the cytotoxic drugs described above comprised the mainstay of cancer chemotherapy for tumors of various histological origins. These agents continue to be widely used in cancer treatment today. Although the fundamental logic of targeting DNA replication and cell division components with drugs would argue that all rapidly dividing cells would be susceptible to these agents, practice has shown that certain agents are effective in specific tumor types and inactive in others. While much of what is known regarding the activity of various agents in specific tumor types has been determined empirically, the lessons have begun to reveal the molecular characteristics associated with sensitivity and resistance allowing clinical oncologists to predict which patients will respond to which treatments. For instance, it was discovered that drug-resistant tumors expressed on their surface molecular transporters (P-glycoprotein) that actively exported drugs from cells. These mechanisms have provided targets for further drug discovery to overcome resistance to therapy [reviewed by Szakacs et al., (2006)].

Today, drug discovery in the field of oncology is driven by our understanding of the disease. The discovery of oncogenes that, when activated, drive inappropriate proliferation of cells and tumor suppressor genes that, when lost or inactivated, allow cell growth to proceed unchecked, has uncovered a number of potential molecular targets for drug discovery. What is unique about the modern approach relative to the traditional cytotoxic approach is that targeting oncogenic changes can provide specificity in cell killing for the tumor cells with limited effects on normal tissues. Furthermore, certain tumor types are frequently driven by similar oncogenic pathways. Pathway-targeted agents can therefore be developed clinically in patients whose tumor types are most likely to respond due to the epidemiologic frequency of the corresponding pathway alterations. Additionally, the use of biomarkers for pathway activation and the associated diagnostic tests to evaluate patients prior to therapy is beginning to allow doctors to choose the best drugs for an individual patient (Trusheim et al., 2007). Today, the co-discovery and development of clinical biomarkers that predict responsiveness to novel therapeutics has become standard practice in pharmaceutical research and development and is likely to continue to grow.

Figure 2.2 summarizes the contrast between historical, empirical drug discovery for cancer and the modern target-based approach. Both paths have proven successful in identifying drugs that are effective in treating patients with cancer. In the past, molecular pathology was used to determine the tumor types in which a particular agent might be useful. For instance, determination of the number of mitotic cells in a pathologic specimen (mitotic index) might predict the likelihood that the patient will respond well to antimitotic drugs such as taxanes or vinca alkyloids. Furthermore, molecular pathology played a significant role in elucidating the mechanisms of empirically discovered anticancer drugs. By contrast, our current understanding of the molecular pathobiology of cancer, the signaling pathways important for its development and maintenance, led subsequently to the identification of a number of candidate cancer targets. This knowledge has been exploited to generate compounds with expected activity against specific cancer types based on known pathology. Many of these targets have resulted in the generation of novel compounds currently used in clinical oncology settings, and others are the subject of intense preclinical and clinical studies to understand their usefulness in treating cancer patients.

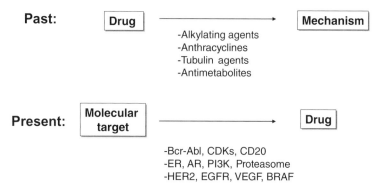

Figure 2.2. Comparison of empirical and target-based cancer drug discovery. Prior to the 1990s drug discovery was an empirical process where drugs were discovered based on effects in disease models. The mechanism of action of the drugs was determined after compounds became drugs. Examples of cancer drug classes discovered prior to elucidation of the molecular targets are shown under the top arrow. Modern drug discovery takes advantage of an extensive knowledge base on the pathobiology of cancer and starts with a target of interest against which a drug compound is identified. This paradigm begins with a hypothesis that a compound with a specific mode of action will be safe and effective against cancer. This is tested both preclinically and in human subjects. Examples of well-established cancer targets against which drugs have been or are being developed are shown under the bottom arrow.

2.3. TARGET-BASED DRUG DISCOVERY

Modern drug discovery relies on a target-based approach where the genes and corresponding proteins involved in the development and progression of the disease are identified. Those genes/proteins whose functions can be modulated by small, organic, druglike molecules or by biomolecules such as recombinant antibodies are considered to be "druggable." Drug targets (usually cellular enzymes or receptors) on which cells rely for maintaining the disease state are the foundation of the pharmaceutical industry today (Imming et al., 2006). In terms of cancer biology, the oncogenes that drive tumor cell proliferation or maintain cancer cell survival, as well as the host proteins required to allow the growth, invasion, and metastasis of tumors, are the major entry point for oncology drug discovery.

The simplified diagram in Figure 2.3 illustrates many of the key signaling pathways implicated in the development and progression of cancer. These include growth factor receptors, which convey growth signals from outside the

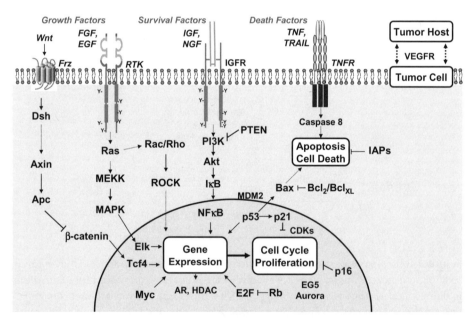

Figure 2.3. Key cancer signaling pathways. The progression of cells from a normal to malignant phenotype involves the activation of growth and survival pathways. Several well-characterized pathways and the proteins known to regulate the transmission of signals through the pathways are illustrated here. Many of the genes/proteins such as EGFR, Ras, β-catenin, Myc, PI3K, BCL2, and so forth function as oncogenes when activated. Other negative regulators of the pathways (e.g., p53, PTEN, APC, p16 and Rb) have been demonstrated to function as tumor suppressors.

cell through key signaling nodes to ultimately direct the cell to divide. In addition, survival signals are transduced in a similar fashion to keep cells alive. In the case of cancer cells, these survival cues are often maintained even under environmental conditions where normal cells would initiate a cell death program called apoptosis. The genes and proteins indicated at the nodes of the signaling pathways can frequently function as oncogenes or tumor suppressor genes depending on whether their role is to promote growth or to inhibit inappropriate cell proliferation signals. Ultimately, the molecular pathways that cells use to transmit growth and survival signals converge on the core components of the cell where the ultimate decision to divide or not (or perhaps to die) is made. Again the key "decision-making" components have been determined to function as oncogenes and tumor suppressors. In addition to integrating signals from outside as well as inside the cell, tumors also adapt to produce signals that cause changes in the surrounding host tissue to support further growth of the tumor. These key oncology signaling pathways and the molecules that participate in them are the mainstay of targeted cancer drug discovery today.

Estrogen and androgen receptors were among the first molecular targets against which effective cancer drugs were developed (Ponzone et al., 2006; Jordan, 2003; Tammela, 2004; Fluchter et al., 2007). Although these proteins do not fit the typical "oncogene" label that many cancer targets fall within, they are critically involved in the normal physiology of the hormone-dependent tissues, and their deregulation can be adopted by tumor cells to gain a proliferative and/or survival advantage. Further, an important characteristic of a cancer drug target is tumor specificity. Because the estrogen and androgen receptors primarily transduce hormonal signals in tissues (ovary, breast, and prostate) not essential for survival of the patient, they can be modulated without producing severe toxicity. Therefore, these hormone receptors are attractive drug targets and synthetic compounds that regulate their activity have been used successfully in treating cancer patients.

Following the hormone receptors, the receptor tyrosine kinases (RTKs) were the next major class of druggable targets to become a focus for cancer drug discovery. Notable success stories in this area are the epidermal growth factor receptors *EGFR* and *HER2* (*ERBB2*) (Mendelsohn and Baselga, 2006). Both *EGFR* and *HER2* are bona fide oncogenes that are overexpressed or activated by mutation in various cancers to drive the malignant progression of epithelial cells from a normal to cancerous state. Because they are protein kinases as well as cell surface receptors, pharmaceutical and biotechnology companies targeted these oncogenes not only with small-molecule drugs including Iressa (gefitinib) and Tarceva (erlotinib) but also with biotherapeutics in the form of antibodies, including Herceptin (trastuzumab) targeting *HER2* and Erbitux (cetuximab) targeting *EGFR*. More recently Tykerb (lapatinib), a small-molecule kinase inhibitor that targets both *EGFR* and *HER2* was approved for treatment of advanced breast cancers that have failed prior Herceptin treatment (Johnston et al., 2006; Dassonville et al., 2007). The specific role that molecular pathology plays in the diagnosis, treatment planning, and disease monitoring of patients potentially eligible for these *EGFR*-targeted drugs will be discussed later in this chapter.

Another recent example of a druggable kinase target that has been successfully exploited for drug discovery is the cytoplasmic tyrosine kinase oncogene, *ABL*. The oncogenic potential of *ABL* is activated in human leukemias by a specific translocation between chromosomes 9 and 22 (Philadelphia chromosome, Ph). The resulting expression of activated *ABL* drives excessive proliferation of bone marrow stem cells and ultimately the development of chronic myelogenous leukemia (CML). Two new drugs, Gleevec (imatinib) and Sprycel (dasatinib), specifically targeting cells with activated *ABL*, have been approved in recent years (Schiffer, 2007). These molecular-targeted agents provide considerable benefit to CML patients whose tumors maintain the Philadelphia translocation. These drugs also provide a perfect example of the impact of molecular pathology to drug discovery, development, and clinical practice. In this case, the drugs were specifically designed to target an oncogene known to play a major role in the development of the pathology of the Philadelphia positive leukemia. The presence of the Philadelphia translocation by polymerase chain reaction (PCR) continues to be used as the critical marker for clinical response to these compounds (Hughes and Branford, 2006). This may be the most striking example of how molecular pathology is impacting drug discovery and development at every step of the process.

In addition to targeting oncogenes that drive proliferation through cellular signaling processes, more recent discoveries of proteins that regulate key cell division processes have provided new targets to selectively kill rapidly proliferating cells. These discoveries have allowed drug discovery scientists to develop new agents that might someday replace the standard cytotoxic chemotherapeutics (Sudakin and Yen, 2007). For example, druggable enzymes such as *EG5*, a kinesin motor protein essential to the cells' ability to segregate chromosomes during cell division, can be inhibited by small molecular agents resulting in death of cancer cells (Duhl and Renhowe, 2005). Another group of antimitotic targets discovered in recent years are the Aurora kinases. These are key regulators of the final stage of cell division that separates the daughter nuclei into two individual cells. When Aurora kinases are inhibited, cells attempting to divide form multinucleated cells that eventually die (Naruganahalli et al., 2006). Both *EG5* and Aurora kinase inhibitors are currently in clinical trials for various cancers. These trials will not only determine their efficacy but will also determine whether the side effects will be reduced (or different) compared to more traditional antimitotics (taxanes and vinca compounds). If they are generally safer, they may replace the older antimitotics entirely. On the other hand, if side effect profiles are markedly different, it may allow these new targeted cytotoxics to be used in drug combinations where the taxanes and vincas could not be utilized.

In addition to directly targeting the cancer cells for therapeutic benefit, much effort in the past decade has been expended to exploit "tumor host" mechanisms to slow the growth of tumors. A highly successful approach has been to attack the tumor's ability to recruit new blood vessels, so-called antiangiogenic therapy [reviewed by Folkman (2007)]. As a mass of cancer cells expands, it will eventually outgrow its supply of oxygen and other nutrients provided by the patient's blood vessels. When this occurs, tumor cells produce signaling molecules such as vascular endothelial growth factor (*VEGF*) to recruit the growth of new blood vessels into the tumor. Several strategies have been taken to inhibit this vascular recruitment by tumors, and one, Avastin (bevacizumab), an antibody that binds to and blocks the action of *VEGF*, has recently been approved for colorectal cancer therapy (Ferrara et al., 2004; Cilley et al., 2007). More discussion on how molecular pathology has contributed to the development and use of antiangiogenic therapies will follow later in this chapter.

In addition to targeting angiogenesis, others have attempted to activate cancer patients' immune systems to attack tumor cells using cancer vaccine and immunostimulatory approaches. While these strategies remain unproven clinically, scientific rationale and preclinical evidence makes them quite promising approaches for future cancer management. The targeted drug discovery approach to date has focused primarily on established oncogenes whose connection to cancer pathology is supported by a wealth of primary literature. To compliment efforts on established molecular targets, drug discovery labs throughout industry and academia have undertaken an enormous effort in the past decade to identify novel targets amenable to small-molecule and/or protein therapeutic modulation.

2.4. UTILIZATION OF MOLECULAR PATHOLOGY IN THE DISCOVERY OF NOVEL CANCER TARGETS

The last 10 years have witnessed the emergence of a variety of genomics technologies that resulted in an overwhelming choice of new gene products to explore as potential oncology molecular targets for drug discovery. These target discovery techniques include bioinformatics target identification approaches based on human genome and expressed sequence tag (EST) efforts, proteomic-based or transcriptional profiling comparisons in tumor versus normal tissues, chemical genomic approaches, and pathway-based genetic screens focused on key tumor suppressor or oncogene phenotypes (summarized in Table 2.1). Each of these target discovery approaches is associated with a key target validation criterion, but each approach is also accompanied by a unique shortcoming that is the focus of subsequent target validation. For instance, novel sequences amenable to small-molecule or protein therapeutic modulation have been readily identified by EST and genome sequencing efforts, yet this group of targets generally requires the most additional research to link the novel gene product to a biological effect of interest. In this section, we will review several of these approaches for oncology target discovery and highlight the importance of molecular pathology analyses within these different methodologies.

The grouping of molecular targets into druggable classes such as kinases, ion channels, proteases, and G-protein-coupled receptors (GPCRs) emerged in the mid-1990s as an approach to identify new gene products for drug discovery

TABLE 2.1. Role of Molecular Pathology in Oncology Target Discovery

Target Discovery Approach	Validation Strengths	Role of Molecular Pathology
Homology-based sequence identification	Novelty Target class selection	Verification of target expression in disease tissue of interest
Transcription profiling and proteomics techniques	Disease-state-associated expression profile	Expansion of disease-associated expression to define breadth and context of target-disease linkage
Model organism genetic screens	Target linkage to a key phenotype in an organismal context	Confirmation of expression in human specimens in appropriate tumor types
Pathway-based RNAi screens in mammalian cell lines	Pathway and cell-based phenotype linkage	Cell line selections, target-tumor expression, RNAi-target knockdown correlations

[reviewed in Lu and Lorenzi (2003)]. This strategy was fueled by large-scale sequencing efforts of the human genome but also through EST sequencing initiatives of different tissue and cell types. The result of these efforts was a wealth of new sequences from a particular target class that were generally novel but frequently lacked supportive biology to place the new sequence within a disease context. A key aspect to validate such sequences as potential oncology therapeutic targets was to document expression of the gene product of interest in the relevant tumor tissue through the use of molecular pathology techniques such as immunohistochemical staining. For sequence-based identification efforts, messenger ribonucleic acid (mRNA) and protein expression in the tissue type was viewed as the key validation parameter needed to support additional research activities. This approach has been used successfully to identify novel members related to apoptotic and proliferative signaling kinase families (Kasof et al., 2000; Lin et al., 2001). An example of differential target expression analysis by immunohistochemistry is illustrated in Figure 2.4. In this example, antiserum specific for a target of interest was generated and used to measure the relative expression of the protein in paraffin-embedded sections taken from cancer patients. These sections were also compared to the corresponding normal tissues for the tumor specimens. In the example shown, the target is expressed at very high levels in lung, ovarian, and pancreatic cancers while expression was much lower in the corresponding normal tissues. Despite advances in techniques for differential expression analysis at both the mRNA and protein levels, it has often proven difficult to provide additional validation data to support a linkage of such novel targets to a particular cancer pathobiology or signaling pathway, which are a general requirement for advancement into further drug discovery research.

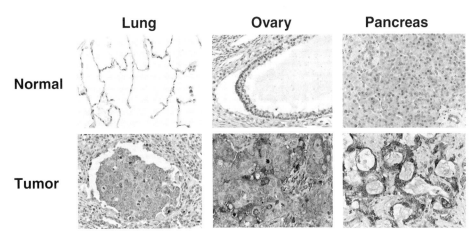

Figure 2.4. Immunohistochemical staining of a candidate cancer target. Differential expression of a protein associated with cancers shown by immunohistochemical staining of the target using specific antiserum on sections from tumor and normal tissue specimens derived from lung, ovarian, and pancreatic tissues. Intensity of staining (dark gray) indicates the relative amount of the target protein in the tissue section. Sections are counterstained with hematoxylin and eosin to visualize cellular and tissue architecture. In the example shown, substantially more target protein is expressed in the tumor tissues for all three histotypes than is expressed in the corresponding normal tissues. An expression pattern like the one shown may indicate that tumors might be more dependent on the target activity than normal tissues. See insert for color representation of figure.

At the other end of the spectrum of oncology target discovery are approaches to identify gene products in an unbiased manner based upon their alteration of a cellular phenotype or pathway endpoint of interest. An advantage of these target discovery techniques is that the target sequence identified is already associated with a critical piece of validation data, the linkage to a phenotype of interest. Such target discovery strategies include model organism pathway-based screens in *Caenorhabditis elegans* and *Drosophia melanogaster*, chemical genetic screens for compounds that can affect a phenotype or pathway of interest, and mammalian-based RNA interference (RNAi) genetic screens (Edgar et al., 2005; Dolma et al., 2003; Ngo et al., 2006). At present, RNAi-based screens are extremely popular approaches to novel target discovery. The diagram in Figure 2.5 shows a common approach to mammalian RNAi screens. Generally, libraries of RNA interference molecules in the form of either synthetic siRNAs (small interfering RNAs) or vectors that produce specific RNAi molecules are assembled. These libraries contain RNAi directed at individual genes and can range in size from several hundred (e.g., those that target the kinases) to many thousands (containing RNAi against every expressed mRNA in the genome). For target identification purposes RNAi libraries contain a number of reagents corresponding to the druggable enzymes in the genome. This simplifies evaluation of hits, focusing only

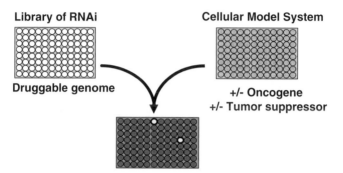

Figure 2.5. RNAi screening for cancer targets. Schematic representation of the systematic evaluation of druggable targets in cancer cell model systems. Libraries of RNAi molecules can be arrayed in multiwell plates and introduced into cell model systems to systematically examine the phenotypic effects of depleting the specific proteins from the cells. RNAi molecules that show a desirable phenotypic effect on the cancer-relevant model are considered as candidate targets for further validation and potential drug screening.

on those that can be followed for direct drug discovery purposes. Using these RNAi libraries, target hunters systematically introduce the RNAi into tumor cells or engineered cells and screen for a desired phenotype, which might be as simple as growth inhibition in a cancer cell line or much more complex (e.g., multiple pathway-specific effects). The RNAi molecules that reverse a cancer-relevant phenotype highlight candidate drug targets for further target validation efforts.

Within these unbiased target screening approaches, molecular pathology methodology takes on a different but yet key role within the validation process. For instance, for genetic screens around a particular tumor suppressor or oncogene pathway, molecular pathology can be used to guide selection of tumor cell lines harboring loss or gain of the pathway of interest, which would be used for a primary genetic screen (e.g., such as in RNAi-based approaches) or for subsequent confirmatory validation experiments (e.g., in the case of the output of model organism-based pathway screens). To highlight this latter point, the search for and validation of new targets that can regulate the c-*MYC* versus *PTEN* versus β-catenin pathways needs to occur in the appropriate tumor cell line genotype context to make informed target selection choices. As such, the characterization of tumor cellular genotypes by immunohistochemistry and direct gene sequencing to identify panels of cell lines that are reflective of clinical tumor specimens is an essential activity for any pathway-based target identification approach as well as a critical general consideration within oncology target validation paradigms (Neve et al., 2006).

Transcriptional profiling and proteomics analysis have been utilized directly as discovery approaches for new oncology target identification. The basis for this reasoning is supported by longstanding observations that oncogenic pathways often are subverted by overexpression of key components through gene amplification or deregulated expression. *EGFR*, *HER2*, androgen receptor, Aurora A, and

MDM2 provide compelling examples of the utility of this approach. However, despite these successes, significant additional work to demonstrate that the overexpression of a given sequence is consequential to a particular tumor phenotype is often difficult. Further, such validation is complicated by overexpression of sequences specific to tumor tissue that can reflect a tumor cell's attempt to dampen growth response rather than an expression event linked to tumorigenesis. This phenomenon is represented by Axin2, which displays prominent tumor versus normal expression profiles in colorectal tumor types harboring constitutively active β-catenin but functionally is a Wnt pathway antagonist (Leung et al., 2002).

Molecular pathology approaches will be a central platform to future oncology target discovery strategies on multiple levels (for summary see Table 2.2). Foremost among its impact will be in validating targets emerging from genomic target discovery strategies such as RNAi and mutational analysis. For example, although RNA interference has become a powerful technique for modulating gene function, interpretation of phenotypes, particularly for oncology endpoints, is frequently problematic due to the cytotoxic off-target activity of small inhibitory RNAs (siRNAs). Because of this feature of siRNAs, the confirmation that target protein knock down is correlated to a chosen phenotype is an essential validation endpoint driven by molecular pathology techniques.

Finally, a challenging feature of oncology drug discovery is determining the appropriate tumor genotype context where a new modulating agent will be most efficacious. To enable target-tumor genotype placements, more extensive analyses of tumor genotypes needs to be developed that link target expression/mutation,

TABLE 2.2. Role of Molecular Pathology in the Drug Discovery Process

	Activities Involved	Potential Molecular Pathology Contribution
Target Validation	Integration of: genomics, proteomics, systems biology, and bioinformatics	Link of target and disease Confirmation of target relevance in clinical samples
Lead ID	Assay development Chemical library HTS Secondary assays	Pathway connectivity Integration of cellular phenotypic data collected in chemical validation assays
Lead Optimization	SAR In silico prediction of druglike characteristics Test in toxicological relevant assays Preclinical evaluation in animal models Pharmacokinetics (PK) / pharmacodynamics (PD) Efficacy models Preclinical toxicology	Confirmation of in vivo effect on target (PD) Confirmation of efficacy at the tissue level Histological characterization of toxicities

chromosomal loss/gains, and transcriptional/proteomic profiling with compound and/or target dependence. To that end, a recent approach to identify relevant molecular targets is the screening of cancer cell genomes for mutations in potential relevant signaling cascades. Several recent studies [among them Greenman et al., (2007)] describe the occurrence of relatively rare somatic mutations in various genes, for instance, kinases that are specific to cancer cells. While at this time it is too early to judge the ultimate importance of many of these mutations for the establishment and survival of tumor cells, it is tempting to speculate that specific drugs can be developed to effectively target these mutated kinases. One difficulty will be the cost-effectiveness of screening the individual cancers of many patients for a large number of mutations, but increasing progress in sequencing technology will make this more feasible in the near future. It is also likely that, over the next decade biologists will have an arsenal of kinase inhibitors effective against a large portion of the kinase repertoire. One can envision a time in the not too distant future where the complement of well-characterized kinase inhibitors will be merged with the knowledge base of cancer-specific kinase mutations. Such integrated data sets will be essential for the more rational placement of targets and their inhibitors and the development of the next generation of oncology therapeutic agents.

2.5. HIT IDENTIFICATION AND IN VITRO LEAD OPTIMIZATION

Once sufficient evidence has been collected that supports a protein or family of proteins as targets with therapeutic utility, in other words once the target has been validated, the next step in the drug discovery process is the search for agents that by acting on the target(s) are efficacious in preclinical models for that specific disease. Those agents can be chemical compounds—synthetic or natural—or biologics (which include engineered protein derivatives and optimized antibodies).

The task at hand in small-molecule drug discovery is to identify among millions of molecules the candidate "hits" that promote the desired effect on the target (inhibition or activation). The primary approach for identifying small-molecule candidates is to utilize a primary screening assay in a medium- to high-throughput manner. Subsequent secondary and tertiary screens select for compounds with added attributes such as cell permeability, effect on the pathway of interest, and selectivity against other targets. Most of the primary high-throughput screens (HTS) are designed as biochemical assays that are reconstituted systems with purified receptor or enzymes. Fewer HTS are performed using cell-based assays due to an increased potential for "off-target" effects. The biochemical assays can be based on different platforms such as those developed for membrane tyrosine kinase receptors, reviewed by Minor (2005). These assays can be either homogenous or heterogeneous (i.e., require separation steps). Examples of the homogeneous methodologies are radioactive (scintillation proximity assay, or SPA), fluorescence resonance energy transfer (FRET), fluorescence polarization (FP), enzyme fragment complementation (EFC), and bead-based or label-free assays. The heterogeneous methods include radiometric, dissociation-enhanced fluorescent immunoassay (DELFIA; PerkinElmer), and enzyme-linked immunosorbent assay (ELISA). For both types of assays, the substrate can be a small peptide containing a consensus tyrosine phosphorylation site or a peptide fragment containing a native peptide sequence (Minor, 2005).

High-throughput cell-based assays are limited to a smaller number of options that include the assessment of cytotoxicity by different methods, the quantification of a reporter gene expression in transfected cells, or the quantification of the secreted proteins (e.g., interleukins). Although these types of assays have been traditionally relegated to secondary assay platforms, the advent of high content cell biology platforms has stimulated a renewed interest in performing screens on cellular assays to identify compounds that regulate a key biological effect. The specific capabilities of the technology are reviewed in the next section. As an example of the potential of the technology in screening, fluorescently tagged *FOXO* transcription factor nuclear translocation, an end product of regulation of the *IGFR/PTEN* signaling, can be imaged robustly with this technology (see Fig. 2.6) and shown to be modulated by inhibitors that modulate different points in the pathway. These types of endpoints illustrate the use of a molecular pathology marker that can be used in early small-molecule drug discovery. Further, when viewed in the context of the tumor suppressor *PTEN*, such pathway-based "hit" identification efforts provide a molecular pathology-defined clinical endpoint for the unbiased identification of modulating agents.

Once compounds or protein therapeutic agents are identified, their activity is confirmed in secondary assays that can also be biochemical or cell based. In general, compounds are tested in secondary biochemical assays for the evaluation of off-target activities or selectivity against close members in the target family. The cell-based secondary assays are useful to confirm the inhibition of the target in a cellular context and to assess the phenotypic consequences of that inhibition. Until recently, most of the cell-based assays used in drug discovery consisted of the treatment of cells with a compound in a range of different concentrations followed by a single readout such as cell number, percent of apoptosis, phosphorylation of endogenous targets (in the cases of kinases), and the like. The introduction of high content screening (HCS) platforms (Paran et al., 2006; Rausch, 2006) has radically changed this trend. HCS utilizes sophisticated image processing algorithms to analyze cell images generated by automated fluorescence microscopy covering a wide range of cell biological parameters allowing measurement of changes in object localization, size, intensity, texture, or shape. This technology adds another level of sophistication since it allows the analysis, in a high-throughput mode, of physiologically relevant cellular events such as cell or protein movements, shape changes, or protein modification. In addition, HCS is now increasingly being used in conjunction with the RNA interference (RNAi) technology for the systematic analysis of phenotypic cellular effects observed in large-scale genetic screens (Krausz, 2007). It is at this point that the perspective of the molecular pathologist provides invaluable input to the drug discovery

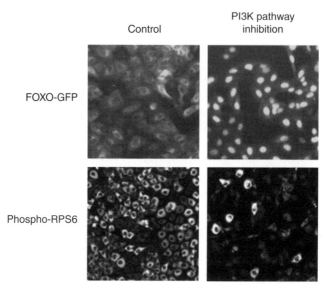

Figure 2.6. High-content pathway assessment. PC3 cells (PTEN mutated) were stably trans-fected with an expression construct encoding GFP-FOXO. High-content GFP imaging of these cells (top panels) revealed predominantly cytoplasmic staining of the GFP-FOXO fusion protein in these cells. In contrast, inhibition of upstream regulators of *FOXO* function (phoshatidylino-sitol kinase, PI3K) revealed a pronounced translocation of the reporter protein to the nucleus. The bottom panels show the same cells stained by immunofluorescence (white) for the phos-phorylation status of the ribosomal protein S6 (RPS6), another downstream effect of PI3K pathway activity. Upon inhibition of PI3K, levels of phosphorylated RPS6 are markedly reduced. High-content biology platforms that combine analysis of multiple pathway readouts such as GFP-FOXO translocation and RPS6 phosphorylation in the case of the PI3K pathway can be used to support both target validation and drug discovery efforts.

process, specifically in the identification of appropriate cellular models that right-fully represent the pathophysiology of the disease or a particular group of patients, and in the interpretation of the large amount of biochemical and cellular morphometric parameters as a result from the high-content screens.

Both biochemical and cell-based secondary assays are part of the chemical validation and provide proof that the agent of interest inhibits specifically the target both in vitro and in cells and, importantly, that there is connectivity between the inhibition of the target, the pathway, and ultimately with the phenotype of interest (e.g., cellular growth inhibition or promotion of apoptosis). Furthermore, these assays provide key information for the development of structure–activity relationship (SAR), which is the understanding of the impact that specific changes made on the original chemical scaffold have on the activity on the target, selectivity, permeability, metabolic stability, and the like. A strong understanding of the SAR is essential for the optimization of compounds and for defining lead candidates.

It is estimated that roughly 40% of preclinical and clinical drug candidates fail in development due to poor pharmacokinetics, deleterious side effects, and compound toxicity (Li, 2001). One discipline that is gaining increasing importance in the drug discovery paradigm is the evaluation of compounds in assays and models that predict metabolic stability and potential toxicities. Several in silico and in vitro approaches have been developed to "weed out" compounds with suboptimal properties before committing to the testing in animal models. For example "virtual test kits" as the ones described by Vedani (Vedani et al., 2006) can predict, in silico, the binding of testing compounds to the estrogen, androgen, thyroid, and aryl hydrocarbon receptors (predictors of endocrine disruption and receptor-mediated toxicity, respectively), as well as on the enzyme cytochrome P450 3A4 (predictor of metabolic transformations and drug–drug interactions). Another example is the in vitro multitier paradigm designed for selecting compounds based on their risk for heptatotoxicity (Dambach et al., 2005). This set of screens assesses the cytotoxic effect of compounds on immortalized human hepatocyte cell lines including parental (control), or expressing several individual CYP450 enzyme isoforms (covering the possibility of the generation of toxic metabolites), or on primary hepatocyte cultures isolated from human donors, or preclinical species. Compounds are profiled further using assays such as reaction phenotyping, CYP450 inhibition and induction, and plasma protein binding. Besides the risk of cytotoxicity, these tests also predict for potential drug–drug interaction (DDI). For example, if drug A is a potent and irreversible inhibitor of a particular CYP450 enzyme, and drug B is metabolized by that particular CYP450, the co-administration of both drugs could lead to the accumulation of drug B to dangerous toxic levels. On the other hand, if drug A is a CYP450 inducer, drug B would be highly metabolized to levels below the ones required for efficacy. In summary, the approach described so far helps to make intelligent choices on which candidate compounds should be progressed to in vivo testing.

The next hurdle for these compounds is to pass a selection based on their in vivo ADME (absorption, distribution, metabolism, and excretion) properties (Singh, 2006). Compounds that are not absorbed or are extensively metabolized or cleared have low chances to be efficacious in vivo. In general, the pharmacokinetic (PK) studies are performed in rodents (mice and rats), and only few advanced compounds are tested in nonrodent species (dogs or monkeys). This selection also takes into consideration that different therapeutic uses require drugs with different PK properties; for instance, an anesthetic should be rapidly cleared while an oncology drug should remain in plasma as long as possible; on the other hand both drugs should reach their target organ/tissue (distribution). A modality that is being followed more frequently is the early incorporation of pharmacokinetic and pharmacodynamic (PK/PD) models in the discovery paradigm. These models provide simultaneous information on both the exposure and the ability of compounds to achieve the desired effect on the target tissue. One example is the determination of both plasma levels and the reduction in the levels of a phosphorylated tyrosine kinase receptor in tumors implanted in nude mice (see below xenograft models) dosed with a small-molecule kinase inhibitor. Knowing the pharmacokinetic properties of selected compounds is crucial for the optimal design of efficacy studies as this information will guide the selection of dose, schedule, and route—oral (po), intravenous (iv), intraperitoneal (ip), or subcutaneous (sc).

Ultimately, the selected compounds will be tested in in vivo efficacy studies. The human tumor xenograft is one of the most widely used experimental models in oncology and consists in the dosing of drugs in immunocompromised mice (e.g., nude mice) bearing subcutaneously human xenograft tumors obtained from patient specimens. The growth of the solid tumors is monitored using in situ caliper measurements, and activity is defined by tumor growth delay, optimal %T/C (T/C, median-treated tumor mass/median control tumor mass) or net log cell kill. Drug-related deaths and body weight loss are used as parameters of toxicity. Although there is some debate regarding the relevance of the xenograft models (specially when implanted subcutaneously), several studies supported their value predicting clinical activity (Suggitt and Bibby, 2005). For example, Fiebig et al., (2004) compared the activity of a set of 12 standard oncological drugs in xenograft models established from primary tumors or metastatic lesions of patients with the clinical outcome of each respective patient. The correct predictive value of the xenograft models was 97% for tumor resistance and 90% for tumor sensitivity.

The current target-driven anticancer drug discovery era is dependent on the selection of the appropriate tumor model as well as the suitable testing modality (e.g., orthotopic, survival, or subcutaneous xenograft models), creating opportunities for the molecular pathologist to contribute to this process by characterizing such xenograft models. Such analyses drive the ultimate decision of moving forward a compound to the clinic and help frame subsequent clinical activities such as tumor expression of the target in the context of tumor genotypes to define patient subtype classifications. Once compounds are progressed based on their efficacy in preclinical in vivo models, they will be subject to toxicological studies that involved single and chronic dosing in at least two species, rodents or nonrodents. As reviewed by Sistare and DeGeorge (2007), a retrospective study of the test in animal experience involving 150 compounds with known clinical toxicities showed that rodent toxicology studies alone "predicted" 43% of human toxicities, nonrodents predicted 63%, and together both species captured only 71% (Olson et al., 2000). It is essential at this point to understand the relationship between the toxicities found and the on-target and/or off-target activities of the compounds being tested. The information gained for toxicology studies will help to make decisions in terms of the future of those compounds and could be fed back to the lead optimization teams for the findings of new safer analogs. Obviously, the molecular pathologist plays a key role in this task by analyzing the physiological, histological, and molecular effects of those compounds on different organs and tissues. Once the toxic exposures are known, it is possible to determine the "no observed adverse effect level" (NOAEL) that together with the "minimum efficacious exposure" (MEE) will allow the calculation of the "therapeutic index" (TI). The TI then represents the difference between the exposures that promote toxicities and the ones that are required for efficacy. Drugs with larger TI will have, in principle, better chances of success in the clinical setting.

The constant advance in the understanding of the molecular basis of diseases together with the rapid development of novel technologies are more than ever creating the right context for breakthroughs in the finding of new therapies. It is foreseeable that the molecular pathologist will play an expanding role at earlier levels in the drug discovery process—for example, target selection and validation, lead optimization, and the like (Table 2.2), which will be added to the well-established roles in patient selection and clinical trial evaluations.

2.6. IMPLICATIONS FOR MOLECULAR PATHOLOGY IN CANCER DRUG DEVELOPMENT AND USE

Clearly, a major objective of current and future cancer treatment and management is pathway-specific therapy. Most tumors develop over a long period of time by accumulating individual genetic mutations resulting in activation of pathways that confer distinct growth and survival advantages to the cells. In many cases specific genes are altered in cancer by large changes in their level of expression. Modern advances in molecular pathology allow clinicians and scientists to detect the deregulation of these cancer-related genes and their corresponding proteins. Techniques such as quantitative PCR, high-throughput transcription profiling (e.g., gene chip analysis) and fluorescent in-situ hybridization (FISH) allow one to detect the gene or its mRNA. Molecular pathology techniques such as immunohistochemistry (IHC) detect the protein products of deregulated genes in the context of the tissue architecture. Today, there are many examples of newly expressed or overexpressed proteins that are themselves the direct target for a specific cancer drug. In these cases, detection of the target in a clinical specimen allows the corresponding drug to be selected for treatment of the patient. In other cases, a biomarker panel of specific antibodies or gene detection probes can allow conclusions to be drawn regarding the activated and inactivated pathways in a given specimen. With this information in hand, drugs that inhibit a target in the activated or disrupted pathway can be selected for the patient. Conversely, biomarker data collected posttreatment can be utilized to gather early information on whether a patient's disease is likely to respond positively over a protracted treatment with a particular drug. For instance, the determination of the presence of the VEGF receptor 2 (*VEGFR2*) and associated blood vessels after treatment with a VEGF pathway inhibitor might be indicative of clinical responsiveness well before measurement of tumor response by radiological methods is possible (Miller et al., 2005; Drevs and Schneider, 2006). The detection of *HER2* (*ERBB2*), a receptor tyrosine kinase involved in the development and maintenance of breast and other cancers, is a prime example of the use of molecular pathology in clinical oncology practice. Amplification of the *ERBB2* gene is thought to be the primary mechanism for overexpression of this oncogene (Akiyama et al., 1986). Therefore, the selection of patients who are treated with therapeutic targeting *HER2*, for example, the humanized anti-*HER2* monoclonal antibody trastuzumab (Herceptin, Genentech, South San Francisco, CA) (Slamon et al., 2001), relies on the identification of *HER2* over-expressing tumors. It may be equally important for other treatment options against this kinase, for instance, in the use of small-molecule dual *HER1/HER2* tyrosine kinase inhibitors. Multitargeted kinase inhibitors present another oppor-tunity for use of molecular pathology in the identification of suitable treatments. A notable example is the use of *ABL* inhibitors such as Gleevec that were ini-tially developed for chronic myelogeneous leukemia in the treatment of gastro-intestinal stromal tumors (GIST). This is possible due to the fortuitous fact that Gleevec is a potent inhibitor of the c-*KIT* receptor tyrosine kinase, which is found to be highly overexpressed and activated in many GIST tumors. Molecular pathology studies can therefore be performed to determine the status of this gene in surgical specimens from GIST patients to determine whether Gleevec might be a treatment option for a given patient (Loughrey et al., 2007). Furthermore, it was recently shown that some colorectal carcinomas also overexpress c-*KIT* and therefore might respond to therapy with Gleevec. Also, colorectal carcinoma cell lines with high expression of nonmutated c-*KIT* show increased apoptosis after Gleevec treatment, independent of its genetic profile, for example, *KRAS* or *BRAF* mutations. Therefore, Gleevec and similar drugs might be an alterna-tive treatment in these cases. Clinical trials will ultimately test this hypothesis (Preto et al., 2007).

While the above examples demonstrate the detection of a target against which a specific drug was developed, future therapy lies in the development of targeted treatment options for very specific patient subpopulations. As a conse-quence this will result in a smaller number of patients taking a particular drug but should offer superior clinical results. Importantly, for the development of substitute biomarkers to identify specific treatment options, immunohisto-chemistry and other molecular diagnostic methods will play a significant role. As an example of pathway-specific therapy, the oncogenic phosphatidylinositol 3-kinase pathway (PI3K) is estimated to be activated in >30% in solid tumors. The identification of new compounds targeting PI3K is an area of intense pre-clinical and clinical development effort throughout the pharmaceutical industry. Activation of the PI3K pathway occurs either by oncogenic alterations of upstream regulators of PI3K (usually growth factor receptors) or by the loss of the *PTEN* tumor suppressor preventing effective regulation of the pathway. However, no reliable test for PI3K pathway activation exists in human tumors. A recent study (Saal et al., 2007) describes the development and validation of a microarray gene expression signature for IHC-detectable *PTEN* loss in breast cancer. While the most significant signature is the absence of *PTEN* itself, some *PTEN* IHC-positive samples exhibited the signature of *PTEN* loss. This corre-lated with a moderately reduced *PTEN* mRNA level and specific types of *PIK3CA* mutations and/or amplification of *HER2*. In this example the expression signature is more sensitive than direct measurement of *PTEN* for the identifica-tion of tumors with pathway activation. Interestingly, stathmin (*STMN1*) is an accurate IHC marker of the signature with prognostic significance for outcome (Saal et al., 2007). The detection of *STMN1* expression might be of special importance in early tumors with a mixed population where only a few cells might be *PTEN* negative and therefore the loss here would be easily overlooked by other methods. Detection of the *PTEN* signature gene stathmin might provide an early indication of the potential for the development of chemotherapy resistance and suggest the co-administration of other PI3K pathway-directed therapies to eliminate these cells. This is but one example where IHC detection of the right marker proteins might have significant influence on therapy selection and potentially patient outcome.

As other signature pathway markers are identified and fine tuned for specific tumor types, it is likely that standard protocols will be developed using specific markers to classify tumors using IHC and related methods with implications for selecting the most appropriate therapeutic strategy, predicting outcome as well as optimal design of clinical trials for new drug development. The industrial use of tissue microarrays (TMAs) will allow relatively inexpensive testing of a tumor sample with a large set of antibodies against specific targets (Sauter et al., 2003). This approach has the potential to identify patients suitable for specific treatments appropriate only in a small percentage of a given tumor type that are currently undetected or not considered due to their rarity.

2.7. SUMMARY AND FUTURE CONSIDERATIONS

Research over recent decades has resulted in an expansion in our understanding of the molecular pathology that underlies diseases of high unmet medical need such as cancer. As a result the way in which scientists approach drug discovery has been transformed from empiricism to a rational, target-based process. Furthermore, the technology and research tools available to drug discovery scientists have expanded greatly and will continue to do so in years to come. The ability to evaluate the role of candidate targets in disease biology with remarkable speed and to screen and test compounds using high throughput and high content techniques makes this an exciting time for pharmaceutical scientists.

Although there are examples of marketed drugs that are tailored to specific and identifiable patient populations based on the molecular characteristics of their disease, the era of personalized medicine is just beginning. Given the broad emphasis on co-development of diagnostic and prognostic biomarkers along with effective therapeutics throughout the pharmaceutical industry, one can only expect to see a rapid expansion of tailored therapies. As molecular pathology continues to subdivide and reclassify diseases, it is anticipated that the medicines of tomorrow will be safer and more effective than ever. Additionally, it seems likely that targeted drugs with associated prognostic biomarkers will be clinically tested in the most appropriate patient populations, increasing their likelihood of regulatory approval and ultimately their availability to the patients who need them.

REFERENCES

Akiyama, T., Sudo, C., Ogawara, H., Toyoshima, K., and Yamamoto, T. (1986). The product of the human c-erbB-2 gene: A 185-kilodalton glycoprotein with tyrosine kinase activity. *Science* 232:1644–1646.

Braña, M. F., Cacho, M., Gradillas, A., de Pascual-Teresa, B., and Ramos, A. (2001). Intercalators as anticancer drugs. *Curr. Pharm. Des.* 7(17):1745–1780.

Cilley, J. C., Barfi, K., Benson, A. B., 3rd, and Mulcahy, M. F. (2007). Bevacizumab in the treatment of colorectal cancer. *Expert Opin. Biol. Ther.* 7(5):739–749.

Cragg, G. M. (2007). DNA intercalators in cancer therapy: Organic and inorganic drugs and their spectroscopic tools of analysis. *Mini. Rev. Med. Chem.* 7(6):627–648.

Dambach, D. M., Andrews, B. A., et al. (2005). New technologies and screening strategies for hepatotoxicity: Use of in vitro models. *Toxicol. Pathol.* 33(1):17–26.

Dassonville, O., Bozec, A., Fischel, J. L., and Milano, G. (2007). EGFR targeting therapies: Monoclonal antibodies versus tyrosine kinase inhibitors. Similarities and differences. *Crit. Rev. Oncol. Hematol.* 62(1):53–61.

Dolma, S., Lessnick, S. L., Hahn, W. C., and Stockwell, B. R. (2003). Identification of genotype-selective antitumor agents using synthetic lethal chemical screening in engineered human tumor cells. *Cancer Cell* 3:285–296.

Drevs, J., and Schneider, V. (2006). The use of vascular biomarkers and imaging studies in the early clinical development of anti-tumour agents targeting angiogenesis. *J. Intern. Med.* 260(6):517–529.

Duhl, D. M., and Renhowe, P. A. (2005). Inhibitors of kinesin motor proteins—research and clinical progress. *Curr. Opin. Drug Discov. Devel.* 8(4):431–436.

Edgar, K. A., Belvin, M., Parks, A. L., Whittaker, K., Mahoney, M. B., Nicoll, M., Park, C. C., Winter, C. G., Chen, F., Lickteig, K., Ahmad, F., Esengil, H., Lorenzi, M. V., Norton, A., Rupnow, B. A., Shayesteh, L., Tabios, M., Young, L. M., Carroll, P. M., Kopczynski, C., Plowman, G. D., Friedman, L. S., and Francis-Lang, H. L. (2005). Synthetic lethality of retinoblastoma mutant cells in the Drosophila eye by mutation of a novel peptidyl prolyl isomerase gene. *Genetics* 170:161–171.

Ferrara, N., Hillan, K. J., Gerber, H. P., and Novotny, W. (2004). Discovery and development of bevacizumab, an anti-VEGF antibody for treating cancer. *Nat. Rev. Drug Discov.* 3(5):391–400.

Fiebig, H. H., Maier, A., and Burger, A. M. (2004). Clonogenic assay with established human tumour xenografts: Correlation of in vitro to in vivo activity as a basis for anticancer drug discovery. *Eur. J. Cancer* 40(6):802–820.

Fluchter, S. H., Weiser, R., and Gamper, C. (2007). The role of hormonal treatment in prostate cancer. *Recent Results Cancer Res.* 175:211–237.

Folkman, J. (2007). Angiogenesis: An organizing principle for drug discovery? *Nat. Rev. Drug Discov.* 6(4):273–286.

Greenman, C., Stephens, P., Smith, R., Dalgliesh, G. L., Hunter, C., Bignell, G., Davies, H., Teague, J., Butler, A., Stevens, C., Edkins, S., O'Meara, S., Vastrik, I., Schmidt, E. E., Avis, T., Barthorpe, S., Bhamra, G., Buck, G., Choudhury, B., Clements, J., Cole, J., Dicks, E., Forbes, S., Gray, K., Halliday, K., Harrison, R., Hills, K., Hinton, J., Jenkinson, A., Jones, D., Menzies, A., Mironenko, T., Perry, J., Raine, K., Richardson, D., Shepherd, R., Small, A., Tofts, C., Varian, J., Webb, T., West, S., Widaa, S., Yates, A., Cahill, D. P., Louis,

D. N., Goldstraw, P., Nicholson, A. G., Brasseur, F., Looijenga, L., Weber, B. L., Chiew, Y. E., DeFazio, A., Greaves, M. F., Green, A. R., Campbell, P., Birney, E., Easton, D. F., Chenevix-Trench, G., Tan, M. H., Khoo, S. K., Teh, B. T., Yuen, S. T., Leung, S. Y., Wooster, R., Futreal, P. A., and Stratton, M. R. (2007). Patterns of somatic mutation in human cancer genomes. *Nature* 446:153–158.

Hoppe, R. T. (1992). Combined-modality therapy for the treatment of Hodgkin's disease. *Front Radiat. Ther. Oncol.* 26:172–180.

Hughes, T., and Branford, S. (2006). Molecular monitoring of BCR-ABL as a guide to clinical management in chronic myeloid leukaemia. *Blood Rev.* 20(1):29–41.

Imming, P., Sinning, C., and Meyer, A. (2006). Drugs, their targets and the nature and number of drug targets. *Nat. Rev. Drug Discov.* 5(10):821–834.

Johnston, J. B., Navaratnam, S., Pitz, M. W., Maniate, J. M., Wiechec, E., Baust, H., Gingerich, J., Skliris, G. P., Murphy, L. C., and Los, M. (2006). Targeting the EGFR pathway for cancer therapy. *Curr. Med. Chem.* 13(29):3483–3492.

Jordan, V. C. (2003). Tamoxifen: A most unlikely pioneering medicine. *Nat. Rev. Drug Discov.* 2(3):205–213.

Kardinal, C. G. (1985). Cancer chemotherapy. Historical aspects and future considerations. *Postgrad. Med.* 77(6):165–174.

Kasof, G. M., Prosser, J. C., Liu, D., Lorenzi, M. V., and Gomes, B. C. (2000). The RIP like kinase, *RIP3*, induces apoptosis and NF-kappaB nuclear translocation and localizes to mitochondria. *FEBS Lett.* 473:285–291.

Krausz, E. (2007). High-content siRNA screening. *Mol. Biosyst.* 3(4):232–240.

Leung, J. Y., Kolligs, F. T., Wu, R., Zhai, Y., Kuick, R., Hanash, S., Cho, K. R., and Fearon, E. R. (2002). Activation of *AXIN2* expression by beta-catenin-T cell factor. A feedback repressor pathway regulating Wnt signaling. *J. Biol. Chem.* 277: 21657–21665.

Li, A. P. (2001). Screening for human ADME/Tox drug properties in drug discovery. *Drug Discov. Today* 6(7):357–366.

Lin, J. L., Chen, H. C., Fang, H. I., Robinson, D., Kung, H. J., and Shih, H. M. (2001). *MST4*, a new Ste20-related kinase that mediates cell growth and transformation via modulating *ERK* pathway. *Oncogene* 20:6559–6569.

Longo, D. L., and DeVita, V. T., Jr. (1992). The use of combination chemotherapy in the treatment of early stage Hodgkin's disease. *Important Adv. Oncol.* 155–165.

Loughrey, M. B., Trivett, M., Beshay, V., Dobrovic, A., Kovalenko, S., Murray, W., Lade, S., Turner, H., McArthur, G. A., Zalcberg, J., and Waring, P. M. (2007). KIT immunohistochemistry and mutation status in gastrointestinal stromal tumours (GISTs) evaluated for treatment with imatinib. *Histopathology* 49(1):52–65.

Lu, J. J., and Lorenzi, M. V. (2003). Identifying and validating oncology therapeutic targets in the post-genomics era. *Curr. Genomics* 4:51–62.

Mendelsohn, J., and Baselga, J. (2006). Epidermal growth factor receptor targeting in cancer. *Semin. Oncol.* 33(4):369–385.

Meresse, P., Dechaux, E., Monneret, C., and Bertounesque, E. (2004). Etoposide: Discovery and medicinal chemistry. *Curr. Med. Chem.* 11(18):2443–2466.

Miller, J. C., Pien, H. H., Sahani, D., Sorensen, A. G., and Thrall, J. H. (2005). Imaging angiogenesis: Applications and potential for drug development. *J. Natl. Cancer Inst.* 97(3):172–187.

Minor, L. K. (2005). Assays for membrane tyrosine kinase receptors: Methods for high-throughput screening and utility for diagnostics. *Expert Rev. Mol. Diagn.* 5(4): 561–571.

Naruganahalli, K. S., Lakshmanan, M., Dastidar, S. G., and Ray, A. (2006). Therapeutic potential of Aurora kinase inhibitors in cancer. *Curr. Opin. Investig. Drugs* 7(12): 1044–1051.

Neve, R. M., Chin, K., Fridlyand, J., Yeh, J., Baehner, F. L., Fevr, T., Clark, L., Bayani, N., Coppe, J. P., Tong, F., Speed, T., Spellman, P. T., DeVries, S., Lapuk, A., Wang, N. J., Kuo, W. L., Stilwell, J. L., Pinkel, D., Albertson, D. G., Waldman, F. M., McCormick, F., Dickson, R. B., Johnson, M. D., Lippman, M., Ethier, S., Gazdar, A., and Gray, J. W. (2006). A collection of breast cancer cell lines for the study of functionally distinct cancer subtypes. *Cancer Cell* 10:515–527.

Ngo, V. N., Davis, R. E., Lamy, L., Yu, X., Zhao, H., Lenz, G., Lam, L. T., Dave, S., Yang, L., Powell, J., and Staudt, L. M. (2006). A loss-of-function RNA interference screen for molecular targets in cancer. *Nature* 441:106–110.

Noble, R. L. (1990). The discovery of the vinca alkaloids—chemotherapeutic agents against cancer. *Biochem. Cell Biol.* 68(12):1344–1351.

Olson, H., Betton, G., Robinson, D., Thomas, K., Monro, A., Kolaja, G., Lilly, P., Sanders, J., Sipes, G., Bracken, W., Dorato, M., Van Deun, K., Smith, P., Berger, B., and Heller, A. (2000). Concordance of the toxicity of pharmaceuticals in humans and in animals. *Regul. Toxicol. Pharmacol.* 32(1):56–67.

Papac, R. J. (2001). Origins of cancer therapy. *Yale J. Biol. Med.* 74(6):391–398.

Paran, Y., Lavelin, I., Naffar-Abu-Amara, S.,Winograd-Katz, S., Liron, Y., Geiger, B., and Kam, Z. (2006). Development and application of automatic high-resolution light microscopy for cell-based screens. *Methods Enzymol.* 414:228–247.

Ponzone, R., Biglia, N., Jacomuzzi, M. E., Mariani, L., Dominguez, A., and Sismondi, P. (2006). Antihormones in prevention and treatment of breast cancer. *Ann. N. Y. Acad. Sci.* 1089:143–158.

Preto, A., Moutinho, C., Velho, S., Oliveira, C., Rebocho, A. P., Figueiredo, J., Soares, P., Lopes, J. M., and Seruca, R. (2007). A subset of colorectal carcinomas express c-*KIT* protein independently of *BRAF* and/or *KRAS* activation. *Virchows Arch.* 450(6): 619–626.

Rausch, O. (2006). High content cellular screening. *Curr. Opin. Chem. Biol.* 10(4):316–320.

Saal, L. H., Johansson, P., Holm, K., Gruvberger-Saal, S. K., She, Q. B., Maurer, M., Koujak, S., Ferrando, A. A., Malmström, P., Memeo, L., Isola, J., Bendahl, P. O., Rosen, N., Hibshoosh, H., Ringnér, M., Borg, A., and Parsons, R. (2007). Poor prognosis in carcinoma is associated with a gene expression signature of aberrant *PTEN* tumor suppressor pathway activity. *Proc. Natl. Acad. Sci. U.S.A.* 104(18):7564–7569.

Sauter, G., Simon, R., and Hillan, K. (2003). Tissue microarrays in drug discovery. *Nat. Rev. Drug Discov.* 2(12):962–972.

Schiffer, C. A. (2007). *BCR-ABL* tyrosine kinase inhibitors for chronic myelogenous leukemia. *N. Engl. J. Med.* 357(3):258–265.

Scott, R. B. (1970). Cancer chemotherapy—the first twenty-five years. *Br. Med. J.* 4(5730):259–265.

Singh, S. S. (2006). Preclinical pharmacokinetics: An approach towards safer and efficacious drugs. *Curr. Drug Metab.* 7(2):165–182.

Sistare, F. D., and DeGeorge, J. J. (2007). Preclinical predictors of clinical safety: Opportunities for improvement. *Clin. Pharmacol. Ther.* 82(2):210–214.

Slamon, D. J., Leyland-Jones, B., Shak, S., Fuchs, H., Paton, V., Bajamonde, A., Fleming, T., Eiermann, W., Wolter, J., Pegram, M., Baselga, J., and Norton, L. (2001). Use of chemotherapy plus a monoclonal antibody against *HER2* for metastatic breast cancer that overexpresses *HER2*. *N. Engl. J. Med.* 344:783–792.

Sriram, D., Yogeeswari, P., Thirumurugan, R., and Bal, T. R. (2005). Camptothecin and its analogues: A review on their chemotherapeutic potential. *Nat. Prod. Res.* 19(4):393–412.

Sudakin, V., and Yen, T. J. (2007). Targeting mitosis for anti-cancer therapy. *BioDrugs* 21(4):225–233.

Suggitt, M., and Bibby, M. C. (2005). 50 years of preclinical anticancer drug screening: Empirical to target-driven approaches. *Clin. Cancer Res.* 11(3):971–981.

Szakacs, G., Paterson, J. K., Ludwig, J. A., Booth-Genthe, C., and Gottesman, M. M. (2006). Targeting multidrug resistance in cancer. *Nat. Rev. Drug Discov.* 5(3):219–234.

Tammela, T. (2004). Endocrine treatment of prostate cancer. *J. Steroid. Biochem. Mol. Biol.* 92(4):287–295.

Trusheim, M. R., Berndt, E. R., and Douglas, F. L. (2007). Stratified medicine: Strategic and economic implications of combining drugs and clinical biomarkers. *Nat. Rev. Drug Discov.* 6(4):287–293.

Vedani, A., Dobler, M., and Lill, M. A. (2006). The challenge of predicting drug toxicity in silico. *Basic Clin. Pharmacol. Toxicol.* 99(3):195–208.

Welch, A. D. (1983). Folic acid: Discovery and the exciting first decade. *Perspect. Biol. Med.* 27(1):64–75.

Wheate, N. J., Brodie, C. R., Collins, J. G., Kemp, S., and Aldrich-Wright, J. R. (2007). DNA intercalators in cancer therapy: Organic and inorganic drugs and their spectroscopic tools of analysis. *Mini. Rev. Med. Chem.* 7(6):627–648.

Zubrod, C. G. (1979). Historic milestones in curative chemotherapy. *Semin. Oncol.* 6(4): 490–505.

3

MOLECULAR PATHOLOGY AND TRANSCRIPTIONAL PROFILING IN EARLY DRUG DEVELOPMENT

Cornelia Liedtke, Lajos Pusztai, and W. Fraser Symmans

3.1. INTRODUCTION

Novel technologies have evoked changes in clinical trial design with regard to target identification and biomarker co-development. Biomarkers serve numerous purposes in the conduct of early drug development and evaluation, such as providing insight into drug pharmacodynamics and mechanism of action or prediction of response. If performed properly, transcriptional profiling technologies allow for the identification of both individual genes as well as coordinated multigene signatures. Consequently, transcriptional profiling technologies have increasingly been incorporated into modern clinical trial design to identify both potential novel targets as well as biomarkers. Novel tools to evaluate pathway activity and small-scale but coordinated changes in gene expression have great potential to define additional targets and biomarkers.

3.2. BIOMARKERS IN CLINICAL SETTING AND IN EARLY DRUG DEVELOPMENT

To date, physicians will find themselves faced with two fundamental diagnostic challenges when deciding about the treatment of newly diagnosed stage I to III breast cancer: (a) They have to predict the individual prognosis (i.e., estimate the

Molecular Pathology in Drug Discovery and Development, Edited by J. Suso Platero
Copyright © 2009 John Wiley & Sons, Inc.

likelihood of cure with surgery alone), which directs the decision of whether to initiate adjuvant (systemic) therapy at all. These parameters, that is, clinical and molecular features of the cancer that allow for estimation of the probability of cure with surgery alone, are commonly called *prognostic (bio)markers*. (b) If physicians decide to administer systemic treatment, they must then select the most appropriate systemic treatment to administer in order to increase the probability of cure. These parameters, that is, clinical and molecular features of the cancer related to a certain type of treatment are commonly referred to as *predictive (bio)markers* (Hayes et al., 1998).

It is important, however, to acknowledge that this dichotomization is not exclusive. In fact, some markers carry both prognostic and predictive features. For instance, the estrogen receptor (ER) is expressed among 60 to 70% of all breast cancers. Patients with ER-negative tumors are at increased risk for early disease recurrence and are at increased risk of visceral metastasis (Hess et al., 2003). Consequently, ER expression is considered a positive prognostic factor. However, since the advent of hormonal therapy by the means of agents such as selective estrogen receptor modulators (SERMs, e.g., tamoxifen) and aromatase inhibitors (AI, e.g., anastrozole, letrozole, and exemestane), ER has also obtained an important role in predicting response to this kind of therapy, as benefit from endocrine therapy seems to be limited to patients with ER-positive tumors (EBCTCG, 2005). Thus, ER expression can be regarded as a favorable prognostic as well as a favorable predictive factor, the latter with regard to response to hormonal therapy.

A marker with both prognostic and predictive capacity, however, can also carry opposite features. For instance, the oncoprotein HER2 is expressed among 20 to 30% of all breast cancers, and HER2 positivity has long been regarded as an unfavorable prognostic parameter (Slamon et al., 1989, 1987). However, since trastuzumab (Herceptin, Genentech, Inc.), a monoclonal antibody directed against HER2, has demonstrated improved survival and quality of life when given in combination with taxanes as first-line therapy to women with metastatic breast cancer (Marty et al., 2005; Osoba et al., 2002; Slamon et al., 2001), and even more so since the demonstration of a survival benefit from the addition of trastuzumab to adjuvant chemotherapy in patients with HER2-positive breast cancer (Piccart-Gebhart et al., 2005; Joensuu et al., 2006; Romond et al., 2005; Slamon et al., 2005), HER2 expression has also assigned a predictive value. Importantly, benefit from HER2-targeting treatment seems to be almost exclusively limited to patients who have HER2-positive tumors. Hence, while HER2 expression in breast cancer is of negative prognostic value in the absence of trastuzumab therapy, it is of positive predictive value in the context of trastuzumab treatment (Ferretti et al., 2007). Recent reports also suggest that HER2 expression might predict for benefit from addition of neoadjuvant taxanes such as docetaxel (Learn et al., 2005) and paclitaxel (Andre et al., 2007b). Figure 3.1 shows how assessment of HER2 may provide guidance in deciding on adjuvant trastuzumab in patients with early-stage breast cancer.

Recent developments in clinical trial design have expanded the term "biomarker" even further, that is, relating to a number of different parameters that

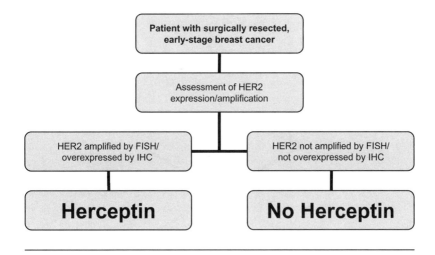

FISH, fluorescence in-situ hybridization
IHC, immunohistochemistry

Figure 3.1. HER2 expression as a predictive biomarker of trastuzumab therapy.

aid in the implementation of a novel compound into clinical practice as well as the conduct of clinical trials (Fig. 3.2). *Pharmacodynamic biomarkers* are biomarkers that are modulated according to the dosage of the drug and are intimately connected to the affected pathway. They consist mostly in the actual drug target or a downstream pathway component and should be indicative of pathway activity/inhibition. They may allow for monitoring of the pharmacodynamic effects of a novel targeted compound in the exposed individual. *Dosage biomarkers* may assist in defining optimal drug dosing and dosing schedule. For instance, a dosage biomarker may be a metabolite whose concentration is correlated to the concentration of the drug itself and may therefore serve as a surrogate marker to find its optimal dosage. *Predictive biomarkers*, again mostly indicating efficacy of pathway targeting, can assist in defining the patient population that might derive the most benefit from a novel component. Optimally, a predictive biomarker should be able to dichotomize a patient population into those individuals who have an excellent chance of response to the drug and those patients who have only a very low chance to benefit and might derive greater benefit from an alternate choice of treatment. *Response/efficacy biomarkers* may be used to identify early effects of therapy in a given individual and may also help understanding the lack of response in a given patient. It has been recognized, for instance, that the occurrence of mild to moderate rash in patients with non-small-cell lung cancer (NSCLC) correlates with improved clinical outcome. Provided that this correlation is further confirmed in independent studies, the biomarker "rash after EGFR-targeted therapy" [epidermal growth factor receptor (EGFR)] might be regarded as a surrogate marker of efficacy of this type of

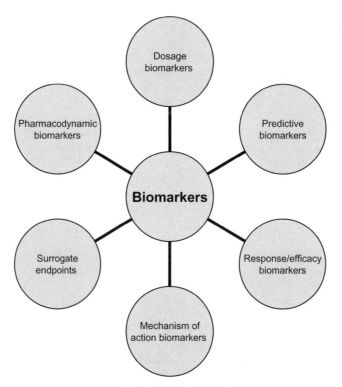

Figure 3.2. Types of biomarkers.

therapy (Perez-Soler, 2006). *Mechanism of action biomarkers* should allow for monitoring if a proposed mechanism that has been proposed from in vitro results is actually met in the in vivo context. This may allow for understanding adverse reactions, as well as emergence of resistance. *Surrogate endpoints* represent accepted clinical endpoints, such as survival parameters or pathologic measurements of response. They should be undoubtedly linked to long-term clinical outcome parameters and should provide clear information on future therapy response. As such, achievement of pathological complete response (pCR), which is broadly defined as lack of any invasive tumor in the specimen obtained at time of definitive surgery, has been demonstrated to serve as an early surrogate marker of the more important endpoint of prolonged overall survival (Fisher et al., 1998; Kuerer et al., 1999). Novel potential surrogate markers have been suggested, most of which can be summarized as "minimal residual disease detection methods," such as quantification methods in hematological diseases such as chronic myelogenous leukemia (CML). Recently, minimal residual disease detection methods have become of interest in solid tumors as well. In breast cancer, for example, circulating tumor cells (CTCs) have been associated with decreased survival in patients with metastatic breast cancer (Dawood and Cristofanilli, 2007).

3.3. ADVANTAGES OF BIOMARKER IMPLEMENTATION

It has been outlined that inclusion of predictive biomarkers into clinical trial design, that is, limitation of study recruitment only to those patients in whom a given predictor is present, may result in a reduction of patients that need to be randomized for the study. Simon and Maitournam (2004) simulated a clinical trial situation in which they compared two different trial designs with regard to the number of patients needed to be (a) randomized and (b) screened in order to demonstrate a certain outcome benefit. An "untargeted trial" design (i.e., patients being randomized regardless of their marker status) was compared against two "targeted trial" settings: (i) a targeted trial design in which an outcome benefit was strictly limited to marker-positive patients and (ii) a targeted trial design in which marker-negative patients did benefit but to a lower extent than marker-positive patients. Overall, the untargeted design required randomization of 75% more patients than both forms of untargeted trial design. However, calculation of the number of patients that would need to be screened in order to identify a marker-positive population revealed an interesting finding: The number of patients needed to be screened in a targeted design, compared to the number of patients needed to be randomized in the untargeted design, was significantly lower only when no benefit would be expected in marker-negative patients. On the contrary, when marker-negative patients derived a partial benefit from the tested agent, more patients would need to be screened in the targeted design than patients would need to be randomized in the untargeted design (Simon and Maitournam, 2004). The importance of implementing patient selection criteria based on biomarkers into clinical study design can be demonstrated persuasively in the context of benefit from HER2-targeted therapy with the HER2-directed humanized antibody trastuzumab. The pivotal trial from Slamon et al. (2001) randomized patients with advanced breast cancer to receive chemotherapy either in combination with or without trastuzumab. Inclusion criteria required HER2 overexpression (immunohistochemical score of 2+ or 3+) for enrollment in the trial. In this patient cohort, addition of trastuzumab to chemotherapy resulted in a statistically significant overall survival benefit (median survival, 25.1 vs. 20.3 months; $p = 0.01$; Slamon et al., 2001). It has been reasoned, however, that if HER2 overexpression had not been an inclusion criterion, no survival benefit would have been observed in the patient cohort of 469 patients as enrolled in the trial (Simon and Maitournam, 2004). If benefit had not been restricted to HER2-positive patients, but patients with HER2-negative tumors also had experienced some degree of benefit (i.e., 50%), as many as 1256 patients would have been required to demonstrate a significant survival benefit. If HER2-negative patients received no benefit at all, as many as 23,586 patients would have been needed for demonstration of a survival benefit. Consequently, it has been demonstrated that when molecular heterogeneity in a given study cohort remains unaccounted for, this may result in lack of sufficient study power to show benefit of a certain intervention that may lead to improved outcome in only a certain subset of study individuals (Betensky et al., 2002). These observations underscore the importance of defining biomarkers of maximal discriminatory performance. Those have the potential to account for patient population heterogeneity that might otherwise obscure small benefits in unselected patient cohorts.

A clinically useful biomarker has to fulfill three requirements: it has to (a) be objectively measurable, (b) indicate the state (i.e., activity) of a biological process, such as a response to therapeutic intervention, and (c) require no more than minimally invasive methods for determination. As of the latter, it becomes obvious that this can be provided well by imaging technologies, examination of tumor tissue when available through tumor biopsy or routine surgery, and serum markers. In this context, gene expression analysis holds the promise of an important tool in the generation of novel molecular targets and biomarkers, as it generates a molecular profile of any given tissue (esp. cancer tissue) consisting of a large number of genes. This provides an invaluable tool to correlate transcriptional tumor features with clinical tumor phenotype and outcome measures. It is important to acknowledge that, especially in the context of signal transduction inhibitors, a large number of potential biomarkers exist, such as various up- and down-stream signaling molecules of that particular pathway. However, the high content of information that could be derived from a detailed pharmacooncologic trial comes at the cost of trial complexity and conflicts with the actual feasibility of biomarker modeling in the clinical trial setting. For example, evaluation of a serum biomarker might require a complex phlebotomy schedule and as such may also come at the cost of decreased patient compliance. Consequently, the design of pharmacooncologic clinical trials requires prioritization of targets based on scientific and technical considerations. However, novel methods, such as transcriptional expression profiling might allow for assessment of a more complex number of potential biomarkers.

Nomograms are a means to combine a set of well-established single predictive factors into a multivariable prediction model and therefore may represent a more appropriate means to address (breast) cancer heterogeneity. They represent mathematical matrices that integrate prognostic information from a variety of sources (Kattan and Scardino, 2002). It is a well-established fact that tumor features such as tumor size, nuclear grade, and estrogen receptor expression status may individually influence the probability of benefit from neoadjuvant systemic treatment. Consideration of clinicopathological features, such as tumor size, grade or nodal status, in concert with molecular markers such as multigene signatures or serum protein profiles may allow for outcome prediction with increased accuracy. Rouzier et al. (2005a) developed a nomogram based on clinical stage, estrogen receptor status, histologic grade, and number of preoperative chemotherapy cycles to predict probability of response to (neoadjuvant) chemotherapy for patients with stage I to III breast cancer. A separate nomogram to predict distant metastasis-free survival (DMFS) was developed using Cox proportional hazards regression model. When testing the model on two independent cohorts of patients, high concordance with actual patient outcome was observed. The nomogram for DMFS had equally high concordance indices and outperformed other prediction tools (Rouzier et al., 2005a).

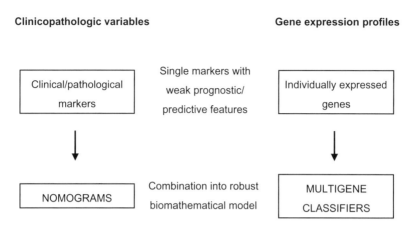

Figure 3.3. Increased information through combination of parameters.

Figure 3.3 demonstrates how the generation of a multivariable nomogram resembles the development of a multigene prediction model. Although both approaches differ with regards to mathematical matrix used to compute them, they both represent the idea that combination of a number of (clinical or molecular) markers may be a more accurate means to classify diseases such as breast cancer with regard to various endpoints.

3.4. CHANGING PARADIGM IN CLINICAL DRUG AND BIOMARKER DEVELOPMENT

Novel technologies have challenged historical approaches to therapeutic target and biomarker identification and validation in the field of oncology. Traditionally, antitumor activity of certain components has been hypothesized based on observations in humans, xenograft, or cell line models. Consequently, these agents were transferred to the laboratory and examined both for suitability as a pharmacological agent and for their mechanism of action, again using mostly cell lines or xenograft models. If in vitro and in vivo efficacy testing yielded promising results and did not cause safety concerns, these agents were allowed to enter the clinical stage. Furthermore, patient selection was mostly based on empirical observations or histological characteristics. Combination of antitumor agents was mostly empirical or at most based on observation of synergistic or at least additive effects in preclinical models. Biomarker development was usually conducted retrospectively rather than prospectively and consisted of examination of archival patient tissue after study closure, when potential biomarkers became imminent based on novel scientific observations.

It should be acknowledged that these approaches have led to the emergence of a number of active antitumor agents. In breast cancer, survival rates have increased significantly over the last two to three decades (EBCTCG, 2005). However, novel approaches might be required to continue this success in drug development. It is increasingly recognized that cancers, even when derived from the same tissue of origin, might still comprise considerable heterogeneity with regard to both disease biology and prognosis (Sorlie et al., 2001; van de Vijver et al., 2002) as well as to response to systemic therapy (Hess et al., 2006). Hence, it is increasingly recognized that novel therapeutic concepts (a) should consist of targeted therapies that benefit a patient subset that carries this target and (b) may require prediction of response based on certain biomarkers that may be derived, for instance, from examination of individual tumor tissue specimens.

Recent approaches in early drug development increasingly meet these concerns. Modern oncology drug development is a complex multistep process. First, a novel target has to be identified and validated. In this context, two major approaches toward identification of a novel target should be distinguished:

1. Screening/correlation analysis of large-scale clinical data sets using high-throughput technology
2. Hypothesis generation based on biological pathway analysis

This step should then be followed by testing the potential target for its suitability through mechanistic research in cell lines and xenograft models. If this is provided, an active agent such as an antibody or a small molecule will be generated and evaluated in vitro for activity in its designated context. The next step comprises the evaluation of the novel agent in preclinical up to clinical phase II studies, before the novel agent will finally be taken into the phase III clinical trial setting to demonstrate its superiority or at least noninferiority against known agents.

An important difference between the classical and the modern trial design are the time points at which biomarker identification and especially validation will be performed. Provided that the target as well as its signaling context is known, implementation of biomarkers, such as representatives of pathway activity, may be included as soon as the novel compound enters the clinical (or even preclinical) stage. Furthermore, it is not only the agent itself that is designed based on a certain scientific rationale. Also, combinatory partners are chosen based on considerations derived from molecular pathology and pathway interactions. As a consequence, development of biomarkers and biomarker assessment is required parallel to the development of the actual compound. Recent trials have met this requirement through subset analyses in which a more detailed evaluation of a subgroup of the total study population is performed.

The increasing importance of side-by-side evaluation of novel drugs and corresponding biomarkers has also been acknowledged by the U.S. Food and Drug Administration (FDA). In 2005, the FDA issued a statement paper (http://www.fda.gov/cder/genomics/pharmacoconceptfn.pdf) in which the importance of "Drug-Test Co-Development" was outlined. The report describes the implementation of novel oncologic products requiring evaluation of both agent efficacy and safety as well as validation of the appropriate biomarker (i.e., test).

3.5. PROMISES OF TRANSCRIPTIONAL PROFILING

Transcriptional profiling refers the simultaneous measurement of the expression of thousands of messenger ribonucleic acids (mRNAs) in a given tissue or cell suspension by the means of oligonucleotide and complementary dioxyribonucleic acid (cDNA) microarrays (Brown and Botstein, 1999; Fig. 3.4). This approach is based on the assumption, that differences in the expression level of a certain number of mRNAs among cells reflects the activity of their corresponding genes and thereby determines their individual phenotype. Shalon et al. (1996) and Lockhart et al. (1996) were the first to describe the experimental background of this technology. Briefly, RNA is isolated from the analytical specimen (i.e., patient tissue, cell lines), is reverse transcribed into cDNA, and again transcribed into cRNA (complementary RNA), thereby introducing a labeling system such as biotinylation. The biotinylized cRNA specimen is then hybridized to the actual

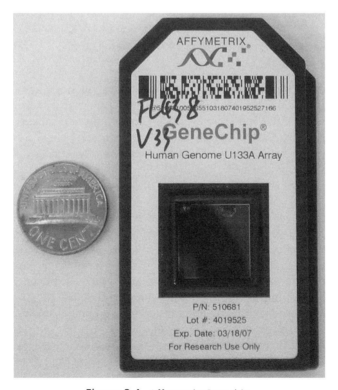

Figure 3.4. Affymetrix Genechip.

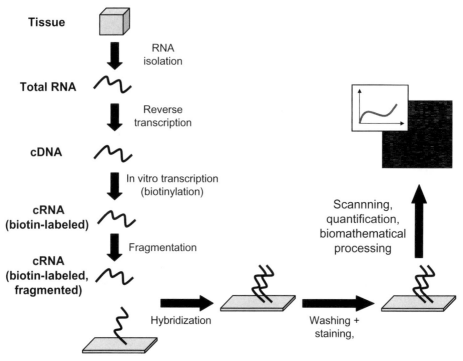

Figure 3.5. Genechip processing.

genechip, which contains complementary genomic sequences bound to a carrier matrix. Depending on the array system used, these can be either cDNA or oligonuecleotides (Pusztai and Gianni, 2004). The amount of (labeled) RNA bound to the array corresponds to the amount of a given gene (probeset) in the test specimen and will be determined using a scanning device (Fig. 3.5). To date, a number of platforms have become available commercially to measure mRNA expression based on its ability to hybridize to corresponding probesets on a given matrix.

Transcriptional profiling technology has become an established feature of a high number of research areas, such as prognostic/predictive biomarker development and characterization of complex molecular pathways. It provides a scientific/diagnostic tool to determine the degree of activity of certain genes in a given tissue (such as tumor tissue). Table 3.1 briefly summarizes the possible implementations of translational profiling in human (breast) cancer research and therapeutic development. First, molecular profiling has assisted to overcome insufficiencies in morphological classification of breast cancer and led to the description of a number of breast cancer subtypes that share a similar transcriptional profile. To date, breast cancer is understood to consist of molecular subclasses such as luminal A, ErbB2-positive, or basal-like cancers (Perou et al., 2000; Sorlie et al., 2003). Interestingly, molecular subclasses do not only serve as a means to capture breast cancer het-

TABLE 3.1. Translational Profiling in Human Breast Cancer Research and Therapeutic Development

Determination of tumor subgroups based on transcriptional differences (i.e., molecular classification of breast cancer) (Perou et al., 2000; Sorlie et al., 2003)

Determination of tumor prognosis based on its transcriptional profile [i.e., 70-gene signature (Mammaprint), 76-gene signature] (van de Vijver et al., 2002; Wang et al., 2005)

Refinement/optimization of known clinicopathologic parameters (i.e., GGI[a]) (Sotiriou et al., 2006)

Prediction of probability of response to a given (systemic) therapy [i.e., 30-gene predictor of response to neoadjuvant T/FAC[b] chemotherapy (DLDA-30[c])] (Hess et al., 2006)

Identification of novel single markers or potential targets (i.e., GABRP[d], tau) (Tordai et al., 2007; Rouzier et al., 2005b)

Identification of pathways indicative of certain tumor subtypes (i.e., five pathway signatures) (Bild et al., 2006)

[a] Genomic Grade Index.
[b] Chemotherapy with paclitaxel followed by 5-fluoruracil, adriamycin, and cyclophosphamide.
[c] Diagonal linear discriminant analysis.
[d] Gamma-aminobutyric acid receptor π subunit.

erogeneity but are also associated with disease prognosis, that is, basal-like and ErbB2-positive breast cancers exhibiting a more unfavorable prognosis than other breast cancer subtypes (Sorlie et al., 2006). In fact, it is increasingly recognized that variations in prognosis as well as response to systemic therapy can be seen among tumors of the same tissue of origin or even the same histological tumor subtype and may be related to different transcriptional features. Two major approaches can be distinguished: (a) identification of patients that may be *spared* from therapy that would have been recommended based on traditional markers but not based on the molecular expression profile and (b) identification of patients that may need *additional* therapy that would not have been recommended based on traditional markers but will be based on the molecular expression profile (Fig. 3.6). Current guidelines in breast cancer treatment recommend the application of adjuvant endocrine and/or chemotherapy in the majority of breast cancer patients (Goldhirsch et al., 2007). Thus, genomic approaches to identify relevant prognostic subgroups among breast cancer patients has been aimed to define patient subgroups whose prognosis is favorable enough to spare them from unnecessary and potentially toxic treatments. Using transcriptional profiles of 295 primary lymph-node-negative breast carcinomas, van de Vijver et al. (2002) were the first to report on the compilation of a 70-gene signature that allowed for dichotomization of the patient cohort into a poor-prognosis and a good-prognosis group: overall 10-year survival rates associated with the good-prognosis signature, as compared to the poor-prognosis signature, were 95 and 55%, respectively ($P < 0.001$). Validation of the prognostic signature in an independent cohort of 307 breast cancer patents

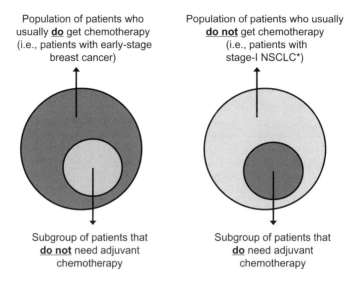

Population of patients who usually **do** get chemotherapy (i.e., patients with early-stage breast cancer)

Population of patients who usually **do not** get chemotherapy (i.e., patients with stage-I NSCLC*)

Subgroup of patients that **do not** need adjuvant chemotherapy

Subgroup of patients that **do** need adjuvant chemotherapy

* Non-small-cell lung cancer

Figure 3.6. Predictive biomarkers may predict or exclude benefit from therapy.

was carried out. It showed that the gene signature contained its significant association with an increased risk of death in the poor-prognosis cohort. Another group has reported on the identification and successful validation of a 76-gene prognostic signature in patients with lymph-node-negative breast cancer (Wang et al., 2005; Foekens et al., 2006). This signature consisted of 60 and 16 genes for ER-positive and ER-negative patients, respectively. The gene profile could identify patients with an increased risk of distant metastases within 5 years and was validated with a sensitivity of 93% and a specificity of 48% in an independent validation set of 171 lymph-node-negative breast cancer patients (Wang et al., 2005). This signature has subsequently been successfully validated in an independent data set representing a more diverse population of lymph-node-negative patients from multiple institutions. Sensitivity and specificity for 5-year distant metastasis-free survival was 90 and 50%, respectively. The positive and negative predictive values were 38% [95% confidence interval (CI), 29 to 47%] and 94% (95% CI, 86 to 97%), respectively (Foekens et al., 2006).

In contrast, current guidelines recommend that the standard of treatment for patients with stage I NSCLC be limited to surgical resection, while adjuvant chemotherapy for this disease stage is thus far not recommended outside of clinical trials (Pisters et al., 2007). However, recurrence rates of as high as 30 to 35% have been reported following initial surgery, indicating that a subgroup among stage IA NSCLC exhibits a particularly adverse prognosis (Hoffman et al., 2000; Mountain, 1997; Nesbitt et al., 1995). It has been suggested that molecular profiling might allow for identification of those patients with stage IA NSCLC who carry a particularly unfavorable prognosis and may therefore need additional therapy. Potti et al. (2006b) identified a gene-expression-based lung metagene model predictive of risk of recurrence in a cohort of 89 patients with early-stage NSCLC. The lung metagene model was shown to predict recurrence significantly better than clinical prognostic factors among all early stages of NSCLC. It could further be validated in two independent patient cohorts and exhibited an overall predictive accuracy of 72 to 79%. Most importantly, the predictor could identify a subgroup of patients with stage IA disease who were at increased risk of recurrence and who might in fact benefit from adjuvant chemotherapy (Potti et al., 2006b). These studies show that gene expression profiling allows for refinement of standard staging systems and thus may assist in tailoring current treatment regimens more appropriately.

Furthermore, transcriptional profiling can be employed to refine or even replace well-established clinical and pathologic markers, such as tumor grade. Sotiriou et al. (2006) developed a panel of 97 genes that were differentially expressed between grade 1 and grade 3 breast cancers and combined them into a "genomic grade index" (GGI). They demonstrated that the GGI is significantly associated with tumor prognosis in several independent data sets. Strikingly, when applying the GGI to grade 2 tumors, the authors demonstrated that grade 2 breast cancers can be subdivided into one group with a similarly favorable prognosis as grade 1 cancers in contrast to another group whose prognosis resemble the one associated with grade 3 tumors. It seems that the GGI comprises a refinement of the classical pathological grading systems especially with regard to grade 2 breast cancers (Sotiriou et al., 2006). However, an important promise of these new high-throughput technologies is their applicability to predict treatment response for two reasons:

1. Transcriptional profiling covers a high number of genes with often unknown biological function. It seems reasonable to argue that among these several individual genes might hold the promise of potential pharmacologic targets and biomarkers.
2. Given the high amount of intra- and intertumor heterogeneity more than a single gene within a tumor alone has to be measured to determine a patient's probability to respond to a given treatment. This provides the rationale for using gene expression profiling, which allows for development of regimen-specific complex transcriptional markers to predict which patients might actually benefit from a given cytotoxic regimen.

3.6. BIOMARKER DEVELOPMENT AND VALIDATION USING MICROARRAY ANALYSIS

However, some degree of both technical and analytical bias still remains to be accounted for. Overall, gene expression data carries the risk of systematical bias when not analyzed properly. Sources of variation when performing gene expression analysis comprise variation between corresponding probes on different arrays for the same sample, between labeling reactions for the same RNA specimen, between specimens for the same individual, and between individuals within a population (Simon et al., 2002).

A number of different gene expression platforms are currently used. However, cross-platform comparison of gene expression profiling results has shown considerable divergence (Kuo et al., 2002; Tan et al., 2003; Yuen et al., 2002), rendering data comparisons difficult. It has been demonstrated that when assigning certain probesets from different platforms to a given gene, there is a strong influence of the method used to match probesets and gene identifications (IDs). Ji et al. (2006) profiled samples from 33 breast cancer patients on two different microarray platforms (Affymetrix and cDNA). UniGene-based gene matching resulted in poor correlations of gene expression results between platforms. In contrast, using RefSeq, a database maintained by the National Center for Biotechnology Information (NCBI), gene matching could be significantly improved (Ji et al., 2006). This demonstrated that gene expression measurements of one gene on different platforms may be highly concordant if the probesets match to the same gene sequence. However, it is important to realize that this is rarely met when expression results between different platforms are compared. Before a novel biomarker is established for routine clinical use, it is essential to demonstrate that it is highly reproducible within and across laboratories. In order to demonstrate the inter- and intralaboratory reproducibility of the Affymetrix gene expression technology, Anderson et al. (2006) profiled 35 cases of fine-needle aspiration biopsies from breast cancer patients in replicates: 17 within the same laboratory, 11 in two different laboratories, and 15 to assess manual and robotic labeling. The average concordance correlation coefficients were 0.978 (range, 0.96 to 0.99), 0.962 (range, 0.94 to 0.98), and 0.971 (range, 0.93 to 0.99) for intralaboratory, between-laboratory replicates, and for manual versus robotic labeling, respectively. When complex multigene models were tested, >90% agreement in replicate data was reached (Anderson et al., 2006). Another potential bias lies within data normalization. The purpose of data normalization as an initial step of gene expression data analysis consists in the reduction of experimental variability (i.e., artificial noise) without influencing biological variability of gene expression (Hegde et al., 2000). A number of methods have been described to accomplish this (Smyth et al., 2003; Kerr et al., 2001; Tseng et al., 2001). However, cross comparison of different data sets that have been normalized using different normalization methods harbors a substantial risk for systematic bias. The FDA has addressed the issue of interplatform and intraplatform reproducibility of transcriptional profiling by conducting a large comprehensive study, namely the MicroArray Quality Control Phase I (MAQC-I) project. The study demonstrated high concordance in determining differentially expressed genes (as the tested variable) when the same specimen was tested on different platforms or repeatedly on the same platform in various testing sites (MAQC Consortium, 2006). Phase II of the MAQC project is currently being planned. MAQC-II has been designed to address the reproducibility of complex gene

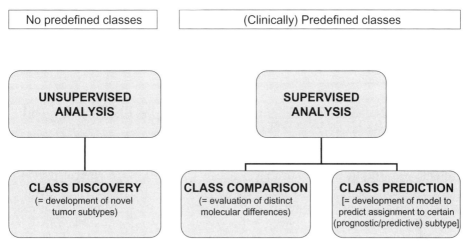

Figure 3.7. Different types of biomarker analysis.

expression profiles rather than single individual genes in interplatform and interlaboratory replicates (http://www.fda.gov/nctr/science/centers/toxicoinformatics/maqc/).

A number of different methods exist that allow for analysis of gene expression patterns and development of classification algorithms in gene expression data sets. Those can broadly be subdivided into three different approaches: (a) class discovery, (b) class comparison, and (c) class prediction (Fig. 3.7).

Class discovery studies are based on the hypothesis that new subclasses of a heterogeneous entity (such as breast cancer) may be discovered de novo using gene expression profiles. Cluster analysis, such as unsupervised hierarchical clustering, are generally applied in these types of studies (Eisen et al., 1998). Unsupervised analysis is understood as an analysis without knowledge of clinical parameters. This type of "blinded" approach does not exclude, however, that correlation with clinical parameters might be performed after the molecular classes have been assigned to test the performance as well as clinical utility of the classification. In contrast, *class comparison* and *class prediction* studies make use of clinical information and are characterized as supervised approaches. Data analysis is carried out with the goal to identify molecular differences between certain predefined groups. Sample classes are identified independently of gene expression data using known clinical parameters such as tumor grade (Loi et al., 2007), *p53* mutation status (Miller et al., 2005), or development of distant metastasis within 5 years (van 't Veer et al., 2002). Class comparison and class prediction are closely linked and often not truly separable. In fact, many supervised studies include both class comparison and class prediction approaches. Class prediction differs from class comparison in that it emphasizes the development of a gene-expression-based multivariate function that may be employed to assign new cases to the distinct classes. This model is usually referred to as the predictor. Class comparison and prediction approaches have been used, for instance, with regard to patient outcome (van 't Veer et al., 2002) or response to neoadjuvant chemotherapy (Hess et al., 2006).

3.7. NEOADJUVANT CHEMOTHERAPY AS AN INTRIGUING MODEL FOR BIOMARKER DEVELOPMENT

To date preoperative chemotherapy is regarded as the standard of care for patients with locally advanced breast cancer. It leads to high clinical response rates harboring the promise of down-staging of tumors, thus rendering a number of previously inoperable tumors suitable for either surgery or even breast-conserving treatment. Importantly, it has been demonstrated that even patients with early-stage breast cancer can benefit from the administration of chemotherapy before rather than after surgery, as patients treated with neoadjuvant chemotherapy may be able to undergo less extensive resection (Boughey et al., 2006). Importantly, clinical long-term outcomes such as disease-free and overall survival in this group of patients do not seem to vary whether chemotherapy is administered before or after surgical treatment (Scholl et al., 1994). The National Surgical Adjuvant Breast and Bowel Project (NSABP) Protocol B-18 was designed to compare four cycles of doxorubicin/cyclophosphamide given preoperatively to the same regimen given postoperatively with respect to overall survival (OS) and disease-free survival (DFS) in patients with breast cancer. Even after 9 years of follow-up, no statistically significant overall differences in OS or DFS between the two treatment groups was observed, with OS at 9 years being 70% in the postoperative group and 69% in the preoperative group ($P = 0.80$). Patients receiving preoperative chemotherapy could undergo significantly more lumpectomies than patients who were randomized to receive a postoperative regimen, especially patients with tumors that had a diameter greater than 3 cm (Wolmark et al., 2001). Several studies have corroborated these results in that even in patients with operable tumors there is no statistically significant difference in survival between those who receive chemotherapy before surgery compared to those who are treated with the same regimen postoperatively (Makris et al., 1998; Mauriac et al., 1991). Application of neoadjuvant as opposed to adjuvant chemotherapy is associated with a number of advantages as well as disadvantages (Table 3.2). Most importantly, however, administration of preoperative chemotherapy and determination of rates of pathological complete response (pCR) as opposed to residual disease (RD) may serve as an excellent tool to develop prognostic or predictive markers while being of no clear disadvantage to the individual patient.

It has been noted, however, that dichotomization into pCR and RD may be too simplistic to completely capture the complexity of response to neoadjuvant chemotherapy in patients with breast cancer. Thus, a novel measurement has recently been introduced: the residual cancer burden (RCB) score (http://www.mdanderson.org/breastcancer_RCB) combines the largest diameter of the inva-

TABLE 3.2. Advantages and Disadvantages of Neoadjuvant Chemotherapy

---

Advantages

Possibility of early response monitoring (option to change the treatment)[a]
Possibility of tumor shrinkage
    Enabling breast-conserving surgery
    Possibility of reduced surgery even in primarily operable breast cancer
Utilization of pathological complete remission (pCR) as an early surrogate marker
    for overall survival
Unique opportunity to identify molecular predictors of chemotherapy response to
    various chemotherapy regimens (with pCR as a surrogate marker and clinical
    endpoint)

Disadvantages

Necessity of surgical/pathological staging in some patients to determine need for
    chemotherapy
Inevitability of frequent consultations:
    To assess patient response
    To avoid unacknowledged tumor progression (occurring in up to 5% of patients)
Necessity to postpone final surgery to several months which may
    Cause increased psychological stress caused by fear of disease spread
    Endanger eligibility for (breast conserving) surgery in case of tumor progression
Difficulty to asses the original tumor bed in the case of excellent response[b]
Reluctance to change the well-established and well-documented standard practice in
    face of lack of improved survival with neoadjuvant schedule
Risk of complications such as neutropenia while on chemotherapy (postponing
    further systemic therapy)
Loss of important prognostic information, such as true pathologic tumor size and
    lymph node status[c]
Fear of increased risk for local recurrences[d]

---

[a] However, no increased response rates when changing to "second-line"-chemotherapy regimen after failure of the prior.
[b] May be circumvented by marking the original tumor site (i.e., tattoo, ultrasound-assisted insertion of a radioopaque marker).
[c] May be counterbalanced by residual tumor size and the number of lymph nodes involved with carcinoma after neoadjuvant chemotherapy.
[d] Which, however, has been supported in neither randomized clinical trials nor large single institution case series.

sive cancer, the percent cellularity of the tumor, the number of lymph nodes involved, and the largest diameter of the nodal involvement into a neoadjuvant chemotherapy response score (Symmans et al., 2007a). This score correlates with survival and can be used to define four distinct pathologic response categories RCB-0 (same as pCR), RCB-I (near pCR), RCB-II (moderate residual cancer), and RCB-III (extensive residual cancer). These RCB categories are predictive of long-term survival; patients who achieve RCB-I pathologic response have similar overall and disease-free survival as the patients achieving pCR (i.e., RCB-0) and those with RCB-III have very poor prognosis, particularly if they have ER-negative disease (Symmans et al., 2007a).

3.8. TRANSCRIPTIONAL PROFILING FOR IDENTIFICATION OF INDIVIDUAL GENES AS BIOMARKERS

The most commonly used approach for individual feature selection from the list of thousands of genes usually produced in transcriptional profiling experiments is to determine genes that are differentially expressed in a given population with respect to a known outcome or clinical parameter. Differential gene expression analysis is based on the assumption that if a gene is significantly higher expressed in one subset compared to the other, it contributes to the clinical or pathological phenotype of the subset and can be employed to assign other cases to this subset. Statistical analysis such as unequal variance t test, nonparametric tests, or Bayesian networks (Efron and Tibshirani, 2002) are appropriate tools to determine differentially expressed genes in a given data set.

Although simple, the search for differentially expressed genes is associated with a number of statistical pitfalls. Lists of differentially expressed genes, especially when rank ordered, are inherently unstable and even more so when they are generated based on small sample sets and the genes they contain have only limited discriminatory value (Pusztai and Hess, 2004). Another major problem when analyzing high-dimensional data sets is that statistical values used for traditional correlative analysis might no longer be valid. This issue has been related to "multiple hypotheses testing" and has to be addressed when the number of variables (i.e., probesets) examined exceeds the number of test individuals (i.e., tissue specimens/patients) (Osier et al., 2004). In this setting, a p value of <0.0001 might not indicate a significant association with sufficient probability. Determination of the false discovery rate (FDR) can assist in determining a truly significant association (Storey and Tibshirani, 2003; Tusher et al., 2001). In multiple hypotheses testing, the FDR indicates the number of false-positive results, that is, the number of associations that may be expected by chance alone. Determination of the FDR is a more stringent parameter that usually reduces the number of genes considered significant compared to the use of the p value alone. Commonly, an FDR of <0.01 is regarded as appropriate to characterize a gene as being significantly differentially expressed. Importantly, the FDR can be used not only to identify the significance of an association between a single probeset and an outcome variable or group assignment but also to determine the significance of a pathway being present in a certain group (see below).

The characterization of the microtubule-associated protein tau as a predictor of paclitaxel chemosensitivity serves as a good illustration of how differential gene expression can be implemented to define new breast cancer biomarkers. Tau has been identified through the use of gene expression profiling (Rouzier et al., 2005b): 82 stage I to III breast cancers from patients who had been treated with neoadjuvant T/FAC chemotherapy (weekly taxol followed by three-weekly 5-fluoruracil, adriamycin, and cyclophosphamide) at the M. D. Anderson Cancer Center were screened using Affymetrix U133A GeneChips. Response to neoadjuvant chemotherapy was dichotomized based on pathological examination of the tissue specimen at the time of surgery into pathologic complete response and residual disease. Comparison of gene expression profiles between these two response groups revealed that tau was the most differentially expressed gene. Consequently, tumors with pCR had significantly lower tau mRNA expression $[P < 0.3 \times 10(-5)]$. In other words, low tau expression was a predictor of response to chemotherapy in this cohort. To validate this finding molecular pathology was used by making tissue microarrays from 122 independent breast cancer cases, which had received similar treatment, and stained them with an antitau antibody. In multivariate analysis, tau-negative status ($P = 0.04$) was an independent predictor of pCR among these cases. Of note, data mining based on gene expression profiling is highly susceptible to false-positive discoveries and is usually carried out independently from the biological background. Hence, it is helpful to provide biological validation as well. In the study we have described above, down-regulation of tau in breast cancer cell lines was performed using small interfering RNA experiments and led to increased sensitivity of breast cancer cell lines to paclitaxel but not epirubicin in vitro. The lack of correlation between tau expression and response to epirubicin alluded that tau may be a paclitaxel-specific predictor rather than predicting general chemosensitivity. To provide a mechanistic model to explain this phenomenon, a tubulin polymerization assay was carried out. Preincubation of tubulin with tau caused decreased paclitaxel binding and reduced paclitaxel-induced microtubule polymerization (Rouzier et al., 2005b). However, the predictive value of tau has not remained unchallenged. Rody et al. (2007) reported on gene expression data obtained from of 50 patients with breast cancer enrolled onto an anthracycline and taxane-containing neoadjuvant chemotherapy trial. No correlation between pCR rate and tau mRNA expression was observed. Another study suggests that the predictive role of tau might exceed that of a predictor of response for taxane-containing neoadjuvant chemotherapy and may in fact also be related to response to adjuvant endocrine therapy as well as to disease prognosis in the absence of systemic therapy (Andre et al., 2007a). Increased tau expression when determined by gene expression analysis predicted significantly decreased risk of disease recurrence at 5 and 10 years ($P = 0.005$ and $P = 0.05$, respectively) in 267 patients treated with adjuvant tamoxifen, indicating a predictive value for endocrine therapy. It also showed a nonsignificant trend toward better prognosis in 209 patients, who received no adjuvant systemic treatment at all (Fig. 3.8).

Another example is the identification of GABRP (gamma-aminobutyric acid receptor π subunit) as a novel gene with particular relevance to ER- and HER2-negative breast cancer (Symmans et al., 2005). Gene expression profiles from ER/HER2 breast cancers were compared to tumors expressing these receptors, using two independent gene expression data sets ($n = 286$ and $n = 82$, respectively). Expression of GABRP expression was significantly higher in ER/HER2 cancers compared to the receptor-positive cancers (mean expression 5758 versus 881, $p < 0.0001$). Cell culture studies provided strong evidence that GABRP mRNA

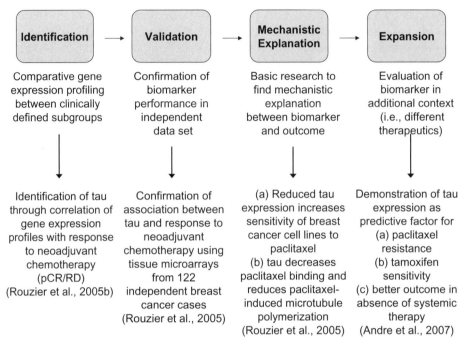

Figure 3.8. Different steps in the development of multigene biomarkers.

expression can be induced through serum deprivation. In contrast, GABRP down-regulation by the means of siRNA (small interfering ribonucleic acid)-mediated knockdown leads to increased cell death. The latter observation provides a strong rationale for the evaluation of GABRP as a potential target for a novel therapeutic approach in patients with ER/HER2 breast cancers (Tordai et al., 2007). Interestingly, GABRP gene expression is increased in breast cancers of immature (undifferentiated) cell type and is also significantly correlated with a shorter lifetime history of breastfeeding and possibly with high-grade breast cancer in Hispanic women (Symmans et al., 2005).

3.9. TRANSCRIPTIONAL PROFILING FOR THE DEFINITION OF MULTIGENE PREDICTORS USING TRANSCRIPTIONAL PROFILING

While determination of differentially expressed genes is a suitable and sufficient tool for the identification of single biomarkers, more advanced approaches are needed for the identification of complex multigene models. Multigene predictors of chemotherapy response have usually been developed without consideration of the biology of the genes they comprise. Instead, genes are chosen solely based upon their association with a short- or long-term variable, such as pathological complete response to neoadjuvant chemotherapy or overall survival.

A number of ways to identify pharmacogenomic predictors have been introduced:

- Correlation of patient response to (neoadjuvant) chemotherapy with gene expression data from tumors obtained from these patients
- Correlation of data on in vitro response of cell lines exposed to cytotoxic drugs with gene expression data obtained from those cell lines
- Correlation of changes between pre- and postchemotherapy profiles with response data

Development and validation of multigene predictor/biomarker is carried out following a certain schema (Fig. 3.9). The initial step consists of the development of the multigene predictor. First, individual genes/probesets have to be identified that will become part of the multigene predictor. This is usually performed through the identification of differentially expressed genes between relevant (pre)clinical subgroups. These genes will then be combined into a multivariable predictor using a biomathematical model. When the model has been developed, a prediction rule and a cutoff will be defined. A number of mathematical models have been proposed, such as diagonal linear discriminate analysis (DLDA), support vector machines (SVM; Ramaswamy et al., 2001), and artificial neural networks (ANN; Khan et al., 2001), some of which are relatively complex. However, increasing model complexity does not necessarily translate into

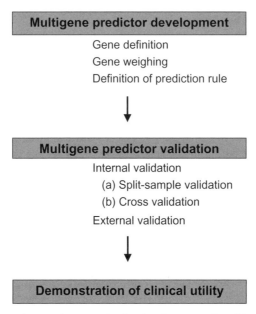

Figure 3.9. Stepwise requirements in the development of multigene biomarkers.

improved model performance (Dudoit et al., 2002). Instead complex models carry the risk of overfitting the data (Simon, 2003). This phenomenon describes the observation that highly complex models may be fitted well to even random variations in a given data set. However, the random variations do not represent true observations and the "overfitted predictor" may be of low predictive ability when tested in an independent data set. Consequently, validation of the results is of high importance. Validation can be carried out as internal validation (i.e., split-sample validation or cross validation) or as external validation. Internal validation is commonly carried out by dividing the initial study population into a training set and a test set, the latter being excluded when the model is developed in order to prevent model overfitting. In contrast, external validation is performed on a completely independent validation set, for instance, from a different institution.

Commonly used terms to describe the performance of a (multivariable) biomarker in an independent data set comprise predictive accuracy, sensitivity, specificity, positive, and negative predictive value (PPV and NPV, respectively). Table 3.3 shows how these five parameters are calculated. It has been emphasized that validation optimally be carried out in an independent data set that shares a high degree of homogeneity compared to the developmental data set; this goal may be achieved best using data obtained as part of randomized clinical trials (Simon, 2002). Unfortunately, this is often disregarded. Dupuy and Simon (2007) analyzed 42 gene expression profiling studies with regard to their analytical quality. They reported that as many as half of them featured one of three major flaws:

1. Lack of description of their method of control for multiple testing or lack of reporting thereof
2. Unjustified claims of a correlation between clusters and clinical outcome
3. Biased estimation of prediction accuracy due to incorrect cross validation

The ultimate step in (multigene) biomarker development and validation consists in the demonstration of clinical utility. No biomarker should find access

TABLE 3.3. Statistical Terms Relevant to Biomarker Validation

Predictive accuracy: Ratio of cases correctly predicted (*true positives and true negatives*) vs. all cases

Sensitivity: Ratio of cases correctly predicted pCR (*true positives*) vs. cases experiencing pCR (*true positives and false negatives*)

Specificity: Ratio of cases correctly predicted RD (*true negatives*) vs. cases indeed experiencing RD (*true negatives and false positives*)

Positive predictive value (PPV): Ratio of cases correctly predicted pCR (*true positives*) vs. all cases predicted pCR (*true positives and false positives*)

Negative predictive value (NPV): Ratio of cases correctly predicted RD (*true negatives*) vs. all cases predicted RD (*true negatives and false negatives*)

to the clinical setting unless it has been demonstrated that patient stratification based on the novel marker leads to increased patient survival (or at least decreased toxicity) in a randomized clinical trial.

Of note, approaches employed to develop a multigene predictor of response to targeted therapies (such as antibodies or targeted small molecules) rather than standard chemotherapy differ from this approach. The majority of standard chemotherapy response predictors represent a so-called bottom-up approach with differences in certain populations being defined without biological input. In contrast, predictors of response to targeted therapies make use of top-down strategies. Provided that the underlying mechanisms of therapy response are often at least partially known, response predictors for targeted agents can be designed while making use of the underlying molecular biology. Another important feature of targeted designs is the prospect of combined targeting of a number of possible targets based on a biologic rationale rather than on an empiric rationale alone. In fact, it is generally conceived that most tumors may depend on more than one signaling pathway alone to promote their growth and survival.

Consequently, a variety of strategies have been proposed to inhibit multiple signaling pathways or multiple steps thereof. This may be provided by the development of multitargeted agents or the combination of single targeted drugs. In the following section we will give examples of the development of multigene predictors of chemotherapy response and multigene predictors of response to a targeted therapy agent.

3.9.1. Multigene Predictors of Chemotherapy Response

It has been outlined that the process of (genomic) biomarker development validation closely resembles the classical three-phase clinical trial design (Pusztai et al., 2005). For instance, the Breast Cancer Pharmacogenomic Discovery Program at the Nellie B. Connally Breast Center of the University of Texas M. D. Anderson Cancer Center has been designed to develop multigene predictive biomarkers for response to (neoadjuvant) chemotherapy in patients with breast cancer. In this three-phase process, phase I was issued to test for feasibility of gene expression profiling from needle biopsies of breast cancer tissue and potential accuracy of the technical approach itself (i.e., interplatform reliability as well as inter- and intralaboratory reproducibility of gene expression data and complex genomic models). In phase II, optimal sample size will be determined and the best marker genomic predictor will be selected and optimized. Phase III is designed to validate the predictor independently and test its clinical utility (Pusztai et al., 2005). In an earlier report from this group, Buchholz et al. (2002) reported on the results of a gene expression study using core biopsy specimens from 21 women obtained before initiation of neoadjuvant chemotherapy for breast cancer. Serial biopsies were obtained before treatment and 24 and/or 48 hours after treatment. Interestingly, not only did the authors observe gene expression changes among serial samples, but they also found that samples from patients with good response had gene patterns that clustered distinctly from those of poor responders

(Buchholz et al., 2002). As outlined above, neoadjuvant chemotherapy offers an intriguing possibility to identify predictors of response to chemotherapy. Achievement of pathological complete response is identified as lack of any invasive cancer following preoperative chemotherapy and is associated with excellent long-term survival (Mazouni et al., 2007). Thus, pCR is regarded as an early surrogate marker of disease prognosis, can easily and relatively early be assessed at the time of definitive surgery after completion of chemotherapy, and thus serves as an excellent target variable in predictive biomarker development. Accordingly, pCR was used as a surrogate marker in the conduction of a subsequent pharmacogenomic study. This time, gene expression profiles from one-time pretreatment fine-needle aspiration (FNA) samples from 24 patients with early-stage breast cancer were utilized to build a multigene model with 74 markers. When validated on an independent data set from 18 patients, the predictor performed with a 78% predictive accuracy, a 100% positive predictive value for pCR, a 73% negative predictive value, a sensitivity of 43%, and a specificity of 100%. Interestingly, no single marker was found to be sufficiently associated with pCR to be used as an individual predictor in this data set (Ayers et al., 2004). This study is regarded as proof of principle that gene expression profiling in the neoadjuvant setting can be employed to develop multivariable genomic markers of therapy response.

The follow-up study comprises the largest pharmacogenomic study in breast cancer to date. Gene expression profiles from 82 breast cancers were used to develop a multigene predictor for neoadjuvant chemotherapy. All patients had been treated uniformly with a neoadjuvant chemotherapy regimen (paclitaxel followed by 5-fluoruracil, adriamycin, and cyclophosphamide, T/FAC), and response was assessed at the time of definite surgery, being either pathological complete response or residual disease. First, differential gene expression was performed using two-sample unequal variance t tests and genes were rank ordered by P values. False discovery rates (FDRs) were estimated using beta uniform mixture (BUM) analysis. Several prediction models as well as various numbers of included genes were tested to define a nominally best predictor. A 30-gene model using DLDA-30 performed best and was successfully validated on 51 independent cases, with a 76% overall accuracy, 52% positive predictive value (PPV), 96% negative predictive value (NPV), 92% sensitivity, and 71% specificity (Hess et al., 2006). Of note, although the DLDA-30 was characterized as the nominally best predictor, the authors demonstrated that different prediction models and a higher and lower number of genes performed comparably well (Fig. 3.10).

As outlined above, there are a number of possibilities to develop predictors of response to cytotoxic therapy. One interesting approach describes the utilization of in vitro chemosensitivity data from 60 cell lines from various human cancers of different tissue origin and corresponding gene expression profiles to develop multigene predictors of in vitro chemotherapy response. These predictors performed with high accuracy in predicting response to cytotoxic therapy when tested on human data sets (Potti et al., 2006a). These and other approaches are interesting and promising; however, correlation of patient response data, as

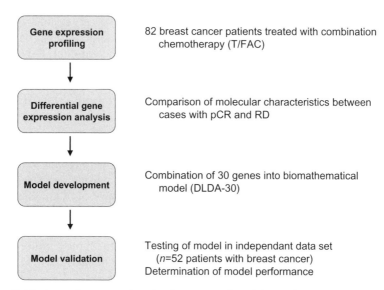

Figure 3.10. Exemplary stepwise development of multigene biomarkers—the DLDA-30 (Hess et al., 2006).

outlined above, remains the most advanced and most established approach to date (Pusztai, 2006).

3.9.2. Multigene Predictor of Response to a Targeted Therapy Agent

The term "targeted therapies" implies that only a fraction of patients, that is, those carrying the target, will benefit from this certain treatment. It is increasingly recognized that not only the target itself but also other parameters (such as pathway components) may be involved in response to the target and thus may be predictive of response. Consequently, determination of pathway activity status has increasingly come into scientific focus (Curtis et al., 2005) and is of high importance in the context of targeted therapies. Components of pathways may serve several purposes, such as monitoring drug pharmacodynamics, surrogate endpoint of clinical outcome, and validation of a drug actually hitting its designated target. Several probabilities to identify predictors of response in the context of targeted therapies have been introduced. To illustrate how many alternative approaches may allow for characterization of a response predictor for a targeted therapy agent, we describe what methods may be or have been employed to predict response to the multityrosine kinase inhibitor Sprycel (BMS-354825). First, Sprycel has been demonstrated to inhibit a number of different protein kinases with high affinity, such as src, kit, and platelet-derived growth factor receptor (PDGFR) (Schittenhelm et al., 2006; Nam et al., 2005; Chen et al., 2006).

It seems reasonable that a combination of weighted average expression values of these targets may allow for calculation of a "Sprycel target index," which may be used to predict the chance of response to Sprycel treatment. Second, Bild et al. (2006) reported on the identification of a "*Src* activation pathway geneset." They compared gene expression profiles from wild-type human mammary epithelial cells (HMECs) versus Src-transformed HMECs (Bild et al., 2006). This Src activation pathway geneset may also be used to predict response to Sprycel treatment. Third, the developing company itself reported on the identification of a candidate Sprycel response predictor from in vitro data: 23 cell lines were exposed to Sprycel in vitro and their sensitivity profile was established. Additionally, gene expression was carried out and both parameters were used to develop an in vitro response predictor of response to Sprycel. A six-gene-model was established and validated with high accuracy in 11 of 12 independent breast cancer cell lines and 19 of 23 lung cancer cell lines (Huang et al., 2007). To date, no patient data are available to validate either of these response indices for the use in the clinical setting. However, pharmacogenomic clinical trials are currently under way to address this issue.

3.9.3. Novel Approaches to Phase II Clinical Trial Design

It has been demonstrated that the probability of successful discovery of novel drug-specific pharmacogenomic response markers in a typical phase II study is small. Pusztai et al. (2007) described a translational trial simulation in which they assumed that HER2 was yet unknown in order to calculate the probability of identifying it de novo as a predictor of benefit from trastuzumab treatment in patients with breast cancer. Gene expression data from 132 patients with newly diagnosed breast cancers were employed in order to simulate 50,000 single-agent phase II trastuzumab studies. It was shown that the vast minority, that is, no more than 4% of the simulated studies, identified *HER2* as the top predictor. In contrast, more than 96% of the simulated studies identified a different gene as the most efficient predictor of trastuzumab response. Furthermore, *HER2* was among the 10 most predictive genes in each simulation in only about 10%. Interestingly, when *HER-2* was a priori suspected as a potential predictor, its overexpression among responders was confirmed in almost all simulated studies (99.6%). The results of this study have important consequences for the design of modern clinical trials. In fact, broad pharmacogenomic screening as part of phase II trials to identify molecular predictors for therapeutic agents that show low overall response rate harbors a high risk of yielding insignificant and irreproducible results. Instead a more productive strategy may be to prospectively test an a priori defined predictor in pharmacogenomic data obtained during a phase II study. One approach may be based on the knowledge of the mechanism of action of the drug. Based on that, it may be possible to propose at least one or more potential response predictors that may then be tested as part of the phase II trial. Another promising approach consists in the identification of predictors in cell line models (Huang et al., 2007). However, the authors themselves proposed a novel phase II trial design: The "tandem, two-step phase II trial" design for rapid marker assessment combines two optimal two-stage phase II trials into a single study. Traditionally, the two-stage phase II trial design has been used for several decades to identify drugs with promising clinical activity while quickly discarding those with low activity. The goal of the phase II clinical trials is to determine whether a new drug has enough clinical activity to warrant larger scale evaluation in a phase III trial. During the first stage of a classic two-stage phase II study, a limited number of patients are entered into the trial. If less than a target number of responses are observed, the accrual terminates for lack of activity. In contrast, when the target number of responses is reached in the limited cohort, the trial continues to accrue the final patient population. If the second stage yields positive results, the drug is recommended for further evaluation (Simon, 2001).

In contrast, the tandem, two-step phase II trial design was designed as a combination of two two-stage phase II trials into a single study (Fig. 3.11). The first stage of the first step starts out as a two-stage phase II trial for unselected patients. Provided that sufficient numbers of events such as clinical benefit rate or response rate are observed as part of the first stage, the study proceeds to the second stage, thus increasing the total study population in order to establish the benefit rate more precisely in unselected patients. If an insufficient number of events occur during the initial stage, the new design demands that the trial not be stopped but remain open for response marker–positive patients only. At this

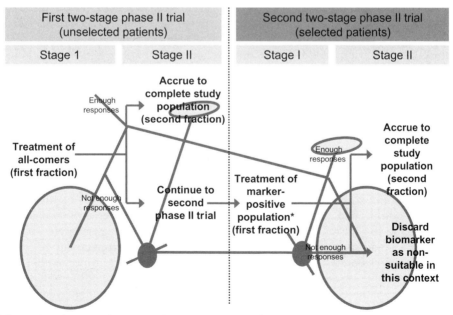

* Several markers can be tested simultaneously.

Figure 3.11. Tandem, two-step phase II trial design.

point a second two-stage trial commences. The rationale for the initiation of the second stage is that it may be very unlikely that the small group of patients who participated in the first phase included a sufficient number of marker-positive cases to draw a conclusion about the activity of the drug in this molecularly defined subset. If in the second two-stage trial an insufficient number of events occur after accruing a target number of marker-positive cases during the second step of the study, the trial marker will be rejected due to lack of predictive performance and the study be discontinued following the early stopping rules. If the target of events is reached, however, the study proceeds to complete accrual of additional marker-positive patients in order to estimate the benefit rate more precisely in this selected population. Importantly, several second-to-stage trials can be run in parallel, allowing for the assessment of several potential biomarkers in one trial only (Pusztai et al., 2007). The authors felt that this type of study design could provide two important options: to allow for the estimation of response rates in both an unselected and a marker-selected patient cohort and to enable simultaneous screening of multiple different predictors for the same drug as well as distinct predictor–drug combination as part of a single, parallel-multiarm trial (Pusztai et al., 2007).

3.10. NOVEL TOOLS FOR PATHWAY ANALYSIS

Several methods exist that can identify altered pathway activity in a given tumor. Pathway analysis tools identify pathways in a given list of genes through the use of a number of gene-expression-based research tools. Such tools are the Gene Ontology (GO) project (http://www.geneontology.org; Harris MA et al., 2004), the Kyoto Encyclopedia of Genes and Genomes (KEGG) (http://www.genome.jp/kegg; Kanehisa et al., 2004), and GenMAPP (http://www.genmapp.org; Dahlquist et al., 2002). In order to determine, whether a given pathway is more common in one tumor subset compared to another, ranked lists of differentially expressed genes are compared to these databases, using classic statistical tests, such as Chi Square or Fisher's exact test. The resulting p values indicate the probability to which a given pathway is in fact overrepresented in a given subset. A variety of software tools can assist in these calculations (Curtis et al., 2005).

It is important to note that individual genes that are identified as being differentially expressed do not necessarily reflect the activity of a given pathway in a tumor. Differential gene expression analysis might miss small-scale but coordinated gene expression differences. Consequently, gene set enrichment analysis (GSEA) has been introduced as a novel tool to characterize complex gene sets that are coordinately up-regulated (i.e., "enriched") in a given population. The particular value of this approach lies in the notion that while differential gene expression methods might gather only high-scale changes, coordinated but small-scale change might be of equal importance. For example, the presence of a given pathway in a given cohort might be missed if no single member of this pathway is overexpressed alone. GSEA requires the availability of predefined gene sets, such as pathway activity profiles, chemotherapy response profiles, or profiles associated with a certain tumor phenotype, such as high tumor grade. Gene sets may be derived through the comparison of cancers with certain characteristics, such as low versus high grade (Sotiriou et al., 2006), *p53* mutation versus *p53* wild type (Miller et al., 2005), or response versus resistance to neoadjuvant chemotherapy (Hess et al., 2006). When performing GSEA, genes are ranked according to a certain measure of expression, such as the fold change in absolute expression or signal-to-noise ratio in descending order. An enrichment score indicates the presence of a given gene set among the tumor samples (Subramanian et al., 2005). However, many genes have not yet been clearly associated with distinct pathways or gene sets, so we presume that many associations are currently unrecognized. Currently, neither technique has been sufficiently standardized so the results from these different methods show only moderate overlap (Curtis et al., 2005).

3.11. IMPLEMENTATION OF BIOMARKERS INTO THE CLINICAL SETTING

A major challenge is the translation of gene expression biomarkers into clinically utilizable tools. Genechips have the advantage of complex and multidimensional gene expression data, however, they come at the cost of complexity, labor intensiveness, and still a high price. Consequently, two major approaches can be distinguished with regard to the impact of gene expression profiling-based discoveries on clinical practice, which are outlined in Figure 3.12. On one hand, it may be possible to replace complex gene expression profiling methods, such as genechip technology, by much simpler methods such as those employed by molecular pathology like such as immunohistochemical (IHC) or molecular biology methods such as reverse-transcription polymerase chain reaction (RT-PCR) ("replacement" strategy). For example, several lines of research have focused on defining subclasses of breast cancer that have initially been identified by gene expression profiling through a panel of IHC markers. Tischkowitz et al. (2007), for instance, have shown that by using a panel of IHC markers, they could in fact refine the prognostic value of the so-called basal-like breast cancer subtype. However, there is a lack of consistency in defining breast cancer molecular subtypes based on IHC markers (Conforti et al., 2007; Rodríguez-Pinilla et al., 2007; Kim et al., 2006). A major obstacle to replacing gene-expression-based classification matrices with models based on immunohistochemistry may be that traditionally IHC approaches represented semiquantitative scoring systems. In contrast, gene-expression-based approaches are based on continuous intensity measurements. Rather than replacing gene expression profiling, another approach may be to exploit the multidimensional nature of gene-expression-profiling results and define more than one (univariable or multivariable) biomarker to answer several questions in parallel ("expansion" strategy). Thus, it has been suggested that gene expression profiling itself, using gene expression platforms as in basic research, may serve as a clinically utilizable tool. The DLDA-30, predicting response to

Step I: Biomarker identification using gene expression profiling

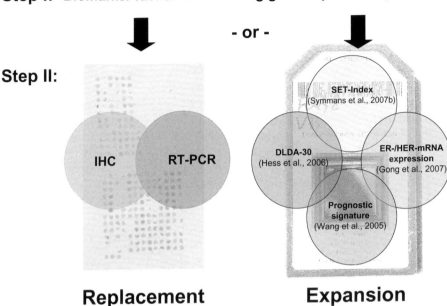

Replacement Strategy

Expansion Strategy

Figure 3.12. Translating gene expression profiling-based discoveries into clinical practice.

neoadjuvant T/FAC chemotherapy, has been developed and successfully validated using Affymetrix U133A GeneChips. Furthermore, Symmans et al. (2007b) have developed a 200-gene signature that predicts response to adjuvant tamoxifen therapy better than ER expression status. This "sensitivity towards endocrine therapy (SET)" index does not contain ER itself, but consists of 200 ER related genes. It has been successfully validated using two independent gene expression data sets (Symmans et al., 2007b). Gong et al. (2007), have recently demonstrated that measurement of ER and HER2 mRNA expression using their corresponding probesets (on Affymetrix U133A GeneChips) correlates well with expression status as determined using immunohistochemistry or FISH, respectively. An ESR1 mRNA cutoff value of 500 exhibited an overall accuracy of 90% (training set) and 88 to 96% (two independent validation sets) in identifying ER-positive cases. For HER2, an mRNA threshold of 1150 identified HER2-positive cases with an overall accuracy of 93% (training set) and 89 to 90% (two independent validation sets; Gong et al., 2007). Finally, Wang et al. (2005) have developed a 76-gene signature, consisting of 60 genes for ER-positive patients and 16 genes for ER-negative patients, that predicts poor prognosis in breast cancer patients as outlined above. These four parameters, namely the DLDA-30, the SET-Index, the ER/HER2 mRNA expression cutoff values, and the 76-gene-signature have been developed and validated using Affymetrix U133A GeneChips. Thus, gene expression profiling of a given tumor sample using this platform would allow for retrieval of these four parameters through one single assay, by this means avoiding the costs of several different assays.

At the M. D. Anderson Cancer Center, this approach will be tested for suitability as a triaging model as part of a novel neoadjuvant systemic therapy trial. Patients with operable early-stage breast cancer, who enroll in the trial, will undergo a fine-needle aspiration (FNA) for their invasive cancer, which will be subjected to Affymetrix GeneChip-based gene expression profiling. Patients gene signatures will then be evaluated with regards to (a) DLDA-30 to determine their individual probability to respond to neoadjuvant T/FAC chemotherapy, (b) (ER and) HER2-mRNA expression values to evaluate their response to trastuzumab, and (c) SET-index to determine their probability to respond to hormonal intervention. Patients will then be subjected to the type of therapy that promised the highest chance of response and receive this in a neoadjuvant setting. The goal of this study will consist in increasing pCR rates in this patient population by the means of *optimal treatment assignment* rather than through *implementation of a novel compound*.

3.12. CONCLUSION

Gene expression profiling is a powerful tool to identify both single biomarkers and complex multivariate signatures, with the promise to classify (breast) cancer patients into prognostic and predictive subgroups. Biomarkers bear many promises, such as the increase of response by definition of certain prognostic/predictive subgroups, the definition of novel exploitable molecular tools, and the decrease of patient populations in clinical trials. It is not yet clear whether gene expression profiling itself will eventually become a diagnostic tool in the clinical setting itself or will rather serve as a means to eventually identify independent and hopefully more easily applicable diagnostic tools.

REFERENCES

Anderson, K., Hess, K. R., Kapoor, M. Tirrell, S., Courtemanche, J., Wang, B., Wu, Y., Gong, Y., Hortobagyi, G. N., Symmans, W. F., and Pusztai, L. (2006). Reproducibility of gene expression signature-based predictions in replicate experiments. *Clin. Cancer Res.* 12:1721–1727.

Andre, F., Hatzis, C., Anderson, K., Sotirou, L., Mazouni, C., Mejia, J. A., Wang, B., Hortobagyi, G., Symmans, W., and Pusztai, L. (2007a). Microtubule-associated protein-tau is a bifunctional predictor of endocrine sensitivity and chemotherapy resistance in estrogen receptor-positive breast cancer. *Clin. Cancer Res.* 13:2061–2067.

Andre, F., Mazouni, C., Liedtke, C., Kau, S. W., Frye, D., Green, M., Gonzalez-Angulo, A. M., Symmans, W. F., Hortobagyi, G. N., and Pusztai, L. (2007b). HER2 expression and efficacy of preoperative paclitaxel/FAC chemotherapy in breast cancer. *Breast Cancer Res. Treat.*

Ayers, M., Symmans, W. F., Stec, J., Damokosh, A. I., Clark, E., Hess, K., Lecocke, M., Metivier, J., Booser, D., Ibrahim, N., Valero, V., Royce, M., Arun, B., Whitman, G., Ross, J., Sneige, N., Hortobagyi, G. N., and Pusztai, L., (2004). Gene expression profiles predict complete pathologic response to neoadjuvant paclitaxel and fluorouracil, doxorubicin, and cyclophosphamide chemotherapy in breast cancer. *J. Clin. Oncol.* 22:2284–2293.

Betensky, R. A., Louis, D. N., and Cairncross, J. G. (2002). Influence of unrecognized molecular heterogeneity on randomized clinical trials. *J. Clin. Oncol.* 20:2495–2499.

Bild, A. H., Yao, G., Chang, J. T., Wang, O., Potti, A., Chasse, D., Joshi, M.-B., Harpole, D., Lancaster, J. M., Berchuck, A., Olson, Jr., J. A., Marks, J. R., Dressman, H. K., West, M., and Nevins, J. R. (2006). Oncogenic pathway signatures in human cancers as a guide to targeted therapies. *Nature* 439:353–357.

Boughey, J. C., Peintinger, F., Meric-Bernstam, F., Perry, A. C., Hunt, K. K., Babiera, G. V., Singletary, S. E., Bedrosian, I., Lucci, A., Buzdar, A. U., Puszlai, L., and Kuever, H. M. (2006). Impact of preoperative versus postoperative chemotherapy on the extent and number of surgical procedures in patients treated in randomized clinical trials for breast cancer. *Ann. Surg.* 244:464–470.

Brown, P. O., and Botstein, D. (1999). Exploring the new world of the genome with DNA microarrays. *Nat. Genet.* 21:33–37.

Buchholz, T. A., Stivers, D. N., Stec, J., Ayers, M., Clark, E., Bolt, A., Sahin, A. A., Symmans, W. F., Hess, K. R., Kuerer, H. M., Valero, V., Hortobagyi, G. N., and Pusztai, L. (2002). Global gene expression changes during neoadjuvant chemotherapy for human breast cancer. *Cancer J.* 8:461–468.

Chen, Z., Lee, F. Y., Bhalla, K. N., and Wu, J. (2006). Potent inhibition of platelet-derived growth factor-induced responses in vascular smooth muscle cells by BMS-354825 (dasatinib). *Mol. Pharmacol.* 69:1527–1533.

Conforti, R., Boulet, T., Tomasic, G., Taranchon, E., Arriagada, R., Spielmann, M., Ducourtieux, M., Soria, J., Tursz, T., Delaloge, S., Michiels, S., and Andre, F. (2007). Breast cancer molecular subclassification and estrogen receptor expression to predict efficacy of adjuvant anthracyclines-based chemotherapy: A biomarker study from two randomized trials. *Ann. Oncol.* 18(9):1477–1483.

Curtis, R. K., Oresic, M., and Vidal-Puig, A. (2005). Pathways to the analysis of microarray data. *Trends Biotechnol.* 23:429–435.

Dahlhquist, K. D., Salomonis, N., Vranizan, K., Lawlor, S. C. and Conklin, B. R. (2002). GenMAPP, a new tool for viewing and analyzing microarray data on biological pathways. *Nat. Genet.* 31:19–20.

Dawood, S., and Cristofanilli, M. (2007). Integrating circulating tumor cell assays into the management of breast cancer. *Curr. Treat. Options Oncol.* 8:89–95.

Dudoit, S., Fridlyand, J., and Speed, T. P. (2002). Comparison of discrimination methods for the classification of tumors using gene expression data. *J. Am. Stat. Assoc.* 97:77–87.

Dupuy, A., and Simon, R. M. (2007). Critical review of published microarray studies for cancer outcome and guidelines on statistical analysis and reporting. *J. Natl. Cancer Inst.* 99:147–157.

Early Breast Cancer Trialists' Collaborative Group (EBCTCG) (2005). Effects of chemotherapy and hormonal therapy for early breast cancer on recurrence and 15-year survival: an overview of the randomised trials. *Lancet* 365:1687–1717.

Efron, B., and Tibshirani, R. (2002). Empirical Bayes methods and false discovery rates for microarrays. *Genet. Epidemiol.* 23:70–86.

Eisen, M. B., Spellman, P. T., Brown, P. O., and Botstein, D. (1998). Cluster analysis and display of genome-wide expression patterns. *Proc. Natl. Acad. Sci. U. S. A.* 95:14863–14868.

Ferretti, G., Felici, A., Papaldo, P., Fabi, A., and Cognetti, F. (2007). HER2/neu role in breast cancer: From a prognostic foe to a predictive friend. *Curr. Opin. Obstet. Gynecol.* 19:56–62.

Fisher, B., Bryant, J., Wolmark, N., Mamounas, E., Brown, A., Fisher, E. R., Wickerham, D. L., Begovic, M., DeCillis, A., Robidoux, A., Margolese, R. G., Cruz, A. B., Jr., Hoehn, J. L., Lees, A. W., Dimitrov, N. V., and Bear, H. D. (1998). Effect of preoperative chemotherapy on the outcome of women with operable breast cancer. *J. Clin. Oncol.* 16:2672–2685.

Foekens, J. A., Atkins, D., Zhang, Y., Sweep, F. C., Harbeck, N., Paradiso, A., Cufer, T., Sieuwerts, A. M., Talantov, D., Span, P. N., Tjan-Heijnen, V. C., Zito, A. F., Specht, K., Hoefler, H., Golouh, R., Schittulli, F., Schmitt, M., Beex, L. V., Klijn, J. G., and Wang, Y. (2006). Multicenter validation of a gene expression-based prognostic signature in lymph node-negative primary breast cancer. *J. Clin. Oncol.* 24:1665–1671.

Goldhirsch, A., Wood, W. C., Gelber, R. D., Coates, A. S., Thurlimann, B., and Senn, H. J. (2007). Progress and promise: Highlights of the international expert consensus on the primary therapy of early breast cancer 2007. *Ann. Oncol.* 18:1133–1144.

Gong, Y., Yan, K., Lin, F., Anderson, K., Sotiriou, C., Andre, F., Holmes, F. A., Valero, V., Booser, D., Pippen, J. E., Vukelja, S., Gomez, H., Mejia, J., Barajas, L. J., Hess, K. R., Sneige, N., Hortobagyi, G. N., Pusztai, L., and Symmans, W. F. (2007). Determination of oestrogen-receptor status and ERBB2 status of breast carcinoma: A gene-expression profiling study. *Lancet Oncol.* 8:203–211.

Harris, M. A., Clark, J., Ireland, A., and Gene Ontology Consortium. (2004). The Gene Ontology (GO) database and informatics resource. *Nucleic Acids Res.* 32: D258–261.

Hayes, D. F., Trock, B., and Harris, A. L. (1998). Assessing the clinical impact of prognostic factors: When is "statistically significant" clinically useful? *Breast Cancer Res. Treat.* 52:305–319.

Hegde, P., Qi, R., Abernathy, K., Gay, C., Dharap, S., Gaspard, R., Hughes, J. E., Snesrud, E., Lee, N., and Quackenbush, J. (2000). A concise guide to cDNA microarray analysis. *Biotechniques* 29:548–550, 552–554, 556.

Hess, K. R., Pusztai, L., Buzdar, A. U., and Hortobagyi, G. N. (2003). Estrogen receptors and distinct patterns of breast cancer relapse. *Breast Cancer Res. Treat.* 78:105–118.

Hess, K. R., Anderson, K., Symmans, W. F., Valero, V., Ibrahim, N., Mejia, J. A., Booser, D., Theriault, R. L., Buzdar, A. U., Dempsey, P. J., Rouzier, R., Sneige, N., Ross, J. S., Vidaurre, T., Gomez, H. L., Hortobagyi, G. N., and Pusztai, L. (2006). Pharmacogenomic predictor of sensitivity to preoperative chemotherapy with paclitaxel and fluorouracil, doxorubicin, and cyclophosphamide in breast cancer. *J. Clin. Oncol.* 24:4236–4244.

Hoffman, P. C., Mauer, A. M., and Vokes, E. E. (2000). Lung cancer. *Lancet* 355:479–485.

Huang, F., Reeves, K., Han, X., Fairchild, C., Platero, S., Wong, T. W., Lee, F., Shaw, P., and Clark, E. (2007). Identification of candidate molecular markers predicting sensitivity in solid tumors to dasatinib: Rationale for patient selection. *Cancer Res.* 67:2226–2238.

Ji, Y., Coombes, K., Zhang, J., Wen, S., Mitchell, J., Pusztai, L., Symmans, W. F., and Wang, J. (2006). RefSeq refinements of UniGene-based gene matching improve the correlation of expression measurements between two microarray platforms. *Appl. Bioinformatics* 5:89–98.

Joensuu, H., Kellokumpu-Lehtinen, P.-L., Bono, P., Alanko, T., Kataja, V., Asola, R., Utriainen, T., Kokko, R., Hemminki, A., Tarkkanen, M., Turpeenniemi-Hujanen, T., Jyrkkiö, S., Flander, M., Helle, L., Ingalsuo, S., Johansson, K., Jääskeläinen, A. S., Pajunen, M., Rauhala, M., Kaleva-Kerola, J., Salminen, T., Leinonen, M., Elomaa, I., Isola, J., and FinHer Study Investigators. (2006). Adjuvant docetaxel or vinorelbine with or without trastuzumab for breast cancer. *N. Engl. J. Med.* 354:809–820.

Kanehisa, M., Goto, S., Kawashima, S., et al. (2004). The KEGG resource for deciphering the genome. *Nucleic Acids Res.* 32:D277–280.

Kattan, M. W., and Scardino, P. (2002). Prediction of progression: Nomograms of clinical utility. *Clin. Prostate Cancer* 1:90–96.

Khan, J., Wei, J. S., Ringner, M., et al. (2001). Classification and diagnostic prediction of cancers using gene expression profiling and artificial neural networks. *Nat. Med.* 7:673–679.

Kim, M. J., Ro, J. Y., Ahn, S. H., Kim, H. H., Kim, S. B., and Gong, G. (2006). Clinicopathologic significance of the basal-like subtype of breast cancer: A comparison with hormone receptor and Her2/neu-overexpressing phenotypes. *Hum. Pathol.* 37(9):1217–1226.

Kuerer, H. M., Newman, L. A., Smith, T. L., et al. (1999). Clinical course of breast cancer patients with complete pathologic primary tumor and axillary lymph node response to doxorubicin-based neoadjuvant chemotherapy. *J. Clin. Oncol.* 17:460–469.

Kuo, W. P., Jenssen, T. K., Butte, A. J., et al. (2002). Analysis of matched mRNA measurements from two different microarray technologies. *Bioinformatics.* 18:405–412.

Learn, P. A., Yeh, I. T., McNutt, M., et al. (2005). HER-2/neu expression as a predictor of response to neoadjuvant docetaxel in patients with operable breast carcinoma. *Cancer* 103:2252–2260.

Lockhart, D. J., Dong, H., Byrne, M. C., et al. (1996). Expression monitoring by hybridization to high-density oligonucleotide arrays. *Nat. Biotechnol.* 14:1675–1680.

Loi, S., Haibe-Kains, B., Desmedt, C., et al. (2007). Definition of clinically distinct molecular subtypes in estrogen receptor-positive breast carcinomas through genomic grade. *J. Clin. Oncol.* 25:1239–1246.

Makris, A., Powles, T. J., Ashley, S. E., Chang, J., Hickish, V., Nash, G., Ford, T. (1998). A reduction in the requirements for mastectomy in a randomized trial of neoadjuvant chemoendocrine therapy in primary breast cancer. *Ann. Oncol.* 9:1179–1184.

Marty, M., Cognetti, F., Maraninchi, D., et al. (2005). Randomized phase II trial of the efficacy and safety of trastuzumab combined with docetaxel in patients with human epidermal growth factor receptor 2-positive metastatic breast cancer administered as first-line treatment: The M77001 study group. *J. Clin. Oncol.* 23:4265–4274.

MAQC Consortium (2006). The MicroArray Quality Control (MAQC) project shows inter- and intraplatform reproducibility of gene expression measurements. *Nat. Biotechnol.* 24:1151–1161.

Mauriac, L., Durand, M., Avril, A., et al. (1991). Effects of primary chemotherapy in conservative treatment of breast cancer patients with operable tumors larger than 3 cm. Results of a randomized trial in a single centre. *Ann. Oncol.* 2(5):347–354.

Mazouni, C., Peintinger, F., Wan-Kau, S., Andre, F., Gonzalez-Angulo, A. M., Symmans, W. F., Meric-Bernstam, F., Valero, V, Hortobagyi, G. N., Pusztai, L. (2007). Residual ductal carcinoma in patients with complete eradication of invasive breast cancer after neoadjuvant chemotherapy does not adversely affect patient outcome. *J Clin Oncol.* 25(19):2650–2655.

Miller, L. D., Smeds, J., George, J., et al. (2005). An expression signature for p53 status in human breast cancer predicts mutation status, transcriptional effects, and patient survival. *Proc. Natl. Acad. Sci. U. S. A.* 102:13550–13555.

Mountain, C. F. (1997). Revisions in the international system for staging lung cancer. *Chest* 111:1710–1717.

Nam, S., Kim, D., Cheng, J. Q., et al. (2005). Action of the Src family kinase inhibitor, dasatinib (BMS-354825), on human prostate cancer cells. *Cancer Res.* 65:9185–9189.

Nesbitt, J. C., Putnam, J. B., Jr., Walsh, G. L., Roth, J. A. (1995). Survival in early-stage non-small cell lung cancer. *Ann. Thorac. Surg.* 60:466–472.

Osier, M. V., Zhao, H., and Cheung, K. H. (2004). Handling multiple testing while interpreting microarrays with the Gene Ontology Database. *BMC Bioinformatics* 5:124.

Osoba, D., Slamon, D. J., Burchmore, M., et al. (2002). Effects on quality of life of combined trastuzumab and chemotherapy in women with metastatic breast cancer. *J. Clin. Oncol.* 20:3106–3113.

Perez-Soler, R. (2006). Rash as a surrogate marker for efficacy of epidermal growth factor receptor inhibitors in lung cancer. *Clin. Lung Cancer* 8(Suppl 1):S7–14.

Perou, C. M., Sorlie, T., Eisen, M. B., et al. (2000). Molecular portraits of human breast tumours. *Nature* 406:747–752.

Piccart-Gebhart, M. J., Procter, M., Leyland-Jones, B., et al. (2005). Trastuzumab after adjuvant chemotherapy in HER2-positive breast cancer. *N. Engl. J. Med.* 353:1659–1672.

Pisters, K. M., Evans, W. K., Azzoli, C. G., et al. (2007). Cancer Care Ontario and American Society of Clinical Oncology Adjuvant Chemotherapy and Adjuvant Radiation Therapy for Stages I–IIIA Resectable Non-Small-Cell Lung Cancer Guideline. *J. Clin. Oncol.* (in press).

Potti, A., Dressman, H. K., Bild, A., et al. (2006a). Genomic signatures to guide the use of chemotherapeutics. *Nat. Med.* 12:1294–1300.

Potti, A., Mukherjee, S., Petersen, R., et al. (2006b). A genomic strategy to refine prognosis in early-stage non-small-cell lung cancer. *N. Engl. J. Med.* 355:570–580.

Pusztai, L. (2006). Development of pharmacogenomic predictors for preoperative chemotherapy of breast cancer. *Adv. Exp. Med. Biol.* 587:233–249.

Pusztai, L., and Gianni, L. (2004). Technology insight: Emerging techniques to predict response to preoperative chemotherapy in breast cancer. *Nat. Clin. Pract. Oncol.* 1:44–50.

Pusztai, L., and Hess, K. R. (2004). Clinical trial design for microarray predictive marker discovery and assessment. *Ann. Oncol.* 15:1731–1737.

Pusztai, L., Symmans, F. W., and Hortobagyi, G. N. (2005). Development of pharmacogenomic markers to select preoperative chemotherapy for breast cancer. *Breast Cancer* 12:73–85.

Pusztai, L., Anderson, K., and Hess, K. R. (2007). Pharmacogenomic predictor discovery in phase II clinical trials for breast cancer. *Clin. Cancer Res.* 13:6080–6086.

Ramaswamy, S., Tamayo, P., Rifkin, R., et al. (2001). Multiclass cancer diagnosis using tumor gene expression signatures. *Proc. Natl. Acad. Sci. U. S. A.* 98:15149–15154.

Rodríguez-Pinilla, S. M., Rodríguez-Gil, Y., Moreno-Bueno, G., Sarrió, D., Martín-Guijarro Mdel, C., Hernandez, L., and Palacios, J. (2007). Sporadic invasive breast carcinomas with medullary features display a basal-like phenotype: An immunohistochemical and gene amplification study. *Am. J. Surg. Pathol.* 31(4):501–508.

Rody, A., Karn, T., Gatje, R., et al. (2007). Gene expression profiling of breast cancer patients treated with docetaxel, doxorubicin, and cyclophosphamide within the GEPARTRIO trial: HER-2, but not topoisomerase II alpha and microtubule-associated protein tau, is highly predictive of tumor response. *Breast* 16:86–93.

Romond, E. H., Perez, E. A., Bryant, J., et al. (2005). Trastuzumab plus adjuvant chemotherapy for operable HER2-positive breast cancer. *N. Engl. J. Med.* 353:1673–1684.

Rouzier, R., Pusztai, L., Delaloge, S., et al. (2005a). Nomograms to predict pathologic complete response and metastasis-free survival after preoperative chemotherapy for breast cancer. *J. Clin. Oncol.* 23:8331–8339.

Rouzier, R., Rajan, R., Wagner, P., et al. (2005b). Microtubule-associated protein tau: A marker of paclitaxel sensitivity in breast cancer. *Proc. Natl. Acad. Sci. U. S. A.* 102:8315–8320.

Schittenhelm, M. M., Shiraga, S., Schroeder, A., et al. (2006). Dasatinib (BMS-354825), a dual SRC/ABL kinase inhibitor, inhibits the kinase activity of wild-type, juxtamembrane, and activation loop mutant KIT isoforms associated with human malignancies. *Cancer Res.* 66:473–481.

Scholl, S. M., Fourquet, A., Asselain, B., et al. (1994). Neoadjuvant versus adjuvant chemotherapy in premenopausal patients with tumours considered too large for breast conserving surgery: Preliminary results of a randomised trial: S6. *Eur. J. Cancer* 30A:645–652.

Shalon, D., Smith, S. J., and Brown, P. O. (1996). A DNA microarray system for analyzing complex DNA samples using two-color fluorescent probe hybridization. *Genome Res.* 6:639–645.

Simon, R. (2001). Clinical trials in cancer. In *Cancer, Principals and Practice of Oncology*. DeVita, V. T., Hellman, S., and Rosenberg, S. A. (Eds.). Lippincott WilliamsWilkins, Philadelphia, pp. 521–538.

Simon, R. (2003). Diagnostic and prognostic prediction using gene expression profiles in high-dimensional microarray data. *Br. J. Cancer* 89:1599–1604.

Simon, R., and Maitournam, A. (2004). Evaluating the efficiency of targeted designs for randomized clinical trials. *Clin. Cancer Res.* 10:6759–6763.

Simon, R., Radmacher, M. D., and Dobbin, K. (2002). Design of studies using DNA microarrays. *Genet. Epidemiol.* 23:21–36.

Slamon, D. J., Clark, G. M., Wong, S. G., et al. (1987). Human breast cancer: Correlation of relapse and survival with amplification of the HER-2/neu oncogene. *Science* 235:177–182.

Slamon, D. J., Godolphin, W., Jones, L. A., et al. (1989). Studies of the HER-2/neu pro-tooncogene in human breast and ovarian cancer. *Science* 244:707–712.

Slamon, D. J., Leyland-Jones, B., Shak, S., et al. (2001). Use of chemotherapy plus a monoclonal antibody against HER2 for metastatic breast cancer that overexpresses HER2. *N. Engl. J. Med.* 344:783–792.

Slamon, D., Eiermann, W., Robert, N., et al. (2005). Phase III randomized trial comparing doxorubicin and cyclophosphamide followed by docetaxel (AC > T) with doxorubicin and cyclophosphamide followed by docetaxel and trastuzumab (AC > TH) with docetaxel, carboplatin and trastuzumab (TCH) in HER2 positive early breast cancer patients: BCIRG 006 study. *Breast Cancer Res. Treat.* 94(Suppl 1):S5.

Smyth, G. K., Yang, Y. H., and Speed, T. (2003). Statistical issues in cDNA microarray data analysis. *Methods Mol. Biol.* 224:111–136.

Sorlie, T., Perou, C. M., Tibshirani, R., et al. (2001). Gene expression patterns of breast carcinomas distinguish tumor subclasses with clinical implications. *Proc. Natl. Acad. Sci. U. S. A.* 98:10869–10874.

Sorlie, T., Tibshirani, R., Parker, J., et al. (2003). Repeated observation of breast tumor subtypes in independent gene expression data sets. *Proc. Natl. Acad. Sci. U. S. A.* 100:8418–8423.

Sorlie, T., Wang, Y., Xiao, C., et al. (2006). Distinct molecular mechanisms underlying clinically relevant subtypes of breast cancer: Gene expression analyses across three different platforms. *BMC Genomics* 7:127.

Sotiriou, C., Wirapati, P., Loi, S., et al. (2006). Gene expression profiling in breast cancer: Understanding the molecular basis of histologic grade to improve prognosis. *J. Natl. Cancer Inst.* 98:262–272.

Storey, J. D., and Tibshirani, R. (2003). Statistical significance for genomewide studies. *Proc. Natl. Acad. Sci. U. S. A.* 100:9440–9445.

Subramanian, A., Tamayo, P., Mootha, V. K., et al. (2005). Gene set enrichment analysis: A knowledge-based approach for interpreting genome-wide expression profiles. *Proc. Natl. Acad. Sci. U. S. A.* 102:15545–15550.

Symmans, W. F., Fiterman, D. J., Anderson, S. K., et al. (2005). A single-gene biomarker identifies breast cancers associated with immature cell type and short duration of prior breastfeeding. *Endocr. Relat. Cancer* 12:1059–1069.

Symmans, W. F., Peintinger, F., Hatzis, C., et al. (2007a). Measurement of residual breast cancer burden to predict survival after neoadjuvant chemotherapy. *J. Clin. Oncol.* 25:4414–4422.

Symmans, W. F., Hatzis, C., Sotiriou, C., et al. (2007b). Ability of a 200-gene endocrine sensitivity index (SET) to predict survival for patients who receive adjuvant endocrine therapy or for untreated patients. ASCO Breast Cancer Symposium, Abstr. 25.

Tan, P. K., Downey, T. J., Spitznagel, E. L., Jr., Xu, P., Fu, D., Dimitrov, D. S., Lempicki, R. A., Raaka, B. M., and Cam, M. C. (2003). Evaluation of gene expression measurements from commercial microarray platforms. *Nucleic Acids Res.* 31: 5676–5684.

Tischkowitz, M., Brunet, J. S., Bégin, L. R., Huntsman, D. G., Cheang, M. C., Akslen, L. A., Nielsen, T. O., and Foulkes, W. D. (2007). Use of immunohistochemical markers can refine prognosis in triple negative breast cancer. *BMC Cancer* 24(7):134.

Tordai, A., Wang, B., André, F., et al. (2007). Screening for expression of novel marker proteins for triple negative breast cancer in breast cancer cell lines. In *American Association for Cancer Research Annual Meeting: Proceedings*. Los Angeles, April 2007.

Tseng, G. C., Oh, M. K., Rohlin, L., et al. (2001). Issues in cDNA microarray analysis: Quality filtering, channel normalization, models of variations and assessment of gene effects. *Nucleic Acids Res.* 29:2549–2557.

Tusher, V. G., Tibshirani, R., and Chu, G. (2001). Significance analysis of microarrays applied to the ionizing radiation response. *Proc. Natl. Acad. Sci. U. S. A.* 98:5116–5121.

van de Vijver, M. J., He, Y. D., van 't Veer, L. J., et al. (2002). A gene-expression signature as a predictor of survival in breast cancer. *N. Engl. J. Med.* 347:1999–2009.

van 't Veer, L. J., Dai, H., van de Vijver, M. J., He, Y. D., Hart, A. A., Mao, M., Peterse, H. L., van der Kooy, K., Marton, M. J., Witteveen, A. T., Schreiber, G. J., Kerkhoven, R. M., Roberts, C., Linsley, P. S., Bernards, R., and Friend, S. H. (2002). Gene expression profiling predicts clinical outcome of breast cancer. *Nature* 415(6871):530–536.

Wang, Y., Klijn, J. G., Zhang, Y., et al. (2005). Gene-expression profiles to predict distant metastasis of lymph-node-negative primary breast cancer. *Lancet* 365:671–679.

Wolmark, N., Wang, J., Mamounas, E., Bryant, J., and Fisher, B. (2001). Preoperative chemotherapy in patients with operable breast cancer: Nine-year results from National Surgical Adjuvant Breast and Bowel Project B-18. *J. Natl. Cancer Inst. Monogr.* (30):96–102.

Yuen, T., Wurmbach, E., Pfeffer, R. L., Ebersole, B. J., and Sealfon, S. C. (2002). Accuracy and calibration of commercial oligonucleotide and custom cDNA microarrays. *Nucleic Acids Res.* 30(10):e48.

4

MOLECULAR PATHOLOGY IN NONCLINICAL SAFETY ASSESSMENT

Richard A. Westhouse

4.1. INTRODUCTION

Nonclinical safety assessment has evolved from a simplistic goal of *identification* of potential safety liabilities to include a more global definition of mechanistic risk assessment, which is increasingly recognized as a means to gain regulatory approval of investigational drugs. While the identification of safety concerns or toxicities will always be the first and primary stalwart purpose of safety assessment, the modern pharmaceutical industry is finding limitless utility in delving deeper into the real relevant risk of such findings. It is within the realm of mechanistic risk assessment that molecular pathology finds its most value.

Nonclinical safety assessment is founded on the principals of toxicology and animal toxicity studies have always been and will always be the mainstay of hazard identification. Without identification, there is no mechanism to investigate. The means to and philosophy of identification can vary, depending on the timing of activity, specifically, if it takes place in drug discovery or development. While the means and philosophy are not mutually exclusive, some generalizations can be made. For the purposes of this chapter, nonclinical *drug development* is defined as the characterization of a safety of a *single* compound or molecule for the

Molecular Pathology in Drug Discovery and Development, Edited by J. Suso Platero
Copyright © 2009 John Wiley & Sons, Inc.

purposes of enabling a clinical study. These activities include animal toxicity studies and in vitro studies that demonstrate to a governmental regulatory agency, and institutional review board, that the proposed clinical study of an investigational drug will not significantly harm the human subject. As such, the design and contents of the package must demonstrate safety with respect to *all* specific aspects of the clinical study design. So, in practice, one must always consider the perspectives of governmental regulators or clinical sites and determine what concerns they may have so as to proactively address these concerns. *Drug discovery* is defined as those activities leading up to drug development, and the goal is to identify the one lead compound or molecule that is selected with the optimized qualities that increases the chances of successful development to culminate in registration.

Again, while the means and philosophy of hazard identification are not mutually exclusive between drug discovery and development, generally in drug development, the philosophy is toward thoroughness and completeness. Safety assessment here involves widespread query in order to identify every potential side effect of investigational drugs. In these studies, postmortem histopathologic evaluation of samples from every organ and tissue ensures completeness. These studies are not hypothesis driven and in a sense are exercises in *fishing* for findings by casting a broad net to capture large quantities of data (not only histopathology but also gross pathology, organ weights, clinical pathology, clinical observations, body weights, to name a few). Sensitivity is generally considered to be high, relatively speaking (specificity and relevance, however, are often equivocal and therein lies the need for mechanistic risk assessment). Study conduct, recording of data, and general integrity must also be of the highest quality. Therefore, the studies must be conducted under the rigorous quality guidelines of good laboratory practices (GLP) under the Code of Federal Regulations (21 CFR, part 58). These studies form the core foundation of regulatory submission packages.

In drug discovery, however, safety assessment is much smaller in size and frequently more focused by scientific rationale. The shear magnitude and financial investment involved in a development-caliber safety study precludes that type of study in discovery. Additionally, the delayed time for reporting of results is impractical. Instead, discovery scientists focus identification of safety concerns based on the target and history. Target validation and the search for target-related toxicities will be further discussed in Section 4.1. Suffice it to say at this point that the purpose of safety assessment is to *find* toxicity or undesirable drug-related effects; so it behooves the investigator to evaluate organs or systems that are known to express the target. Additionally, focus can be directed by historical knowledge. Chemical libraries of individual companies may demonstrate a higher incidence of toxicities affecting a specific organ or system based on the library chemical space and an overabundance of certain core structures in that library. Retrospective analysis of preceding safety studies may highlight specifics. Lastly, evaluation of major organs or systems is always a good place to start for safety assessment in drug discovery.

While molecular pathology techniques can be utilized in safety assessment in either drug discovery or development, it is within the scope of mechanistic risk assessment that it is most utilized. In mechanistic risk assessment, the investigator attempts to determine the *significance* of an identified finding and the propensity of a patient to develop the same effect. Armed with this perspective, pharmaceutical companies have had greater success in gaining governmental regulatory acceptance for clinical programs of investigational drugs, even in the face of significant animal expression of toxicity! These studies may focus on the mechanism of action of a toxicological finding, species relevancy, risk attenuation, differences in animal and human metabolism, or any other hypothesis that serves to mitigate concern for human risk.

These types of investigational approaches can be initiated either within nonclinical development or in drug discovery, but the real factor dictating the timing of these investigations is knowledge of an effect through first-tier identification. Although it may seem obvious to some, earlier identification of a potential liability of concern is more advantageous than later. This allows more time for investigational risk assessment studies. Because of this, at least *some* degree of safety assessment is increasingly being practiced in modern drug discovery. As such, the purpose of safety assessment in drug discovery is similarly to identify drug-related toxicities, but because the identification is early in the process, it can be used to drive lead optimization (an effort to minimize the potential for expression of the toxicity through chemical substructural alterations) or to enable more thorough mechanistic risk assessment.

This chapter will discuss how molecular pathology techniques have been used in nonclinical safety assessment studies, specifically in routine safety studies of drug development and in drug discovery as part of target validation, lead candidate optimization, and also in investigative, hypothesis-driven studies for the purposes of improved risk assessment and identification of mechanism of actions of toxicities. Finally, special consideration will be given to the role of molecular pathology in the safety assessment of biotechnology-derived products.

4.2. DRUG DEVELOPMENT

The bulk of nonclinical safety assessment takes place in drug development. These are the studies that enable the initiation and continuation of clinical trials. In order to conduct a first-in-human study or continuation of clinical dosing for longer durations, a relevant safety profile must support every specific aspect of the clinical plan. As such, relevant parallel safety must be demonstrated with respect to the clinical subject enrollment, duration and route of dosing, active pharmaceutical ingredient, and the like. For example, if the clinical plan is to enroll women of child-bearing potential in a one-month study, then the nonclinical safety must include at least a one-month in vivo general toxicity study and studies to address the potential for reproductive, embryo and fetal effects, genotoxicity, adverse safety pharmacology, and also acute toxicity. In a sense, the simpler or more selective the clinical plan, the simpler the nonclinical safety assessment package will need to be.

Because in vivo toxicity studies of drug development are submitted to governmental regulatory agencies for the purpose of demonstrating safety of the clinical study of an investigational drug, the main purpose of these studies will always be identification of potential liabilities. There is frequently little latitude, motivation, or even tolerance to collect *nonessential* endpoints. Therefore, molecular morphology-based special techniques do not typically play a large role. Strong scientific rationale, however, may dictate expansion of the typical endpoints, to include special molecular pathology techniques, as long as the collection of such does not negatively impact the integrity of the first and primary purpose: *identification*. Modern pharmaceutical companies are becoming increasingly flexible in their philosophy of the conduct of these studies and less risk averse to generating what may have previously been considered extraneous or superfluous data. In fact, as stated above, the generation of much of this data is increasingly considered abundantly beneficial.

While molecular pathology techniques can be built into the study protocol proactively, thoughts of these techniques are more typically an afterthought and do not occur during the initial planning of the study design. In such cases, only the routine formalin-fixed, paraffin-embedded tissues are collected, and this significantly limits the molecular techniques that can be applied. Again, the ability to provide forethought to the study protocol depends on the prior knowledge gained from activities in drug discovery. Fortunately, however, these studies are so heavily weighted with pathology endpoints that it is standard at least to collect samples from every tissue of the animal for routine histopathology. In those studies that included only routine collection of tissues for histopathology (i.e., formalin-fixed, paraffin-embedded tissue), immunohistochemistry (IHC) is frequently the only reasonably useful molecular pathology technique that can be utilized. One can be fairly confident of high-quality sample collection and fixation, as opposed to the frequently unknown conditions of sample handling of clinical samples. This is because of the rigorous controls and documentation over the study, as mandated through good laboratory practices. The conduct of all study activities must be in accord with a study protocol and institutional standard operating procedures (SOP). The study protocol proactively guides the specific experimental design, parameters for evaluation, and analysis of data. The SOPs outline how to perform each specific task or operate each specific instrument. According to GLP, each SOP must be routinely reviewed and updated as needed. This ensures that the SOPs reflect current techniques and generally reflect an optimized procedure. Additionally, all deviations from such must be documented. Because of all these constraints, the tissues collected in these studies are either optimally handled or deviations from such are documented. Additionally, because histopathology is such a critical component of the study, the cycle time (and correspondingly fixation time) is short (but adequate, nonetheless). Therefore, antigen retrieval techniques are frequently not necessary.

4.2.1. Immunohistochemistry in Drug Development

Immunohistochemistry is mainly used in general toxicity studies in drug development to further characterize drug-related findings that were previously identified by routine histopathologic evaluation with hematoxylin and eosin (H&E) stained slides. Further characterization of findings can be used to confirm equivocal findings, provide insight into potential mechanisms of action, drive further investigative studies, and the like. Other techniques that frequently assist in characterization in these studies include special histochemical stains and ultrastructural evaluation.

An example of using immunohistochemistry in a toxicity study is the following; In a one-month toxicity study of a vascular endothelial growth factor receptor (VEGFR) inhibitor in rats, routine histopathologic evaluation of H&E-stained sections revealed a drug-related renal glomerulopathy. The finding was characterized by increased eosinophilia in the glomerular mesangial matrix, associated with a relative decreased density and number of cell nuclei. Eosinophilic material of this nature could be a number of different specific things, specifically, fibrin thrombi, collagen, amyloid, immunoglobulin complexes, or protein. A definitive characterization for the eosinophilia was necessary because each of these differential diagnoses carries with it a different implication with respect to potential mechanisms or pathogenesis. For instance, if the material was fibrin microthrombi, then the development of the side effect may be controlled in the clinic with anticlotting therapy. Thrombi, collagen, and amyloid, however, were ruled out via the use of special histochemical stains, such as phosphotungstic acid–hematoxylin (PTAH), trichrome, and Congo red, respectively. Immunoglobulin and protein were investigated by the use of immunohistochemistry. An antibody to albumin labeled the material (Fig. 4.1). Positive labeling was characterized by globular, punctate, and granular deposits in the glomerular mesangia. Critical evaluation of the substructural labeling detail revealed staining in vehicle-treated control animals. This staining, however, was within capillary loops lining the endothelium, representing circulating albumin. Additionally, proximal tubules had positive labeling on the brush boarder and within the cytoplasm of tubular epithelial cells, representing reabsorption of excreted albumin. Some eosinophilic tubular casts were also positive. The characterization of this glomerulopathy served to refine and narrow hypotheses for testing in investigative studies for the purpose of identifying a mechanism.

Another common application of IHC is to identify specific subpopulations of lymphocytes by cluster of differentiation (CD) markers. Mature nonplasmacytic lympocytes have little differentiating morphologic features by H&E staining, and effects in lymphoid tissues by either activity at the drug target or off-target may be limited to a specific lymphocyte subpopulation. Target-related pharmacologic effects, however, are more frequently subpopulation specific, while off-target effects tend to be more promiscuous. Sometimes, subpopulation effects can be identified with hematoxylin and eosin based on structural changes, however, sometimes changes in one population may be masked by compensatory changes

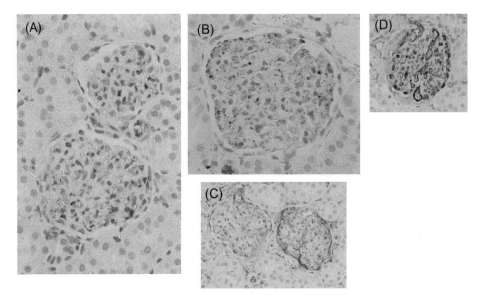

Figure 4.1. Kidney from a rat treated with VEGFR2 kinase inhibitor. Immunohistochemical label for albumin demonstrated globular (A) and punctate (B) deposits of positive material with glomerular mesangium, which correlated with increased mesangial eosinophilia. Additionally, positive labeling was present in the uriniferous space (C). Some glomeruli from vehicle-treated controls (D) demonstrated positive material lining endothelium of capillaries. See insert for color representation of this figure.

in another. Pharmacodynamic effects of notch inhibitors, for example, produce effects on specific lymphocyte subpopulations. Pharmaceutical intervention in notch receptor signaling is a lucrative target because activation of this pathway has been associated with various human malignancies. Signaling through the notch receptor, however, also plays a significant role in B-lymphocyte proliferation, differentiation, and maturation (Wu et al., 2007). Administration of Notch inhibitors to rats produces reduced width of spleen marginal zones. Immunohistochemistry was used to demonstrate that this effect was specific to IgM$^+$, IgD$^-$, CD8$^-$ B-lymphocytes specific to the marginal zone (Fig. 4.2). Metallophilic macrophages also present within the marginal zone, as identified by a silver stain, were not affected. Furthermore, there was no effect on IgM$^-$, IgD$^-$, CD8$^+$ T-lymphocytes in the periarterial lymphoid sheaths (PALS), nor on the IgM$^+$, IgD$^+$, CD8$^-$ B-lymphocytes of the lymphoid follicles. This extensive IHC characterization of the H&E finding was compelling evidence that the effect was indeed target related, as opposed to an off-target effect. A target-related effect of this nature can be used as a biomarker of pharmacodynamic activity to demonstrate that the target exists in the animal model and that it is indeed affected by drug administration (which further validates the animal model as being relevant for assessment of human safety). Additionally, some target-related effects identified in animals can be developed for use in the clinics as surrogate biomarkers for activity.

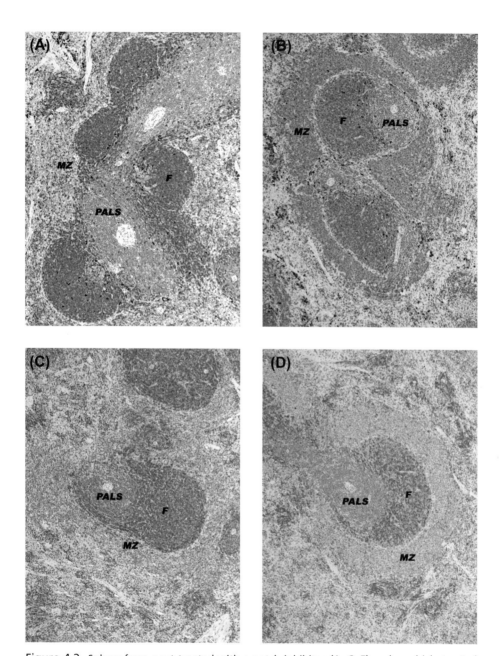

Figure 4.2. Spleen from a rat treated with a notch inhibitor (A, C, E) and a vehicle-treated control (B, D, F). Immunohistochemical stains for IgM (A, B), IgD (C, D), and CD8 (E, F). Target-related effects include decreased marginal zones, which in rats, is uniquely prominent and distinct from the PALS and follicles. (Legend: PALS = periarteriolar lymphoid sheath, MZ = marginal zone, F = lymphoid follicle.) See insert for color representation of this figure.

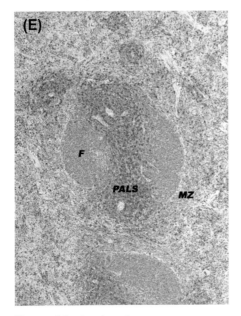
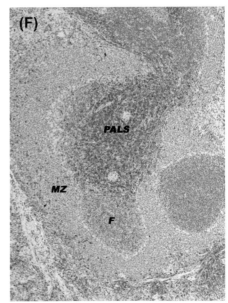

Figure 4.2. *Continued*

4.3. DRUG DISCOVERY

Nonclinical safety assessment that takes place in drug discovery frequently has more applications for molecular pathology than techniques in drug development. In nonclinical drug development, investigations of the mechanisms of toxicity are predominantly used to gain perspective on the actual relative risk that the toxicity or side effect will manifest in the clinical trials. For various obvious reasons, sometimes drug-related effects in animals do not accurately predict the occurrence in humans. Investigations for this purpose are generally categorized as mechanism-based risk assessment, and the purpose is to gain regulatory acceptance for the clinical investigative study. In drug discovery, however, the data from a similar study might be used to drive the discovery process, a portion of which includes target validation and lead optimization. Molecular pathology techniques play a significant role in both of these endeavors.

4.3.1. Target Validation and Target-Related Safety Concerns

As part of overall target validation, the identification of potential safety liabilities should also be considered and investigated, and this query should take place at the earliest stages of drug discovery. While the value of target validation for the purposes of efficacy is widely recognized, target validation from the perspective of safety assessment is, unfortunately, all too frequently an afterthought that does not receive adequate attention. From the perspective of safety assessment, the purpose of target validation is to identify how therapeutic intervention through that target will affect normal tissues that are unrelated to the pathogenesis of the disease process. The perfect *druggable* target is one that is expressed solely on the diseased tissue and perturbed only in the disease state. So, theoretically, there would be no undesirable side effects if a pharmaceutical agent were to be perfectly specific for that target. One example of this would be agents against infections diseases that target specific prokaryotic structures. If a pharmaceutical agent interacts *only* with an infectious agent, then there would be little concern for any side effects. In reality, however, therapeutic agents, especially small-molecule chemical entities, are *never* perfectly specific so as not to interact with other molecules and cause effects from those interactions. Such interactions are called *off-target* safety liabilities and tend to be exposure or dose related; specifically, higher concentrations of the drug will result in more proclivity toward off-target effects.

Most, if not all, potential druggable targets, however, are expressed in normal tissue as well as those tissues related to the disease process. Pharmacological intervention with the target in the normal tissues may have significant implications, especially if that target is involved in normal function or homeostatic processes. For example, antiangiogenic therapy for the treatment of cancer will inhibit blood vessel growth in tumors, as well as in normal tissue. Superficially, perhaps, the target appears to be lucrative from an efficacy and marketing standpoint, however, the potential for target-related effects in normal tissue must also be considered. Angiogenesis is necessary for a number of normal physiologic processes, such as wound repair, development of ovarian follicles and corpora lutea, mineralization of the physes of long bones, and also elongation of teeth. While these effects are readily apparent based on historical knowledge and can be adequately evaluated from a thorough literature search, the potential effects of *novel* targets are rarely so obvious.

Evaluation of a target from a safety perspective usually begins with a search of published literature and may proceed to proactive investigative work. A thorough search of the published literature should include information regarding phenotyping of relevant genetically engineered animals (knockout or transgenic mice; inducible, conditional, tissue specific, etc.), tissue expression profiling, potential human genetic diseases associated with relevant mutations of the target, and the like. In the absence of published information of this nature, such as for recently identified or proprietary targets, studies with normal animal and human tissues should be considered.

To fully validate a target with respect to safety, the presence and/or activity of the target or signaling pathway can be identified in *normal* tissues. Molecular pathology techniques of IHC and in situ hybridization (ISH) are used to identify the presence of a protein target and its corresponding messenger ribonucleic acid (mRNA) message, respectively. While these can be identified at the tissue level using homogenized samples, knowledge of the cellular localization of a target can frequently provide insight for the potential significance (i.e., better define the relative risk). Demonstration of the target itself in a tissue is more definitive than the mRNA message because some mRNAs are not translated to proteins and the identification of only the message may leave questions as to the real significance. Even demonstration of the target itself does not confer an absolute concern, for the experimental therapeutic still may not interact with the target in that specific cell population or tissue for some reason. The definitive answer will be gained from nonclinical toxicity studies.

Tissue Microarrays. The use of tissue microarrays (TMAs) provides a higher throughput approach to this endeavor. TMAs that are used for this type of target localization or tissue distribution are comprised of normal tissues from humans and also the relevant animal species that will be used in the nonclinical regulatory toxicity studies. Tissue distribution in normal human tissues is obviously the main concern for safety, but knowledge of similar or different expression in the nonclinical animal species could predict the potential penetration of findings in the toxicity studies or provide risk assessment based of species differences. If an effect is identified in a nonclinical study that is linked to the expression of the target, but the target is not expressed in those cells in humans, then the potential concern is reduced. For example, p38 inhibitors have long been generally recognized to cause gastrointestinal findings in dogs but not in other species. While dogs were recognized as outliers for this toxicity, it was not known which species would be a more relevant model for human penetration of the finding. Does a human react more like a dog or the other species. Similarly, if one nonclinical species shows a specific sensitivity for expression of the finding at lower exposures, relative to other species, which relative sensitivity would more adequately predict that of human? It was later demonstrated that dogs uniquely express p38 on B-lymphocytes and that the clinical signs in dog toxicity studies resulted from hemorrhagic necrosis of Peyer's patches in the ileum. Knowledge of the expression of the target in nonclinical species can help in mechanistic risk assessment. In this example, the finding was associated with the tissue distribution of the target, and then species differences in localization of the target provided information on relative risk assessment. Additionally, this information can provide an initial direction for further hypothesis-driven mechanistic studies.

Tissue microarrays can also be used to identify relevant animal species for toxicity studies. Relevant toxicology animal species are those that express the target in a rather similar tissue and cellular distribution as humans. This is especially important for biotechnology-derived molecules with high specificity for the intended target (see Section 4.4) because supraphysiologic effects of potential drugs must be identified. However, demonstration of mRNA by in situ hybridization or protein by IHC does not always translate into actual activity. Confirmation of these findings with in vivo activity is always recommended.

Because of the small size of the tissue cores, multiple cores of an organ are likely to be necessary in order to capture every cell type in that organ. In the example above, the cores of ileum would have had to contain Peyer's patches in order to identify that potential association. Similarly, organs with a corticomedullary architecture will need a core from the cortex and another from the medulla. An extreme case of subgross anatomical local uniqueness is the brain with all its nuclei and fiber tracts. In these cases, one can only make his best attempt to sample the most relevant structures to provide a quality screen. Lastly, cores must be periodically evaluated to confirm that the core contains the relevant tissue structures because extensive microtoming of a block may enter into a section of a tissue that is different than originally intended.

Genetically Engineered Mice. Target validation from the perspective of safety may also involve analysis of natural or engineered alterations on the target. While the bulk of this type of data is generally accumulated from published sources, some activities in genetically engineered mice (GEM) may be done proactively. If a human condition or disease exists that has been linked to somatic mutations of the target by genetic linkage analyses, this information may provide useful information on target-related effects. The pathology observed in these patients may reflect the effects that will be manifest from pharmaceutical inhibition of the target. Similarly, phenotypic characterization of a knockout mouse may prove useful. Inducible knockouts may be necessary if the GEM is embryonically lethal. Additionally, inducible knockouts frequently are more relevant to modeling for safety because the timing of knockout can be focused. This is important especially if there are life span differences in the effects observed in the GEM and the patient population, such as the knockout of the gene produces developmental abnormalities, and the patient population is mature. By controlling the timing of the knockout to a mature mouse, the animal model is more relevant. Regardless, genotyping of the GEM for confirmation of the genetic composition is recommended. While, immunohistochemistry and/or in situ hybridization can be used for this purpose, tissue homogenization techniques are more generally practiced.

Biomarkers. While an early thorough investigation of the potential target-related effects can provide an early perspective on the potential safety liabilities, it also provides a basis for the development of potentially useful biomarkers of activity. Activity biomarkers are increasingly recognized as valuable surrogates for efficacy in clinical trials. For example, these biomarkers can give an early indication of future success or failure for regression. Oncology clinical studies frequently have a long lag time from initiation of treatment to signs of regression, based on the typical means of imaging. A biomarker for activity could indicate successful interaction at the target very soon after start of dosing, and, if that interaction properly translates into activity at the tumor, development teams can base decisions to accelerate specific programs that have a higher probability of impending success. How to find some of these biomarkers by means of toxicogenomics is further explained in the next chapter.

4.3.2. Off-Target Effects

Manifestations of toxicities that are unrelated to target (off-target) are generally more challenging from a risk assessment perspective. For small-molecule pharmaceutical agents (as opposed to biotechnology-derived products), the activity is never as specific as desired, such that the new chemical entity will interact with other endogenous molecules (in addition to the target) resulting in toxicities. Data or information that explains the mechanism of action of particular toxicological findings is utilized differently in drug development and drug discovery. In drug development, this information is used to provide robust risk assessment to determine if the toxicity will be expressed in human clinical trials and at what dose (as described above). In drug discovery, however, less effort is spent on risk assessment and more on chemical structural modification to reduce the probability of producing the effect altogether.

In drug discovery, pharmaceutical chemists attempt to minimize off-target effects by substructural modifications to the molecule to increase specificity for the target alone. While this can be done empirically by trial and error (specifically, synthesize a chemical analog and dose an animal to determine expression of the finding), a more fruitful endeavor involves knowledge of the mechanism of action of the toxicity. Such endeavors generally develop more robust structure–activity relationships that have a more rationale and scientific approach to optimizing a compound for success (lead compound optimization). Mechanistic knowledge not only leads to better science but also is more frugal due to refinement of screening assays. Refined screening assays are generally more relevant and specific models also have higher throughput to allow for faster development of structure–activity relationships. Molecular techniques that maintain microscopic structural architecture and cellular morphology are indispensable in studies that seek to identify mechanisms of toxicity.

Compound-related histopathologic changes can be the result of a direct interaction of the compound with the cell that demonstrates the histopathologic change or through indirect mechanisms. The ultimate objective of mechanistic risk assessment investigations is to identify not only the primary cell involved but also the primary molecular mechanism in that cell. Sometimes, if not frequently, this seemingly simple task of identifying a change as primary or secondary is anything but simple or easy. It is more difficult to dissect primary from secondary changes in complex histopathologic findings; and generally, chronic repeat dose studies have more complex histopathologic changes. For instance, in studies of longer than one-month duration, histopathologic findings will have varying components of changes that would be interpreted as secondary, such as attempts at repair and regeneration, or attempts at compensation for inadequacies of function. Even more simplistic than that, it is not intuitive whether a change characterized as necrotizing and inflammatory started as primary parenchymal cell degeneration and necrosis or as primary inflammation.

Time-course studies with interim periodic sacrifices of groups of animals may demonstrate not only the progression of the lesion over time but also the initial primary morphologic change. In toxicology, findings generally manifest at lower doses (or exposures) over chronic repeat dose studies, so higher doses may be necessary for shorter term time-course studies. One must recognize, however, that higher doses (and exposures) may result in new interactions with molecules and potential mechanisms that were not present at lower doses.

For an administered pharmaceutical agent to have a primary effect on a specific cell, the agent must interact directly with that cell. Therefore, the demonstration of the presence of the administered compound (or a metabolite) associated with that cell would provide supporting evidence of the primary effect. These approaches are especially valuable and rewarding for certain cytomorphological changes that suggest compound accumulation, such as hypertrophy, vacuolation, tinctorial changes, and the like. Direct identification of administered drug is sometimes possible with simple hematoxylin and eosin staining, such as with gene therapy. The administration of genetic material as therapy is frequently associated with granular eosinophilic intracytoplasmic material in proximal convoluted tubules of the nephron (Fig. 4.3), which is widely accepted to be the nucleic acid sequences themselves. More commonly, however, the cytomorphological changes are not easily identified as accumulated compound with routine staining. For example, a finding of intracytoplasmic vacuoles within enterocytes as a manifestation of an orally administered drug may be actual drug accumulation or a secondary manifestation of cellular physiology (Fig. 4.4). While special stains could be used to rule out some possibilities, that is, oil red-O for lipid, positive identification as drug may still be necessary. Lastly, other cytomorphologic changes that do not suggest compound accumulation may also benefit from the identification of the compound. For example, centrilobular coagulative necrosis in the liver may be due to a primary effect of a compound (or metabolite from

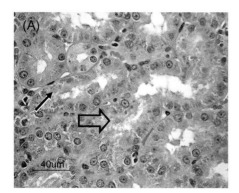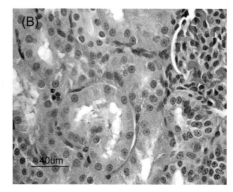

Figure 4.3. Kidney from a cynomolgus monkey treated with structurally modified oligonucleotides (A). Small basophilic granules are more numerous and darker (small closed arrow) and likely represent phagosomes, while larger, paler, droplets (large open arrow) likely represent phagolysosomes within the proximal convoluted tubules of the renal cortex. Proximal convoluted tubules of the renal cortex from a vehicle treated monkey (B).

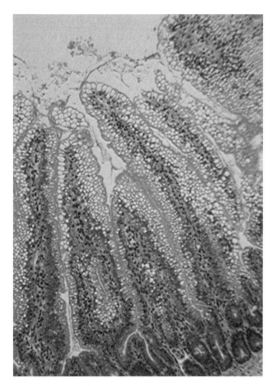

Figure 4.4. Duodenum from a rat treated with a small-molecule kinase inhibitor. Enterocytes at the tips of mucosal villi have intracytoplasmic clear round vacuoles that stain positive for neutral lipid with oil red-O. Drug substance or metabolites may be complexed with the lipid within vacuoles.

a zonal cytochrome P450 with a zonal distribution) or from chronic passive congestion. The demonstration of the presence of the compound in the centrilobular hepatocytes (prior to actual coagulative necrosis) would provide compelling evidence that the effect would have been primary on these hepatocytes.

Localization of Off-Target Effects. There are a number of methods that can be used to demonstrate drug substance in tissue. While tissue can be homogenized and analyzed by chromatography followed by mass spectrometry to demonstrate a pharmaceutical compound, molecular pathology techniques are more valuable for hypothesis testing for the determination of primary effects. Microscopic image-guided techniques allow cellular mapping and localization of drug substance and metabolites where tissue homogenates are limited by heterogeneous cell populations. Imaging-based techniques, such as microautoradiography, image-based matrix-assisted laser desorption/ionization–mass spectrometry (MALDI-MS) and laser capture microdissection followed by chromatography–

mass spectrometry have demonstrated utility for the mapping and localization of small-molecule pharmaceutical agents or their metabolites at the cellular level.

Microautoradiography is perhaps the most frequently used technique in the pharmaceutical industry overall, especially to investigate pharmacokinetics and biodistribution, probably because it has the longest history and employs more readily available equipment. For pharmacokinetic and biodistribution studies, resolution need not be very high and data are usually sufficient at the organ level, via whole-body imaging. For use in mechanistic toxicological investigations, however, resolution must be high and at the cellular level. It is most optimal to have the resolution to differentiate the presence of radiolabeled compound in neighboring cells. The absolute clear discrimination of one cell from the next, however, may not be necessary if the tissue structural architecture lends itself to aid in this determination. For example, if the radiolabeled compound is present in the mucosal epithelium of the intestine, the resolution must only demonstrate a uniform layer on the luminal surface, not necessarily absolute cellular presence. However, higher resolution would be necessary in order to conclude that the labeled compound was present in only neutrophils and not lymphocytes or macrophages in an inflammatory lesion. In the latter circumstance, this high level of resolution for microautoradiography requires special considerations and still may not be sufficient to achieve one's needs.

While there are a number of different methods for high-resolution microautoradiography, the method most suited to maintain fidelity of compound localization should be utilized (Stumpf, 2005). The methods for high resolution are generally more technically challenging than low-resolution techniques and usually entail snap-freezing of tissues, cryomicrotomy, and dry-mounting onto photographic emulsion or emulsion-coated slides without any fluid treatment or thaw. Fluid treatments and thawing tend to result in compound diffusion because the small-molecule drug candidates are not *locked* in place within subcellular components. Whichever method is employed, fidelity of compound localization so as to avoid diffusion of the radiolabeled compound and loss of specificity is of utmost importance.

Radiolabeled drug candidates with the label in the appropriate molecular locations are essential to the process. Typical radioisotopes include tritium (^{3}H), ^{14}C, and ^{125}I. Each offers advantages and disadvantages with regard to resolution and ease of use, but other factors should also be considered, such as location of label on the molecule. The location of the label on the molecule will dictate whether the parent compound and/or metabolite(s) are visualized. Knowledge of specific metabolic pathways is needed so as to place the radioisotope in a relevant location based on the needs of the study. Radioisotopes placed in the core structure will likely be present in most metabolites (as well as the parent structure), whereas isotopes located peripherally in the molecule in metabolically active functional groups could more readily be hydrolyzed off and not be visualized. This may be a desirable situation if the interest is localization of only the parent molecule. Additionally, inherent differences in the radioisotopes should be considered, such as resolution of various isotopes. For instance, carbon-14

(^{14}C)-labeled compounds provide a lower autoradiographic resolution than the others.

In some respects, the utility of high-resolution microautoradiography in the pharmaceutical industry may be limited because of the amount of resources necessary for these studies. The greatest resource commitment is from synthetic chemistry. Even if a synthetic process has been optimized, the process to introduce a radiolabel in a specific location and maintain it there is frequently no simple task. If the location of the label is in the core molecule, standard starting materials may not be able to be utilized because the label is attached to the starting molecule. Therefore, earlier synthetic steps may need to be introduced just to get to the starting point of a derived process. Additionally, protecting groups frequently need to be introduced so as to prevent exchange for an unlabeled molecule. While these tasks are not insurmountable, the factor that is most significant to hindering its use in the pharmaceutical industry is the up-front work needed for *each* molecule of investigation. The resources for synthesis of a single radiolabeled compound are disproportionate for the investigation of only one single mechanism. Because each compound in question will consume similar up-front resources, the tool lacks the broad-based application that newer technologies offer (see below). Additionally, long exposure times of weeks to months are less than desirable in the competitive pharmaceutical marketplace. Therefore, as a tool for mechanistic investigation of toxicology, its utility is limited.

The value of MALDI (matrix-assisted laser desorption/ionization) imaging mass spectrometry for determining cellular distribution of pharmaceuticals is increasingly becoming apparent (Hsieh et al., 2007; Wang et al., 2005). Although the somewhat lower spatial resolution of approximately 100 μm and the high up-front cost may be significant disadvantages for some, the significantly shortened cycle time and additional data generated (see discussion below) are invaluable for many, as compared to microautoradiography.

The concept of MALDI imaging mass spectrometry was introduced by Caprioli and co-workers in 1997. The foundation of analysis relies on the general principles of mass spectrometry as with any liquid or solid biological sample, in short, the identification of the mass-to-charge ratio of ions and construction of a mass spectrum. The basic parts of any mass spectrometer are an ion source, mass analyzer, and detection system. Briefly, an ion source ionizes molecules within the sample, and then these ions are transported to the mass analyzer where they are separated according to their mass-to-charge ratio by various algorithms. The theory, briefly, involves static or dynamic, electrical or magnetic fields that influence the time and direction of flight throughout the mass analyzer. The detector simply records the effect of this influence. While the method is inherently qualitative, quantitative data can be derived from the generation of a standard curve from analysis of known quantities of the analyte.

Matrix-assisted laser desorption/ionization (MALDI)-MS is a specialized application for mass spectrometry that utilizes a *soft* ionization source. The soft ionization allows for the analysis of biomolecules, such as peptides and proteins.

In non-image-based MALDI-MS, a suitable matrix solution is applied to a solid tissue sample, and the molecules of interest leach out of the tissue on to a specially designed MALDI plate. The appropriate matrix solution is dependent on the molecule of interest (analyte) and to a lesser extent the tissue sample. On the MALDI plate, the solvents vaporize, leaving co-crystallized matrix and analyte. Ions are produced by a laser beam directed at the MALDI spot via transfer of energy to the analyte molecule. The matrix is thought to protect analyte molecules from the disruptive energy of the laser.

The theory behind the ionization of biomolecules in *image-based* MALDI mass spectometry is similar to the above, but the analyte molecules are maintained in a structurally complex solid tissue sample, and the structural details are reconstructed in association with the mass spectrum so as to localize specific components of the spectrum with specific structural or cellular components of the tissue. In order to achieve this, matrix solution is sprayed onto the cryopreserved solid tissue section, which extracts molecules into the surface of the tissue and forms co-crystals (as opposed to complete extraction of molecules out of the tissue for non-image-based MALDI). A soft laser ion source is applied to the tissue section, resulting in ionization of analytes as above, but the laser is focused and travels across the tissue in a raster pattern until the whole section has been analyzed. Each focus of the laser generates ions that are similarly processed by a mass analyzer according to general spectrometry principles. The resulting mass spectrum is stored along with the spatial coordinates of the laser, and the resolution of the reconstructed image is relative to the width of the beam. A two-dimensional digital image is reconstructed that consists of the tissue morphology along with the relative expression of the analytes. The spatial tissue image is maintained digitally via the positioning of the beam in the raster pattern for purposes of image reconstruction.

With all these applications of spectrometry, tandem mass spectrometry (MS-MS) can be used to further analyze and define molecular structure. After a separation of molecular ions through one mass analyzer, these ions can be fragmented and the fragments separated by a second mass analyzer. Successive cycles of fragmentation and mass-to-charge separation allow reconstruction of the molecular structure of the drug, metabolites, and/or biomolecules. Prior knowledge of the structure of these components can aid in directing the mass spectrometry investigation, but it is not absolutely required. Fragments can be produced by a number of different methods, but most involve collision of some sort.

The main limitation of image-based MALDI-MS in the pharmaceutical industry for the localization of small-molecule drugs is the limit of resolution, approximately 100 μm. While individual cell localization is beyond the limit of resolution, the system can be adequately used for structural localization, such as within epithelia, specific lobular distributions in the liver (centrilobular, midzonal, periportal), renal glomeruli, periarterial lymphoid sheaths in the spleen, islets in the spleen, and so forth. The system could not be used to identify analytes in single cells, such as in inflammatory cells scattered throughout a tissue, or very small clusters or small numbers of connected cells, such as alveolar type II cells or Clara cells in the lung.

Toxicogenomics. The *-omics* revolution has proven to be very useful in nonclinical drug development and toxicology from many perspectives (Gatzidou et al., 2007; Pognan, 2007). The value of -omics research is that whole sets of macromolecules can be probed for thousands of specific changes. In drug development and toxicology, the use of transcriptomics, proteomics, and metabonomics to identify drug-related changes in the transcriptional message (mRNA), protein, and metabolites, respectively, has proven valuable. In general, -omics data can broadly be used for either predictive or mechanistic queries. For the purposes of illustration, toxicogenomics (or transcriptomics) will be discussed in these capacities.

In predictive toxicogenomics, the goal is to identify a *signature* of expression changes in the transcriptome that is associated with a specific drug-related toxicological change. A signature is comprised of expression changes in a *set* of specific genes. If the composition of the signature is solely based on statistical power of drug-related changes, the signature can become quite large because of the shear number of genes analyzed. Therefore, it is usually most advantageous to provide some scientific and rational reason for including specific genes based on known associations of that gene with the mechanism of drug action or mechanism of toxicity. Certainly, some genes with uncertain function may be added to the signature based solely on statistical power (Foster et al., 2007). For these analyses, bioinformatics and computational analyses are of utmost importance and a number of formats are commercially available.

Genomic and proteomic analyses in mechanistic toxicology, on the other hand, scrutinize drug-related changes in specific individual genes or proteins for the purpose of identifying mechanisms by which toxicities develop. As opposed to identifying sets of components for prediction, changes in individual components may provide insight to the potential mechanisms involved. While toxicogenomic analyses on tissue homogenates can be used for this purpose, investigators are increasingly using a focused collection of specific cells at the microscopic level for analyses. Potential clues that might indicate that specific components have significant involvement in the mechanism might be an overabundance of components in converging signaling pathways, components that are known to play some role in the normal tissue or in the altered tissue morphology. A closer look at the methods employed in toxicogenomics will be discussed in the next chapter.

The motivation to identify mechanisms of actions of toxicologic findings broadly involves risk assessment. Knowledge of the mechanism can give perspective on the relative risk that the finding will manifest in clinical trials. Mechanistic information can also provide a platform for identifying potential biomarkers of toxicity or if the effect is target-related, biomarkers of pharmacodynamic effect. Lastly, this information can potentially be used in drug discovery as a screening tool for the selection of back-up compounds.

In vitro Methods. The analysis of pure samples composed of only cells or structures of interest can lead to *cleaner* signals and deliver a higher potential for the successful outcome of the investigation. One obvious and most common means of obtaining a pure sample of cells is through in vitro culture of cells. From this perspective, in vitro toxicological investigative studies will involve multiple cell cultures that are incubated in the presence of varying concentrations of the compound of interest and no compound as a negative control. Cultured cells can be either immortal cell lines or primary cell cultures from a relevant species. For general toxicologic investigation, primary cell cultures are usually the most relevant; however, if immortalized cell lines must be used, they should be closest to the normal phenotype with respect to metabolism, protein expression, and the like. There are specialized instances where specific genetically engineered cell lines or lines with known genetic alterations are more relevant and desirable.

These systems lack the obvious complexity of in vivo approaches to toxicological investigation. In vitro systems do have the advantage of a much focused approach and also ability to make comparisons across species regarding potential direct effects on specific cell types. This is uniquely valuable for determining risk assessment based on the potential for species specificity. If liabilities have been identified in nonclinical species that manifest as a direct primary drug–cell interaction, the potential (or risk) that humans will develop the same liability can sometimes be determined based on in vitro cultures of that specific cell type from various nonclinical species and human.

Imaging Methods. Imaging-based methods allow a more refined focus of investigation as opposed to the traditional homogenization of tissues, which deliver a heterogenous cell population. Heterogenous cell populations not only dilute signals from -omics investigations but also can frequently confound the degree or significance of these potential signals. Dilutional effects can occur due to the shear number of irrelevant versus relevant cells in the tissue. For instance, if 50% of the cells in the tissue are not affected by the drug, then the signal intensity will theoretically be diluted by one-half. In other words, if there is a drug-related signal in cells of interest, but there is a similar number of cells with no change in the parameter, the volume analyzed will be twice that needed, so the signal will be one-half what it would have been with a pure cell analysis. Similarly, *noise* of extraneous irrelevant cells can confound data. Various cell populations or loci may have a specific intensity of a drug-related signal, and other cell populations or loci may have a different degree of or even an inverse (i.e., increased versus decreased) signal. This noise may adversely impact the ability to identify potential signals, especially when trying to investigate a morphologic change in a specific cell population.

If, however, one desires the multisystemic influence and complexity of an in vivo model, then image-based techniques for isolation and collection of specific cell types and populations from the heterogenous cell populations in organs are generally more valuable. These image-based techniques are MALDI imaging mass spectrometry and laser capture microdissection. For their use in ex vivo histological localization of protein and transcriptional profiling in complex tissues, their utility goes well beyond that of IHC and ISH. IHC and ISH are routinely used for probing with known individual proteins and transcriptional sequences, while MALDI imaging mass spectrometry and laser capture microdissection offer the potential for simultaneous analysis of many molecular species present in the tissue.

While image-based MALDI mass spectrometry for the purpose of identifying small-molecule drug chemical entities has been presented above, the original purpose for its invention was for proteomics (Meistermann et al., 2006; Reyzer and Caprioli, 2007; McDonnell and Heeren, 2007; Chaurand, 2006). Further recently developed platforms for the technology include lipid profiling (lipidomics) (Woods and Jackson, 2006). While the limitations of image-based MALDI mass spectrometry are similar as presented above, the wealth of data in its use for proteomics is similar to that achieved from microarrays.

Another image-based molecular method for the cellular localization of administered drug is through the use of laser microdissection (LM) and mass spectrometry. In laser microdissection, a laser beam is used to microdissect specific cells from a cryopreserved tissue section via a light microscope. There are essentially two means of achieving this (through the use of two different commercially available units). One involves the use of a polymer affixed to a microcentrifuge cap and is called laser capture microdissection (LCM). The polymer surface is apposed to the top of the tissue section on a glass slide. While visualizing the tissue under a microscope and manipulating the location of the slide similar to any other light microscope, the user accentuates a pulsed laser beam onto the tissue–polymer interface, which bonds the cells of interest to the microcentrifuge cap. The capture process does not damage these macromolecules because the laser energy is absorbed by the polymer film. The slide, tissue, and cap are moved to the next cell or location of interest for collection, and collection proceeds in a similar fashion. The laser beam can be "focused" so as to achieve appropriate beam diameter and optimal bonding strength. Currently, the beam can be focused to a 30- or 60-μm diameter. After completion of the microdissection from the tissue section, the cap is removed with adherent collected tissue. The slide with remaining noncollected tissue, as well as the cap with adherent collected tissue, can be independently viewed through the microscope to evaluate efficiency of sample collection. Even the cells that are adherent to the polymer retain morphologic features, so fidelity of collection can be evaluated (Fig. 4.5).

The second method for collecting only specific cells or structures of interest while visualizing through a light microscope involves a noncontact methodology and is commonly referred to as laser microdissection and pressure catapulting (LMPC). This method uses a laser beam to essentially *excise* cells or tissues of interest. Cryopreserved tissue is sectioned by a microtome and placed on a membrane that is suspended by a frame of similar size to a microscope slide. A pulsed laser beam interfaced within the microscope is used to encircle the cells and structures of interest for excision from the tissue of noninterest. The beam is focused to a spot size of less than 1 μm, thus there is a corresponding cut gat

(B)

(A)

(C)

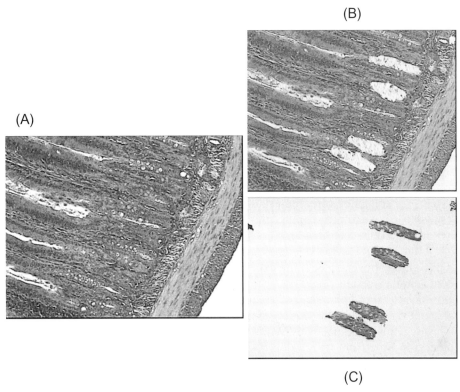

Figure 4.5. Laser capture microdissection of crypt epithelial cells of the intestinal mucosa. Section before microdissection (A), section after microdissection (B), and cap with adherent crypt epithelial cells that have been collected for further molecular analysis (C).

between the tissue of interest and adjacent material. After microdissection, the isolated specimens are *ejected* out of the tissue and catapulted into a collection device, typically a microcentrifuge tube. By this means, there is no contact of the collected tissue with the laser beam, and there is no interaction of the collected tissue with extraneous substance.

Each of the two systems for collection of microdissected tissue has advantages and disadvantages. LCM involves direct contact with a laser and addition of a polymer, both of which the manufacturer claims will not compromise the tissue for transcriptomics and proteomics. The method for collection of LCM is well suited for collection of single nonconfluent individual cells, such as infiltrating inflammatory cells, while the method of LMPC is better suited for collection of larger structural areas, such as whole acini, layers of epithelium, whole glomeruli, and the like. In either case, integrity of tissue is of the utmost importance. Tissue preservation and collection methodology should depend primarily on the stability and properties of the analyte. It is claimed that starting materials can be either cyropreserved or routinely fixed in formalin (or ethanol) and paraffin embedded. While paraffin-embedded tissues theoretically allow for the use of archived materials, in the author's experience, these materials tend to deliver unreliable data and, for toxicology investigations, it is easier to design specialized prospective nonclinical studies for focused investigations involving toxicogenomics and/or proteinomics via laser microdissection (which would also lend itself to MALDI imaging mass spectrometry). Once the cells or structures of interest have been collected by either method, the samples can be used for various molecular profiling methods involving gene expression or differential protein expression for the purposes of mechanistic toxicological investigation. In theory, any method of molecular profiling that is performed on fresh homogenized tissue may be applied to cryopreserved microdissected tissue, and manufacturers of the two systems for collection offer materials as well as guidance on obtaining successful results. It is beyond the scope of this chapter to detail all the specific molecular uses for microdissected tissue.

While the image-based microscopic collection of specific cells and structures as presented above can be quite expensive due to the need for specialized equipment, similar results may be achieved from toxicogenomic or proteinomic approaches using homogenized tissue and subsequent confirmation of the cellular relevance of genetic sequences or proteins by in situ hybridization or immunohistochemistry, respectively. While the up-front cost savings may be significant, the cost in time from two in-depth serial processes as opposed to one may also be significant, especially when dealing with novel, esoteric, or recently discovered gene sequences or proteins.

4.4. BIOPHARMACEUTICALS

A biopharmaceutical therapy can be broadly defined as any therapy that is the product of biotechnology. In this section, we will discuss how molecular pathology techniques are necessary for the nonclinical development of macromolecules, such as monoclonal antibodies, recombinant ligands, immuno- and protein conjugates, and the like. While many aspects of nonclinical safety for biopharmaceuticals are similar to chemical entities (as discussed above), there are certain additional concerns for biopharmaceuticals, and molecular pathology plays a critical role in some of these. First and foremost is the selection of a relevant species in which to evaluate desired pharmacologic effects. Relevant nonclinical species will not only express the target but also parallel the density, tissue, and cellular distribution and the homology of the human target.

While it may seem obvious and even an academic exercise, demonstration of the presence of the target in the nonclinical species is perhaps the most important. Depending on the nature of the target, this can be usually done by fairly straightforward means or even through a thorough literature search. While pure qualitative measures do confirm presence, quantitative measures are much more meaningful. If the target is a receptor, density of the receptor on the cell or tissue can be used to provide perspective on activity and even dosing. For instance, if the receptor is expressed in both humans and monkeys, but humans have a much higher density, then it is conceivable that the in vivo activity will also differ. This can be illustrated considering receptor occupancy. Similar doses of a number of biopharmaceutical particles may produce a similar effect in humans and monkeys, but in the above example, escalation of the dose to the level of full receptor occupancy in monkeys will result in no further effect beyond saturation. In humans, on the other hand, further escalation could yield effects that were not predicted in the nonclinical safety studies.

Similar to target density, species differences in target cellular localization are frequently meaningful. Immunohistochemistry and/or in situ hybridization are most meaningful in these endeavors, and the use of tissue microarrays (as discussed above) are advised for efficiency. While these data can be used to gain perspective on nonclinical safety findings, they can also be used to select the most relevant nonclinical species, that is, that species mimic the distribution, density, and homology of that in humans. For species selection, tissue microarrays from the various potential nonclinical species (mouse, rat, dog, and monkey) and even nonstandard species may be used.

Another comparison for species relevancy is homology of the target in the nonclinical species. If the target is a protein, even single amino acid differences among species can result in profound three-dimensional conformational differences that affect binding of the biopharmaceutical agent. This is especially important because these agents are highly specific for the human target. While off-target liabilities are minimal because of this specificity, most of the agents do not have activity in some nonclinical species due to differences in target homology. Frequently, this leaves only the monkey as the relevant nonclinical species. In reality, much of the above information is most frequently gleaned from literature sources.

Subsequent investigations of this nature involve assessments of the actual biopharmaceutical agent, and the above information is used to make a preliminary decision on relevant animal species. Because these studies can be fairly labor intensive, it is advisable to let published data drive preliminary decisions and do prospective studies to confirm that the proper nonclinical species was selected. These studies use molecular pathology to confirm binding and activity of the biopharmaceutical agent. Binding assays using tissue microarrays are frequently mandatory for regulatory submission in order to confirm relevancy. The most readily available method of evaluating tissue cross reactivity is via immunohistochemistry. Even if one uses published data on target homology, density, localization, and the like, it is prudent to run a pilot study to assess a few selected tissues of all various species that could potentially be used for nonclinical development and compare results to binding in human tissues. This can be done using immunohistochemistry (as with the definitive studies) or using flow cytometry with relevant cells for higher throughput. Once preliminary indications of species relevancy are obtained, the definitive study entails a more stringent design with all 32 tissues (FDA, 2006) from both the selected relevant species and humans.

Binding in human tissues is usually part of the nonclinical package submitted to regulatory agencies. These data are necessary for comparison to nonclinical species and are also used to indicate the potential for unanticipated (or nonselective) binding. Generally, however, the process of discovery and optimization process of biopharmaceutical agents is effective in delivering a very selective agent, and the manifestation of these nonselective agents is exceedingly rare.

Tissues must be from at least three individuals in the event that there are polymorphisms and must be from both males and females. The tissues must be of the highest integrity. Cryopreserved tissue is recommended to ensure integrity and exposure of the antigen or target. Tissues also must be complete in that they contain all different structures in the organ, such as lung must contain alveoli as well as airways, and kidney must contain all portions of the nephron. At least two scientifically relevant concentrations of biopharmaceutical should be evaluated. Additionally, a negative control and a positive control must be included in the assay. Negative controls should be as close a representation to the biopharmaceutical molecule as possible without the target binding moiety. Positive controls should be labeling of an endogenous molecule, with the same amplification system as used for the biopharmaceutical molecules.

Special considerations will need to be taken in some circumstances. Scientifically sound rationale will dictate the conduct of these studies. For instance, for therapies that are targeted to interact directly with only stimulated cells, microorganisms, or other targets that are not expressed in normal tissue, typical binding studies will not deliver any meaningful data. Regardless, attempts should be made to demonstrate binding in the nonclinical species in an artificially created expression of the target. Sometimes this may involve conducting an in vivo study that stimulates the expression of the target. Other drastic cases may involve demonstration of binding and biological activity, or even safety, in the efficacy model.

These studies are used to demonstrate the presence of the orthologous target in the species used in the nonclinical safety studies. Some biopharmaceutical molecules have such high tissue species specificity that there will not be binding to any nonhuman tissues, except for the closest homolog, which is usually a primate. In cases where no nonhuman species tissues will bind the biopharmaceutical, that is, if the orthologous target is not present in animals, special measures might entail xenograft models, which introduce cells expressing the human target into immunodeficient mice, or transgenic models expressing the human target may be employed. However, such data should be interpreted with caution, in light of the artificial surrogate model. Transgenic mice may express the target in tissues or patterns that do not reflect the same in humans. There are numerous guidance documents available from the various governmental regulatory agencies (see recommendations for further reading); however, it is always prudent to consult the specific agencies for input prior to initiating such studies.

Demonstration of in vivo biological or functional activity offers further confirmation of species relevancy. Proof of activity is most easily demonstrated by knowledge of the downstream signaling of the target and ultimate expected tissue response. For example, if a receptor is the target and the targeted mechanism is inhibition of that receptor, confirmation of biological activity of the pharmaco-logic intervention might include demonstration of changes in phosphorylation status of the receptor itself or downstream signals. This could be accomplished by quantitative immunohistochemistry if antibodies are available that are specific for activated and deactivated status of these signals. Similarly, image-based tech-niques such as laser microdissection or MALDI imaging mass spectrometry could also be used, as well as techniques that employ homogenized tissue if cellular localization is not necessary.

In vitro functional assays can sometimes provide valuable risk assessment information. When a specific potential liability is discovered in nonclinical safety studies, tissue cultures of animal origin and human origin may be compared for similar molecule-related effects. Initially, animal origin tissue treated with the molecule should elicit molecular signaling similar to that identified in vivo. These measures will validate the system such that in vitro effects can replicate in vivo. Then, the response in human tissue culture can be compared to that of animal tissue cultures in an attempt to demonstrate the potential for development in clinical trials.

4.5. SUMMARY

Molecular pathology techniques have extensive utility in nonclinical pharmaceu-tical development. As with any technique, the quality of the data is inherently dependent on the quality of the sample for analysis. Sometimes the samples will be retrospective queries and involve archived tissue from previous studies, similar to most of the clinical samples from human patients or volunteers. Archived tissues from nonclinical safety studies tend to be more useful than clinical samples because of the highly controlled details of collection technique, sample handling, fixation type, and fixation duration.

Molecular pathology and image-based technologies are very useful platforms for mechanistic risk assessment investigations in nonclinical safety assessment. The utility is mainly a consequence of the fact that basic nonclinical safety assess-ment tends to be pathology- and morphology-centric, and the investigation of a liability should involve the avenue through which that liability was discovered.

REFERENCES

FDA (2006). Guidance for Industry and Reviewers: Nonclinical Safety Evaluation of Biotechnology-Derived Pharmaceuticals. U.S. Dept of Health and Human Services, Food and Drug Administration, August.

Caprioli, R. M., Farmer, T. B., Gile, J. (1997). Molecular imaging of biological samples: localization of peptides and proteins using MALDI-TOF MS. *Anal Chem.* 69:4751–4760.

Foster, W. R., Chen, S. J., He, A., Truong, A., Bhaskaran, V., Nelson, D. M., Dambach, D. M., Lehman-McKeeman, L. D., and Car, B. D. (2007). A retrospective analysis of toxicogenomics in the safety assessment of drug candidates. *Toxicol. Pathol.* 35:621–635.

Gatzidou, E. T., Zira, A. N., and Theocharis, S. E. (2007). Toxicogenomics: A pivotal piece in the puzzle of toxicological research. *J. Appl. Toxicol.* 27:305–309.

Hsieh, Y., Chen, J., and Korfmacher, W. A. (2007). Mapping pharmaceuticals in tissues using MALDI imaging mass spectrometry. *J. Pharmacol. Toxicol. Methods* 55:193–200.

McDonnell, L.A., and Heeren, R. M. A. (2007). Imaging mass spectormetry. *Mass Spectr. Rev.* 26:606–643.

Meistermann, H., Norris, J. L., Aerni, H. R., Cornett, D. S., Friedlein, A., Erskine, A. R., Augustin, A., Ruepp, S., Suter, L., Langen, H., Caprioli, R. M., and Ducret, A. (2006). Biomarker identification by imaging mass spectrometry: Transthyretin is a biomarker for gentamicin-induced nephrotoxicity in rat. *Mol. Cell Proteomics* 5:1876–1886.

Pognan, F. (2007). Toxicogenomics applied to predictive and exploratory toxicology for the safety assessment of new chemical entities: a long road with deep potholes. *Prog. Drug Res.*, 64:217, 219–238.

Reyzer, M. L., and Caprioli, R. M. (2007). MALDI-MS-based imaging of small molecules and proteins in tissues. *Curr. Opin. Chem. Biol.* 11:29–35.

Stumpf, W. E. (2005). Drug localization and targeting with receptor microscopic autoradiography. *J. Pharmacol. Toxicol. Methods* 51:25–40.

Wang, H. Y. J., Jackson, S. N., McEuen, J., and Woods, A. S. (2005). Localization and analyses of small drug molecules in rat brain tissue sections. *Anal. Chem.* 77:6682–6686.

Woods, A. S., and Jaskson, S. N. (2006). Brain tissue lipidomics: Direct probing using matrix-assisted laser desorption/ionization mass spectrometry. *AAPS J.* 8:E391–E395.

Wu, L., Maillard, I., Nakamura, M., Pear, W. S., and Griffin, J. D. (2007). The transcriptional coactivitor Maml1 is required for Notch2-mediated marginal zone B-cell development. *Blood* 15:3618–3623.

5

TOXICOGENOMICS IN DRUG DEVELOPMENT

Wayne R. Buck and Eric A. G. Blomme

5.1. INTRODUCTION

Toxicogenomics is the discipline of using comprehensive gene expression data to predict or characterize cell and tissue damage due to exposure to chemical agents. Some authors use the term more loosely to include the use of other comprehensive analysis technologies, such as proteomics, metabolomics, and global kinase analysis (kinomics); however, this chapter will not explore these branches of toxicology. In toxicogenomics, gene expression data are gathered using high-density microarray technologies wherein thousands of gene transcripts can be quantified in parallel. Experimental design usually compares one or more doses of a compound against a vehicle-only control data set, but the particular microarray method will dictate whether samples and controls are paired or hybridized individually. Studies may investigate the effects of a compound on cells or organs in culture, or the effects of a compound on tissues taken from a treated animal. Considerations for building hypotheses and designing experiments, such as bioavailability and biotransformation, apply to toxicogenomics as in any area of toxicology. Statistical analysis of the data sets, and therefore the calculation of group sizes, requires a distinctly different approach, however. The greatest danger in applying genomics analysis to toxicology is poor study designs, where heaps

Molecular Pathology in Drug Discovery and Development, Edited by J. Suso Platero
Copyright © 2009 John Wiley & Sons, Inc.

of data are generated that have no practical value in assessing or predicting the potency or mechanism of toxicity of a particular test compound. To its credit, toxicogenomics has successfully accelerated the discovery of mechanisms of toxicity and defined subsets of genes (referred to as gene expression signatures) whose expression predicts particular toxicities in defined experimental models.

The purpose of this chapter is to provide a brief overview of the technologies and methods relevant to toxicogenomics. We will limit this discussion to the perspective of small-molecule drugs, although the application of genomics technology to assess toxicity for biologicals has been recently reviewed (Gay et al., 2007). An overview of the drug discovery and development process is provided elsewhere in this book. For clarity, however, Table 5.1 defines a short list of terms that we will use in this chapter to refer to the drug development process. The remainder of this chapter will be organized from considerations specific to methods to more general issues. First, a brief overview of the microarray technologies and platforms will be provided. Second, methods of analysis of these

TABLE 5.1. Glossary of Drug Discovery and Development Terms

Discovery	Describes the initial part of the process, where disease mechanisms are explored, putative therapeutic targets identified, compound libraries screened, and "hits" identified and optimized to result in development candidates
Hit to lead	Process of creating molecular variations upon a core molecule identified in a screening process (the "hit") with the aim of discovering compounds with high affinity and specificity ("leads") and druglike physicochemical and pharmacological properties
Lead optimization	Generation of compounds with modifications to the core structure of the lead compound to improve characteristics of the drug (such as absorption, distribution, metabolism, excretion, or toxicity, also referred to as ADME-T)
Development candidate	Compound with good affinity for the target and druglike properties that is selected for future nonclinical and clinical studies
Dead compound	Compound that will not be further pursued in discovery or development due to serious drawbacks such as development-limiting toxicity
Development	Regulated processes (GLP/GMP/GCP) initiated after the discovery process where compounds are characterized and tested for safety and efficacy in nonclinical to clinical studies, and where chemical methods are developed for mass manufacturing
GLP/GMP/GCP	Good laboratory, manufacturing, and clinical practices that must be followed according to stringent oversight as dictated by law

information-rich data sets will be introduced. Third, the value of toxicogenomics in either predicting toxicity of a compound or in elucidating mechanisms of toxicity will be detailed. Fourth, considerations for experimental design, such as in vitro drug exposure and cross-species comparison, will be discussed. Fifth, particular examples of successful implementation of toxicogenomics will hopefully encourage the pharmaceutical toxicologist to incorporate toxicogenomics in an effective manner. We shall find that the application of toxicogenomics to the development of new medicines has brought new tools to an industry that is increasingly pressured to deliver new, safer medicines to patients in less time and at a lower cost.

5.2. BRIEF OVERVIEW OF LARGE-SCALE GENE EXPRESSION TECHNOLOGIES

The objective of gene expression technologies is to measure the relative abundance of individual transcripts within a biological sample of ribonucleic acid (RNA). The technical details of global gene expression methodology must be understood to avoid invalid data arising from faulty samples or poorly performing reagents. In homogeneous samples, degraded RNA, and inefficient labeling reactions will still hybridize to microarrays, and the failure of the method to reflect true gene expression may not be immediately evident, even after data analysis. Therefore, quality control in sample processing is indispensible to assure consistent and reliable data.

5.2.1. RNA Quality

Any method that purports to measure the quantity of messenger RNA (mRNA) expressed from a particular gene must rely upon isolation of a representative, intact sample of RNA. The "stability" of RNA is impacted by the chemical and enzymatic environment in which it exists. Nonenzymatic hydrolysis of RNA in the presence of divalent magnesium cations and Tris buffer begins at pH > 7.5 and temperatures above 37 °C (AbouHaidar and Ivanov, 1999). In practice, the greatest culprit in RNA degradation is the enzymatic activity of renatured ribonucleases, which are hardy proteins with high processivity (Peirson and Butler, 2007). Extraction methods typically use strong chaotropic agents (guanidinium) to denature ribonucleases prior to separation of RNA from other biomolecules, either by phase extraction or retention on silica-based substrates. Degradation of RNA has a significant negative impact on the validity of microarray data; therefore, it is important that every RNA sample be evaluated for integrity prior to use in microarray analysis (Copois et al., 2007; Strand et al., 2007).

The classical method of RNA visualization is agarose gel electrophoresis, optionally with additives that denature RNA secondary structure. However, microgram quantities of RNA are typically needed, and the procedure is time consuming and labor intensive. Visualization of sharp single bands of a particular mRNA probed by northern blotting remains the only direct method to assess mRNA quality but is so technically demanding as to be impractical for routine mRNA quality assessment. Ultraviolet (UV) absorbance at 260- and 280-nm wavelengths can be used to quantify nucleic acids, and interfering absorbance caused by proteins or other molecules will skew 260/280 absorbance ratios to flag impure samples. However, UV absorbance does not detect scission of RNA molecules and is highly dependent upon the pH and ionic strength of the sample (Wilfinger et al., 1997). Microfluidic applications of capillary electrophoresis have gained stature as the new standard method for RNA quality assessment. While mRNA is the source of microarray data, it accounts for less than 5% of total RNA. Therefore, mRNA quality is inferred from more abundant 28S and 18S ribosomal RNA (rRNA) sequences (5 and 2 kb in length, respectively). In theory, these rRNAs are present in equimolar amounts, and the difference in resolved 28S and 18S rRNA fluorescence is due to differences in mass with a theoretical 28S:18S ratio of approximately 2.7 to 1. In practice, 18S rRNA degrades more slowly than 28S rRNA, and for a time the 28S:18S peak area ratio was proposed as a measure of RNA degradation. Better quantitative measures of RNA degradation (e.g., RNA integrity number, RIN) have recently been devised that are on par with subjective interpretation of capillary electropherograms (Strand et al., 2007). The RNA integrity number is a weighted score based on electrophorectic fluorescence peak heights or peak areas ratioed to the total integrated fluorescence and evaluates features of the electropherogram profile in addition to the 28S and 18S peaks (Schroeder et al., 2006). The "degradometer" and RNA quality scale are similarly performing scales of RNA quality based on the electropherogram (Copois et al., 2007). In our laboratory, every sample is evaluated with an Agilent microfluidics electrophoretic bioanalyzer (Agilent Technologies, Santa Clara, CA) before inclusion in microarray experiments. The Agilent bioanalyzer is illustrated in Figure 5.1 with electropherograms of high quality and degraded RNA.

5.2.2. Hybridization Platforms

A number of methods have been developed to allow high-density quantitation of specific transcript abundance (Table 5.2). In general, the RNA sample is reversed transcribed using oligo(dT) and then linearly amplified by in vitro transcription. The amplified sample is labeled with a fluorophore by incorporation of labeled nucleotides or primers during the amplification step, made single stranded, and then hybridized to capture sequences on a solid substrate that can be imaged with a light source and detector. Differences between technologies at each of these steps have an impact on the susceptibility of the method to error. For instance, methods using oligo(dT) priming of the sample mRNA are inherently susceptible to RNA degradation, and partial degradation of transcripts results in a bias for detection of probes in the 3′ region of transcripts. The bead array method uses random primed reverse transcription and is promoted as less susceptible to RNA degradation. The most important difference between microarray

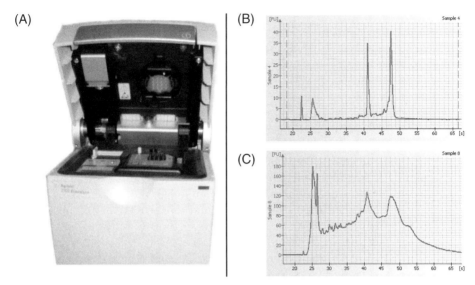

Figure 5.1. RNA quality analysis by microcapillary electrophoresis. (A) Agilent Bioanalyzer 2100 system is able to analyze up to 12 samples in about 30 minutes. (B) Electropherogram of a good quality RNA sample showing distinct peaks for 5, 18, and 28S ribosomal RNA. (C) Electropherogram of poor quality RNA with indistinct peaks.

TABLE 5.2. Gene Expression Technology Platforms

Technology	Affymetrix GeneChip(R)	Spotted microarrays		Bead array
Methodology	Photolithographic synthesis of oligonucleotides on solid support	Oligonucleotides synthesized on solid support by directed deposition of reagents	Contact transfer of nucleotide probes to solid support	Ligation of oligonucleotide probes to silica beads
Manufacturer	Affymetrix	Agilent		Illumina
Simultaneous probe set sizes	~30,000/chip			~2,000/well
Transcript-specific probe length (nucleotides)	25	50–120		50
Sample total RNA requirement	3–5 µg			50–100 ng
Fluorescent probe	Phycoerythrin	Cy3 and Cy5	Cy3 and Cy5	Cy3
Reference	Rouse and Hardiman (2003)	Lausted et al. (2006) and Heller (2002)	Dufva (2005)	Kuhn et al. (2004) and Gunderson et al. (2004)

technologies is in the design of the transcript-specific probes themselves. Affymetrix uses relatively short (25 nucleotides) gene-specific probes that bind to labeled complementary RNA (cRNA), which have been thermally fragmented to lengths of 50 to 120 nucleotides. Spotted microarrays and bead arrays use longer gene-specific probes (50 to 120 nucleotides) that bind to full-length complementary deoxyribonucleic acid (cDNA), which may be kilobases long. The Illumina bead microarray uses 50-nucleotide probes in pairs that bind to short regions of cDNA and are consumed in a ligation step prior to polymerase chain reaction (PCR) amplification. In each case, the probe design for each gene must discriminate the target mRNA from all other sequences at the same hybridization temperature. As the probe length increases, the sensitivity of detection increases due to the greater free energy of hybridization of longer sequences. For example, a 60-nucleotide oligomer detects at 8 times greater sensitivity than a 25-nucleotide oligomer (Chou et al., 2004; Kreil et al., 2006). At short (25-nt) oligonucleotide probe lengths, a single nucleotide mismatch suppresses hybridization more effectively than with longer (>60-nt) probe lengths. Depending upon one's point of view, this characteristic makes longer probes either more "forgiving" of single nucleotide polymorphisms or less "specific" in distinguishing closely related genes. The Affymetrix solution has been to capitalize on the high density of their array by synthesizing 11 perfectly matched and 11 mismatched probes for every gene on the array. The gene expression signal is derived as a composite value of the perfect match probe signals, either with or without subtraction of the mismatched probe signals. The choice of probe sets that are combined to estimate the expression of a single gene is the major variable in the "calibration" of gene expression using the Affymetrix platform (Harrison et al., 2007).

Longer oligonucleotide probe formats usually incorporate one or a few probes per gene, which may be replicated in several spots on the microarray. Variation in signal may result from manufacturing processes causing the amount of oligonucleotide synthesized or spotted on the array to vary within or between arrays, and the shape and intensity of signal may vary within a single probe spot. Methods for averaging out individual probe spot intensities and evaluating exclusion criteria for individual spots have been reported (Glasbey and Ghazal, 2003). Recommendations for ensuring quality manufacture of spotted microarrays have been published but will not generally be a direct concern for the toxicologist (George, 2006). However, the design of studies using two-color microarrays requires the toxicologist to choose between common reference, loop, and balanced incomplete block replicate designs (Karakach and Wentzell, 2007). In the common reference design, one RNA sample is hybridized in one color channel for all analyses and the other color channel is used for each sample (Schena et al., 1995). This method is easy to understand and execute. In the loop design, samples are hybridized in pairs following a sequence where each sample is hybridized once to the previous sample in sequence and once to the next sample in sequence (Kerr and Churchill, 2001). The advantage of the loop design is efficiency in that each sample is hybridized twice, once in each channel color, using the same number of microarrays as in the common reference design. This results in higher precision in the data collected due to replication but requires more complex analysis to deconvolute the gene expression data (Vinciotti et al., 2005). The reader is referred to the in-depth reviews of microarray experimental design by Yang and Speed (2002) and Churchill (2002) for further discussion.

The reliability of any microarray data is dependent upon the quality of the probe sequences designed into the array. Probes are uniquely designed by each manufacturer, should not cross-hybridize with conserved sequences between genes, and are species specific. Initial recommendations for microarray transcriptional profiling called for confirmation of interesting signals by reverse transcriptase (RT)-PCR because of the potential for interference between transcripts and the greater dynamic range of quantitation with RT-PCR (Tan et al., 2003; but see a critical analysis of the same data in Shi et al., 2005a). Experience with microarrays over the past several years has generally found good concordance between microarrays and RT-PCR. For instance, many genes of particular toxicologic importance, such as cytochrome P450 expression, have already been validated by RT-PCR assays in several publications for specific platforms (Takahashi et al., 2005).

5.3. ANALYSIS OF MICROARRAY DATA

The ideal microarray platform would report the copy number of each transcript in the sample with a high degree of accuracy over several orders of magnitude. Technology continues to make steps toward this ideal, although routine calibration of microarray data in terms of absolute transcript copy number is currently not attempted (Dudley et al., 2002). Even if it were, the total amount of RNA used as the sample is usually not related back to cell number, so transcript abundance remains relative to the expression of all transcripts in the sample. The use of external RNA controls for quality control of microarray data has been the focus of the MicroArray Quality Control consortium (Shi et al., 2006; Tong et al., 2006). In practice, raw microarray data are fluorescence intensities reported in arbitrary units that have no reference to absolute quantities. Analysis consists of first determining whether a signal is present or absent, taking into account detector noise. Then fluorescence intensities are compared for each gene between samples. Because a ratio cannot be calculated if the reference sample does not express the gene, a number of data transformations have been employed by manufacturers and authors to calculate a normalized measure of gene expression intensity for this purpose.

5.3.1. Normalization and Filtering

The purpose of normalization, also called scaling, of microarray data is to eliminate the effects of systematic bias introduced by variations at any level in the experimental conditions to facilitate between-sample comparisons (Fan and Niu, 2007). Examples of bias in a single chip can include regional variation of intensities across a chip or slide array, background intensities, and saturation of fluorescence at higher signal levels. In two-color platforms, three simple methods of normalization for dye intensity effects are (1) normalizing each spot intensity by the total integrated spot intensities for the entire array (Kroll and Wolfl, 2002), (2) building a linear regression curve relating intensity in one channel versus the other (requiring hybridization of an identical sample in both channels), and (3) integrating the spot intensities of a select group of "housekeeping" genes, on each array and each channel, which are not supposed to change with treatment (Hegde et al., 2000). More sophisticated methods have been advanced, resulting in a wide number of described statistical normalization methods. Several of these normalization models have been applied to single-channel microarrays as well. Multiple statistical reports have attempted to assess the comparative value of these normalization methods, but the complexity and controversy regarding normalization of microarray data is an indication of the need for collaboration with biostatisticians in the design and analysis of microarray experiments (Fan and Niu, 2007; Barash et al., 2004; Liu et al., 2006; Seo and Hoffman, 2006; Khondoker et al., 2007; Quackenbush, 2002).

Filtering of microarray data is intended to remove uninformative data points from the microarray data set, such as genes where expression is absent in all treatment groups and spots with unusual shape or poor edge definition (Karakach and Wentzell, 2007; Brown et al., 2001). Removal of these data points before statistical testing for difference between treatment groups eliminates the chance that they will be incorrectly flagged as different when they really are not (Calza et al., 2007). Intensity filtering eliminates data points whose intensity is below an arbitrary threshold and is simple and widely used (Quackenbush, 2002). The lack of correlation between replicate spot intensities within a single microarray can also be used as exclusion criteria (Kadota et al., 2001).

5.3.2. Analyzing for Differences between Experimental Samples

The purpose of toxicogenomics is to predict a toxic effect or elucidate a mechanism of toxicity. Once microarrays have been evaluated to determine the transcript abundance for each sample, it is necessary to compare between samples to determine which transcripts are up-regulated, down-regulated, or not regulated by treatment. The list of regulated genes, along with their relative change, becomes the expression profile, a kind of fingerprint, of a compound at a particular dose in a particular tissue. Logarithmic transformation of nonzero values is commonly performed to facilitate ratio calculations, to compress dynamic range, and to simplify error estimation (Karakach and Wentzell, 2007). Then, either pairwise comparison tests between treatment and control are made for each gene or genes are ranked by the magnitude of change from control. Statistical testing of pairwise comparisons typically uses Student's t test, although calculation of the variance can be problematic. Tusher and colleagues (2001) reported modification of the calculation of the variance in their t test, which they called statistical analysis of microarrays, and a number of other approaches have been designed (Jeffery et al., 2006). Genes for a particular treatment group are ranked by magnitude of change from the control group or by pairwise test statistical p values, from greatest change to least change. Then, a threshold is set to designate those genes that are considered differentially expressed within a defined level of confidence.

5.3.3. Familywise Error Rate

Because 10,000 or more genes may be represented on a microarray, the chances of incorrect classification of at least one gene, termed the *familywise error rate*, is multiplied. In small studies analyzing a single gene, the type I error rate (the rate of false positives, designated α) is usually set to $p = 0.05$, meaning that 95% of positive tests should be due to real differences in the sampled population means. The large number of tests in microarray experiments can result in a substantial number of false positives. The *false discovery proportion* is the number of false positives divided by the number of positive test results, but this cannot be calculated when the number of true positives versus false positives is unknown. Instead, a *false discovery rate*, which is an estimate of the false discovery proportion, is typically used for microarray studies. If a microarray experiment testing 10,000 genes has 200 apparently differentially expressed genes (positive test results), then we would expect that 5%, or about 10 in this example, of these genes are incorrectly classified. The familywise error rate, or the probability of at least one incorrectly classified gene, would be essentially 100%.

The simplest statistical method to control the false discovery rate is the Bonferroni correction. The Bonferroni correction reduces the type I error rate by dividing by the number of tests, so our $p = 0.05$ for one test becomes $p = 0.000005$ for each of 10,000 tests. The Bonferroni is overly conservative and would often result in no statistically significant findings in experiments where changes in gene expression are clearly evident. Therefore, a number of statistically sound corrections to control the familywise error rate have been described (Farcomeni, 2007); however, a consensus on best statistical practices for microarray analysis remains elusive.

5.3.4. Resampling

Analysis of microarray data is complicated by typically low sample sizes (perhaps as low as three samples per treatment group), which may not match a calculable statistical distribution, such as the normal distribution. Estimating a 95% confidence interval for a descriptive statistic, such as the mean or median, becomes a problem. Resampling is a statistical approach commonly used in microarray analysis to determine the standard error and/or confidence intervals of a descriptive statistic of the sample (Hesterberg et al., 2006). Bootstrap resampling involves recalculation of the descriptive statistic (it could be the mean, median, or any other derivative of the sample data) using a random sample drawn from the original sample data, maintaining their treatment group identities. Bootstrap resampling is done with replacement, meaning that the original data can be selected multiple times during resampling, and the group of resampled numbers may be any size. Permutation resampling is a different approach, where the individual data from different treatment groups are mixed together and randomly resampled (without replacement) into two new groups. The difference in means between these two new groups should be zero, on average. A plot of the difference in means calculated over many repetitions forms an exact distribution curve of the resampled data, from which 95% boundaries can be defined. If the difference in mean values between the original treated and control group lies outside of this 95% confidence interval, then the sampled populations are considered significantly different. In either case of resampling, an empirical, nonmathematical estimate of the distribution of a sample statistic is obtained that allows boundaries to be set, outside of which the null hypothesis can be rejected with a known degree of certainty.

5.3.5. Expression Profile Analysis

The list of differentially expressed genes, along with the direction and magnitude of their change, constitutes the gene expression profile induced for a compound at a particular dose. In toxicogenomics, expression profiles form the basis for further analysis. Mechanisms of toxicity can be investigated by grouping altered genes according to functional annotations found in databases. The test compound can be clustered according to its similarity with reference compounds that have known toxicological characteristics and whose profiles have been stored in reference databases. Finally, sophisticated evaluation algorithms can be trained, by weighting the up- or down-regulation of particular genes, to classify a particular gene expression profile. Biological data is accumulating at an ever increasing pace, including sequencing of whole genomes, characterization of protein–protein interactions, and biochemical or structural functions of individual proteins. Gene expression profiles may be linked back to these databases to reveal a dizzying amount of information that rapidly becomes overwhelming for an individual to evaluate. Therefore, microarray annotations include general classifications of gene function, such as transporters, transcription factors, signal transduction pathways, cell cycle proteins, and the like. When a compound is known to exert a toxic effect, the presence of numerous changes in gene expression within certain pathways can direct the investigation. For example, Andrew and colleagues (2003) reported effects of low and high doses of sodium nitrite in cell culture, finding that stress–response genes were activated at the high dose but not lower doses. Such findings are consistent with toxicological experience where a threshold of exposure is associated with a change in cellular responses leading to toxicity.

5.3.6. Pathway Analysis

In some cases, such as the expression of transporters or drug metabolizing enzymes, the impact of altered gene expression has a clear interpretation on the effect of drug treatment and the potential for toxicity. However, the effect of up- or down-regulation of most transcripts does not directly indicate toxicity, and instead inductive reasoning generally predicts that the more genes modified in a pathway, or the more markedly the expression of those genes is modified, the more likely a chemical entity mediates toxicity through that pathway (Foster et al., 2007). Visualization of these pathways can help show the hierarchy of the altered gene expression by organizing the data into simple branched linear diagrams based on known protein interactions (Bell and Lewitter, 2006). Public and commercial databases are continually updated with protein–protein interaction information derived from a variety of sources so that these pathways may be reconstructed, including all key proteins (Yue and Reisdorf, 2005). A number of software programs draw these pathways in legible form and incorporate gene expression data simultaneously. It is not always apparent whether up- or down-regulation of genes in a particular pathway are adaptive or toxic changes, but experience coupled with more definitive evaluation of cell function can further address these questions.

5.3.7. Gene Expression Databases

Generation of gene expression profile databases from compounds known to be toxic or nontoxic provides a reference for mechanistic association of new entities with well-understood compounds. A great number of variables impact every toxicological study, such as species, strain, age, sex, dose, duration, and route. Gene expression has even been reported to vary by liver lobe (Irwin et al., 2005). Meaningful use of such databases has required the collection of details of study design and methods of data analysis. Standardization of database structure to include information critical for interpretation and comparison of genomic data is not unique to toxicology. The European Bioinformatics Institute developed the Minimum Information about a Microarray Experiment (MIAME) standard to guide the formation of such databases (Brazma et al., 2001). Public genomic data repositories exist in Europe, North America, and Japan that contain datasets linked from published articles. Specialized databases have been developed by the European Bioinformatics Institute, the U.S. National Institutes of Health, and the U.S. Food and Drug Administration to store toxicogenomics information relevant to ecotoxicology and pharmaceutical development. In addition, commercial toxicogenomics databases containing extensive related histopathological, clinical pathological, and methodological information have been developed that facilitate cluster analysis and genomics comparisons to reference compounds with toxic or nontoxic effects of known mechanism. One example is the DrugMatrix database from Iconix Pharmaceuticals (Mountain View, CA), which contains data from over 600 different compounds (Ganter et al., 2005).

5.3.8. Analyzing Relatedness of Gene Expression Profiles

Cluster Analysis. Cluster analysis is a method to evaluate similarity between samples with multiple variables. Clustering can either be supervised or unsupervised. In unsupervised clustering, gene expression is the only factor used to associate samples. Clustering can either organize microarray data in a hierarchical format, comprised of a treelike dendrogram, or it can divide the data into an arbitrary number of groups without ranking members within the group. In either case, each sample, with its multiple gene expression values, is considered a multidimensional vector. Vectors are compared pairwise, by some measure of their similarity (such as the Pearson correlation, Spearman rank correlation, or mathematical distance between vectors) and then associated according to similarity (Gollub and Sherlock, 2006). Pairwise comparisons between a vector and a group of vectors may use the group average, the most or least similar vector from the group, and the like in order to represent the group. When data are partitioned into groups using unsupervised methods such as self-organizing maps or k-means clustering, the number of groups or shape of the relationship map must be specified at the start of the algorithm. The groups are seeded either randomly, or according to principal component determination, and then vectors are swapped between groups based on iterative measurements of group homogeneity or another measure of model fit. An overall fit parameter of the model is typically asymptotic when plotted against the number of groups in the model. Therefore, determination of the model's fit across a number of grouping schemes can be performed to find the optimal grouping scheme.

Cluster analysis, in combination with data in genomics databases, can be used to group the new chemical entity's gene expression profile with those of well-defined toxicants and nontoxic compounds. This approach can be used to investigate the mechanism of toxicity. For example, if a test compound has a gene expression profile that clusters with those of activators of the aryl hydrocarbon nuclear receptor, it is logical to hypothesize that the aryl hydrocarbon nuclear receptor pathway is involved in the toxic mechanism of the test compound. In this regard, microarray data are powerful survey tools for generating hypotheses regarding mechanisms of toxicity that can be pursued in follow-up studies. Figure 5.2 illustrates how cluster analysis is able to distinguish hepatotoxicants from nontoxic compounds based on gene expression profiles.

Dimension Reduction. Two mathematical transformations can simplify microarray data into fewer dimensions: principal component analysis (PCA) and wavelet analysis (Duda et al., 2001a; Lio, 2003). PCA is essentially a least-squares fit line drawn in n-dimensional space, where n is the number of genes in the array. PCA can be extended to any number of additional principal components, each of which is the best least-squares fit line for the data distance to the previous principal component lines. The value of PCA is that data can be visualized and grouped based on the differences in gene expression that account for the majority of the differences between samples. An exact description of the microarray data would require as many principal component dimensions as genes on the array; however, using a few (usually less than 10) principal components, the data are accurately described and data noise is reduced. Figure 5.3 illustrates PCA per-

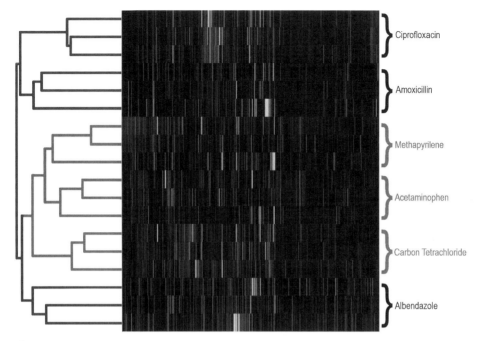

Ciprofloxacin

Amoxicillin

Methapyrilene

Acetaminophen

Carbon Tetrachloride

Albendazole

Figure 5.2. Cluster analysis. Rats in groups of three were treated with three hepatotoxins (methapyrilene 100 mg/kg, acetaminophen 972 mg/kg, carbon tetrachloride 400 mg/kg) and three nonhepatotoxic compounds (ciprofloxacin 72 mg/kg, amoxicillin 1100 mg/kg, albendazole 62 mg/kg) for 5 days except that carbon tetrachloride was a 7-day treatment. The figure shows a heat map of gene expression (red increased, green decreased expression) with the clustering hierarchy of compounds to the left. Gene expression for individual compounds clearly cluster together, and hepatotoxicants form a single cluster within the hierarchy (red). See insert for color representation of this figure.

formed on gene expression profiles of rat liver after exposure to five compounds. Wavelet analysis, which is mathematically similar to Fourier transforms and JPEG compression, similarly fits a function to the data by shifting and stretching the function for a best fit in multiple data dimensions. Wavelets are more complex functions than PCA, and therefore the fit is more precise. As in PCA, where the first component explains most of the variation in the data, a series of wavelets is produced where subsequent wavelets provide additional levels of detail. The reduction of gene expression profiles classified by treatment or toxicity into a few wavelet parameters can extract the most useful information, reduce the level of noise in the data, and facilitate clustering of compounds. Unfortunately, while both wavelet and PCA reduce the dimensions of data to something more manageable, the biological meaning of each component (calculated by mutliplying each genes expression value by a weighting constant

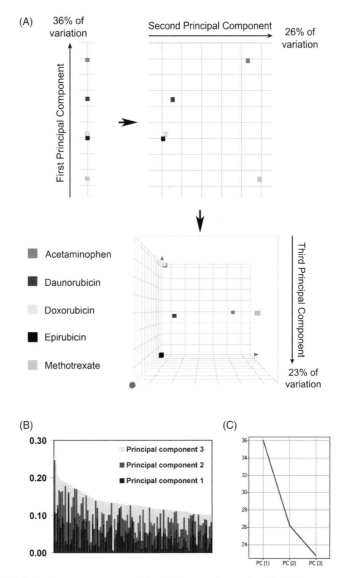

Figure 5.3. Principal component analysis. Rats were treated with five compounds at toxic doses for 5 days and microarray analysis on RNA isolated from liver was performed. (A) The first principal component (top left) represents 36% of all variation between the sample profiles and separates methotrexate and acetaminophen by the greatest difference. The second principal component (top right) represents 26% of all variation and distinguishes daunorubicin, doxorubicin, and epirubicin profiles from other gene profiles. The third principal component (bottom) represents 23% of all variation and separates the profiles of doxorubicin and epirubicin. (B) The relative weighting for each principal component for the top most weighted 100 genes out of a total of 2289. Note that individual genes may contribute to all three principal components. (C) Graph showing the relative contribution of each principal component to the total variation in the data set. The first three principal components describe 85% of the variation in the data set. See insert for color representation of this figure.

for that gene and component) is difficult to decipher from the individual weights of the genes.

Supervised Analysis. Whereas unsupervised analysis of microarray data groups compounds based on the entire gene expression profile (profile → groups), supervised analysis of microarray data is useful for starting with experimentally defined groups of gene expression profiles and then determining which members of the expression profile distinguish the groups (groups → profile). These approaches are all distinguished by requiring training data sets for each classification before they analyze and classify new data. A number of approaches exist for finding the criteria that best discriminate two sets of microarray data, which could, for example, be liver gene expression after exposure to toxic and nontoxic substances. Logistic regression calculates the logarithm of the odds ratio (e.g., the proportion of toxic outcomes, given a particular level of gene expression) and derives a best-fit equation for predicting outcomes based on the data. Linear discriminant analysis is similar to PCA except that instead of a least-squares fit of the data, a boundary vector is fit that minimizes some measure of misclassification (Duda et al., 2001a). These approaches tend to work best where a large number of samples are available to fit the model (Bushel et al., 2002). Naive Bayesian classification quite simply figures the probability of a particular classification by multiplying the separate probabilities of the class for each bit of gene data in the data set. While it theoretically requires independence of the expression data for each gene, which we know is not really the case, it is a robust classifier and relatively straightforward to apply (Thomas, 2001). Artificial neural networks are similar to multiple layers of logistic regression, with parameters produced from one logistic regression feeding into the next layer (Bishop, 1995). Iterations of fitting the model are performed using the training set; thereafter, the neural network can be used to calculate a classifier for a particular set of gene expression data. Figure 5.4 illustrates the concept of training, testing, and using machine learning algorithms in toxicogenomics. Finally, support vector machines are an interesting, relatively new method where the dimensionality of the data is actually *increased* prior to defining boundaries between supervised groups (Duda et al., 2001b). Once these boundaries are found, the algorithm attempts to maximize the distances from the boundary to nearest group members, which are termed the support vectors. Determining which vectors are the support vectors is computationally intensive, but the increased data dimensionality prior to setting boundaries can allow groups to be separated that would otherwise overlap. Supervised array analysis allows training of an analysis model using microarray data collected from compounds with a known classification scheme, such as hepatotoxicity. Once trained, new data can be analyzed and the classification is predicted by the model. In order to determine the confidence in the model's operation, it is necessary to test or validate the trained model with additional classified data. Typically, a large classified training data set is randomly split into training and validation groups and the model is trained and then tested over multiple iterations (Simon, 2003). The performance of the model is then reported in terms

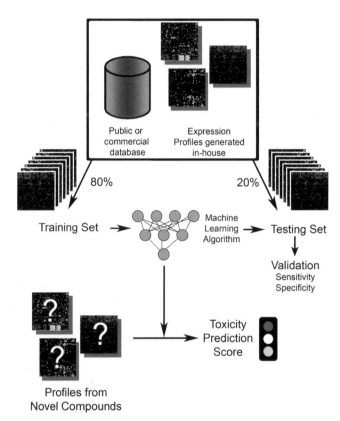

Figure 5.4. Signature generation and testing. Gene expression profiles from compounds of known toxicity are used from databases or are generated in the laboratory. These profiles are randomly divided into a training set and a testing set (here shown divided as an 80/20 split). The neural network or other machine learning algorithm is first trained to profiles classified as toxic or nontoxic. The testing set is used to determine the accuracy of the trained algorithm. Gene expression profiles from new compounds of unknown toxicity are evaluated by the trained algorithm to predict their toxicity.

of the average and variance observed in its positive and negative prediction accuracy. One potential problem, which is particularly evident with neural networks, is overfitting of the model. This is akin to a student memorizing old test answers without understanding the content of the questions and answers. When new gene expression patterns are analyzed by the trained model, they may be misclassified at a high rate, just as a test with entirely new questions will flunk the student. Models with fewer parameters tend to detect more general indicators of toxicity and perform better when compounds of a different class are introduced. This also underlies the importance of training predictive algorithms with gene expression profiles from compound collections that vary as much as the new compounds to be classified. In general, support vector machines and artificial neural networks are more useful in complicated systems that may involve multiple mechanisms that cause toxicity (like a general hepatotoxicity score), as compared to a simpler classification scheme, for example, the presence or absence of oxidative stress.

5.4. APPLICATION OF TOXICOGENOMICS IN DRUG DEVELOPMENT

Toxicogenomics can be usefully applied at multiple steps in drug discovery and development. The earliest opportunity is in discovery, where toxicological evaluation of inhibition or stimulation of a potential therapeutic target can be evaluated for on-target toxicity. The ability to prioritize targets according to toxicity would theoretically increase chances for successful development of a marketable drug. Gram quantities of a tool compound for the purpose of evaluating on-target toxicologic effects could be used in rat dosing studies to evaluate target tissue gene expression. Application of toxicogenomics to this stage of discovery is not well reported in the literature and is complicated by the difficulty in differentiating on-target gene expression changes that are therapeutic from those that are indicative of toxicity. Toxicogenomics must be applied with care not to prematurely discontinue research on promising new targets since targets for drug development are finite.

5.4.1. Discovery

Toxicogenomics has been widely implemented in discovery during the lead identification and optimization stages, where multiple compounds are evaluated for potency, pharmacokinetics, and safety. Since in vivo drug exposure for 3 to 7 days results in reproducible changes in gene expression, short-term studies using gram quantities of drug in small in vivo rat studies can be performed to evaluate toxicity of multiple compounds before scaling up of synthesis and investment in more expensive good laboratory practices (GLP) safety studies (Ganter et al., 2005). The strength of in vivo toxicogenomics is detection of gene expression changes that predict toxicity which only manifests after longer treatment or treatment at higher doses (Fielden et al., 2005). Predictive algorithms, such as those discussed above, are effectively employed at this stage in the drug development pipeline when study design is comparable between new compounds and reference compounds. Typically, doses in these short-term studies are many multiples of the expected therapeutic drug exposure to enhance the sensitivity of early detection, although development of toxicity may be nonlinear according to drug exposure. Histopathology, clinical pathology, organ weights, and in-life observations (clinical signs, food consumption, body weight) remain by far the most economical methods for evaluating toxicity in short-term studies. However, toxicogenomics is useful when findings by these standard methods are inconclusive or no indication of toxicity is found. Toxicogenomics data is usually only collected on a few tissues (e.g., liver, heart, kidney), balancing expense against the likelihood of development of toxicity for those cases where no target tissue is identified by histopathology or clinical pathology.

5.4.2. Safety Testing

Preclinical or clinical testing may reveal toxic changes that were not detected in short-term preclinical studies. At this stage of the pipeline, investment has expanded to include at least preclinical GLP safety studies. Toxicogenomics can be useful to rescue a particular program by investigating potential mechanisms of toxicity, followed by determination of the relevance of these mechanisms for human toxicity and the development of assays to identify backup compounds that do not have these toxic liabilities. Reasons why short-term studies in rats fail to identify toxic effects at this stage of development are often related to the duration of exposure, the tissue in which the toxicity developed, and the difference in species (dog, monkey, or human) being evaluated. This also provides the company with an important opportunity to learn of new toxic mechanisms that may be incorporated into earlier stages of toxicology testing. Most compounds exert a toxic effect given a sufficiently high exposure. Lead compounds and drug candidates, which have a narrow therapeutic window, typically require monitoring for toxicity as a prerequisite for human trials. In some cases, toxicity may be monitored by well-established biomarkers such as clinical pathology; however, in those cases where toxicity monitoring is not possible by noninvasive techniques, toxicogenomics might represent a solution. Gene expression in peripheral blood, typically in the peripheral blood mononuclear cell (PBMC) fraction, has been shown to be highly sensitive and responsive in a number of disease states (Rockett et al., 2004). PBMCs have the potential to serve as sentinels of toxicity even though they only circulate through toxicologically relevant tissues because they are a readily available sample for transcriptional profiling. Development of PBMCs as a valid indicator of toxicity in humans will require preclinical studies to establish the correlation, sensitivity, and specificity of expression profiles in preclinical species coupled with the invasive methods that expression profiling will replace. Such monitoring might be feasible in particular circumstances during early dose escalation studies where safety and tolerability are being determined in human volunteers but would probably not be economical in larger phase II or III studies.

5.4.3. Idiosyncratic Toxicity

Finally, while preclinical safety testing is quite effective at protecting humans from unsafe compounds (Olson et al., 2000), a small proportion of drugs are found to exert toxic effects by poorly understood mechanisms that occur in a small minority of patients. These idiosyncratic reactions in the clinic are typically non-dose-dependent and can lead to human suffering and fatalities and costly failures for drug companies. Toxicogenomics offers hope of understanding the mechanism(s) of these reactions by detecting gene expression changes that occur uniquely with drugs having idiosyncratic effects. This is particularly the case where drugs having similar therapeutic targets have dissimilar susceptibility to idiosyncratic reactions. One potential mechanism of an idiosyncratic drug reaction is free radical injury, which occurs when the liver is preconditioned by exposure to increased levels of bacterial lipopolysaccharides (LPS) (Liguori et al., 2007). In these cases, a clear difference in gene expression has been reported for compounds that have a clinical history of idiosyncratic drug reactions (Waring et al., 2006). While toxicogenomics may help explain the mechanisms of toxicity for some of these idiosyncratic reactions, it is hoped that identification of gene expression profiles predicting these human toxicities in preclinical species will avoid human injury and market withdrawal before clinical trials have begun.

5.5. CONSIDERATIONS FOR TOXICOGENOMIC STUDY DESIGN

5.5.1. In Vitro Studies

In lead optimization, a number of chemically similar compounds are synthesized in small amounts, and their characteristics are evaluated to select the most promising compound for scaled-up synthesis and in vivo testing. The quantities of compound available may be less than the 1 to 2 grams required to run a short-term (e.g., 5-day) rat study to provide an early indication of toxicity problems. Cell culture experiments can often be used to answer specific questions regarding the effect of the compound on xenobiotic response pathways, such as cytochrome P450 induction and nuclear receptor activation (Thum and Borlak, 2007). Gene expression profiling of cell cultures exposed to reference toxicants, such as carbon tetrachloride, ethanol, and acetaminophen, successfully distinguished the mechanisms of toxicity (deLongueville et al., 2003; Harries et al., 2001). Cell culture gene expression profiling has also successfully identified gene sets that predict the presence of particular toxic liabilities, such as DNA damage-mediated genotoxicity or peroxisome proliferation (Fielden et al., 2007; Yang et al., 2006). In the future, it might be possible to use gene expression analysis of cultured cells to routinely predict specific toxic endpoints.

Dose. Gene expression profiling of cultured cells or tissues has a number of obvious advantages: lower compound requirements, decreased use of animals, rapid generation of data, reproducible testing conditions, and the ability to use cells and tissues from preclinical species and humans. One principal limitation of cell culture techniques is the relevance of the drug exposure level to plasma or tissue levels in the living animal (Blaauboer, 2001). Toxicity is always defined by dose, and the delivery of a compound to a tissue depends on protein binding, hydrophobicity, active and passive transport, metabolism, and the like. Typically, the test compound is added directly to the cell culture medium at a known concentration and allowed to incubate with the cells for a defined period of time. The distribution of the test compound into the target tissue and the plasma/target tissue concentration ratio are often not known during lead optimization and are difficult to predict, further obscuring the relevant concentrations for drug exposure in culture experiments. Because primary cells and tissue preparations cannot be maintained indefinitely in culture (Farkas and Tannenbaum, 2005), test compound concentrations are sometimes increased to compensate for shorter exposure times. Genomic analysis over a range of doses for a particular compound might theoretically reveal a threshold in vitro dose for generating a toxic signature; however, the relation of such a threshold to plasma levels would remain uncertain.

Development of Focused Assays. As currently implemented, in vitro toxicogenomics is not reliable for the quantitative estimation of safety margins but is more often used to hypothesize potential mechanisms of toxicity and to cluster new compounds with prototypical toxicants. Subsequent development of focused microarrays, or multiplexed RT-PCR assays, could then be used to screen many compounds across several doses for activation of these signature genes at lower cost than running complete genomics analysis. Because cell culture assays require much less compound, toxicity evaluation can be implemented along with potency, selectivity, and bioavailability during the selection of lead compounds.

Cell Culture Systems. The choice of culture and assay method is influenced by the ease of performing the assay and the consistency in results. When compared against gene expression from whole liver, for example, remarkable differences are seen between slice cultures, primary hepatocyte cultures, and cell lines (Jessen et al., 2003; Boess et al., 2003; Olsavsky et al., 2007). The effects of the culture conditions on expression of inducible genes of toxicological significance also may impact the ability to detect important effects of the test compound. Because of these differences, only a portion of the gene expression changes identified in tissues from whole-animal dosing may actually have meaning in cell culture systems. An empirical approach to this problem is to dose the culture system with a variety of toxicants to derive new signatures of toxicity; however, this requires a substantial investment and rigid adherence to the method. In the case of organ slices and primary cell cultures, donor peculiarities may affect the results as they would in whole-animal studies (Olsavsky et al., 2007). Because of the many uncertainties in the design of relevant in vitro toxicogenomics studies, it has been easier to establish data sets from whole-animal studies.

5.5.2. In Vivo Studies

Group Size. Toxicogenomics analysis of tissues from animal studies has the advantages of determination of plasma and tissue drug levels, correlative classical toxicological assessment such as clinical pathology and histopathology, and available reference databases. However, large group sizes become costly to establish. Early reports on group size analysis often cited a group size requirement of 10 to 14 to obtain false detection rates controlled below 0.05. Jeffery and colleagues (2006) found that the quality of the signatures derived from sample sets of 5 and 10 replicates was somewhat reduced in the smaller sample set. Page and colleagues (2006) reported a method to estimate the probability of true negatives, true positives, and the average power across all genes in the microarray, which they termed the expected discovery rate. Their methods showed that, for one example dataset, the probability of a positive being a true positive was approximately 80% for $p < 0.05$ and a sample size of just 3. Furthermore, the method can use a laboratory's own microarray data to customize the estimation of power for a microarray experiment. Alternatively, Seo and Hoffman (2006) presented a method to subselect only those probe sets from a microarray that demonstrate adequate statistical power based on specified parameters. They demonstrated that within rat microarray experiments using only three replicates, between 50 and 90% of probe sets were adequately powered depending upon the statistical test performed. Thus, recent statistical reports have shown that even small group sizes can produce a large amount of useful information, and new methods to select only adequately powered probe sets may improve subsequent analysis.

Tissue Heterogeneity. Experiments utilizing tissues derived from compound-treated animals must also consider tissue heterogeneity when samples are collected. Liver is relatively exceptional in its structural homogeneity, whereas differences in gene expression would be expected in kidney, depending upon sampling from the cortex or medulla. Genomics studies of tumors containing a mixture of neoplastic and nonneoplastic tissue have clearly shown the value of microdissection techniques, including laser capture microdissection (Fuller et al., 2003). The ability of RNA amplification methods to provide sufficient material for microarray analysis from such small samples promises a better understanding of mechanisms of toxicity by removing the contribution of irrelevant cells to the gene expression data (Viale et al., 2007). In our experience, even gross dissection methods such as scraping the small intestinal mucosa away from the muscular tunics has resulted in less variable and more useful gene expression data.

The majority of pharmaceutical development is for eventual use in humans. Olson and colleagues (2000) found that together, the rat, dog and nonhuman primate predicted most human drug-related toxicities and validated these preclinical species for drug safety testing. However, a number of toxicities found in preclinical species, particularly the rat, are not observed in humans. For example, fibrates induce liver tumors in rats but not humans due to the differences in the response of peroxisome proliferator-activated receptor-α (PPAα) (Hays et al., 2005). Improvement of toxicology testing models, such as using human tissue in culture or genetically modified animals with humanized genes of toxicological significance, will hopefully allow findings in models to be more easily translated into risk for human toxicity.

Toxicogenomics may also be employed in the investigation of mechanisms of toxicity discovered in preclinical species to evaluate their relevance for humans. For example, cyclosporin nephrotoxicity is observed in rats but not humans. The rat lesion has been associated with regulated calcium binding proteins that are differentially regulated in the presence of cyclosporin compared to humans (Wu et al., 2004). Discovery of mechanisms of toxicity in preclinical species that are not predictive for human toxicity should reduce the number of unnecessarily discontinued promising drug candidates.

5.6. OVERVIEW OF MAJOR REGULATORY DEVELOPMENTS RELATED TO USE OF TOXICOGENOMICS IN DRUG DISCOVERY AND DEVELOPMENT

Toxicogenomics is a technology that has the potential to improve safety assessment. Because of their unique role in developing and enforcing standards for drugs, regulatory agencies can promote the use of novel technologies that can positively impact the toxicological evaluation of experimental medicines. Most current toxicogenomics data are exploratory in nature and usually not at a stage sufficiently mature to be part of the regulatory approval process. This is, however, rapidly evolving and in an effort to promote the use of genomics technologies in drug development and to familiarize regulatory authorities with these emerging technologies, several draft or final guidance or position documents have been issued in the last few years. Here, we provide a brief overview of some documents relevant to toxicogenomics that have been issued by regulatory authorities.

5.6.1. Data Submission

The Food and Drug Administration (FDA) has recognized the potential of pharmacogenomics in general, and toxicogenomics in particular, to maximize the effectiveness and minimize the risk of novel medicines. As a result, it has issued guidance in March 2005 for the regulatory submission of pharmacogenomic data (http://www.fda.gov/cder/guidance/6400fnl.pdf) and has created a Genomics at FDA webportal (http://www.fda.gov/cder/genomics/). This website provides up-to-date regulatory and background information on genomics, and the reader is highly encouraged to regularly visit this resource. The guidance reflects an effort to foster the use of genomic technologies in drug development and is also designed to enhance the agency's knowledge of these emerging technologies.

During preparation of the guidance, the FDA has openly cooperated with the various stakeholders using public consultation and organized appropriate forums to focus on the major issues and principles that the document should cover. Summaries of the outcomes of these various public forums can be found in recent publications (Leighton et al., 2004; Lesko et al., 2003; Salerno and Lesko, 2004a, 2004b; Trepicchio et al., 2004). The guidance clarifies the policy of the agency on the use of pharmacogenomic data in the drug application review process and covers the application of genomic concepts and technologies to nonclinical, clinical pharmacology, and clinical studies. More specifically, it provides guidelines to sponsors on pharmacogenomic data submission requirements, the format and procedure for data submission, and how the data will be used in regulatory decision making. In general terms, genomic data for which formal submission is required include 1. data used for decision making within a specific trial; 2. data used to support scientific arguments about mechanism of action, dose selection, safety, or effectiveness; 3. data that will support registration or labeling language; and 4. data generated on previously validated biomarkers. Useful algorithms are provided as appendices in the guidance to help evaluate whether or not submissions are required for investigational new drug applications (INDs), new drug applications (NDAs), or biologic license applications (BLAs).

5.6.2. Voluntary Genomic Data Submission

An objective of this guidance was also to encourage sponsors to share genomic data in a voluntary process outside the formal regulatory mechanism. The agency acknowledged that most genomic data are exploratory in nature and would therefore not be part of formal regulatory submissions. Because of the perceived growing role of genomic data in drug development, the FDA recognized the need to prepare its staff to future submissions. The voluntary genomic data submission (VGDS) process provides a mechanism by which genomic data can be submitted outside the formal regulatory approval process. VGDSs can be used for any type of genomic data generated and applied at all stages of the drug discovery and development process. They are reviewed by a cross-center Interdisciplinary Pharmacogenomic Review Group (IPRG) that does not include staff involved in an associated formal submission. VGDS data are not distributed outside the IPRG without prior agreement of the sponsor and are not used for regulatory decision making. In general, the VGDS experience appears to be a success for both sponsors and the FDA. VGDS have allowed the FDA to gain access to many genomic data that otherwise would not have been available and have enabled sponsors to learn about the regulatory decision-making process and expectations involving genomics data. A recent summary of the FDA's experience with VGDS can be found elsewhere (Orr et al., 2007).

It is noteworthy that as part of a wider process of collaboration between the FDA and European Medicines Agency (EMEA), joint meetings can now also be held for voluntary submissions. Additional information can be found at the following URL: http://www.fda.gov/cder/genomics/FDAEMEA.pdf.

In August 2007, the FDA released a draft guidance that is intended to be utilized as a companion guidance to the pharmacogenomic guidance (http://www.fda.gov/cder/genomics/conceptpaper_20061107.pdf.). This document is based on the agency's experience with VGDSs as well as with its review of numerous protocols and data submitted under IND, NDA, and BLA applications. The recommendations provided by the guidance are intended to facilitate the use of pharmacogenomic data in drug development. This document provides details regarding a variety of technical and analytical aspects, such as laboratory proficiency testing, methodological issues associated with microarray data, and format for data submission. This guidance is strongly influenced by the work and experience of FDA scientists at the National Center for Toxicological Research (http://www.fda.gov/nctr/). Some of this work has been published elsewhere (Tong et al., 2006; Han et al., 2006; Shi et al., 2004, 2005b).

5.7. SUMMARY

In this chapter, we have provided an overview of the principles and methods of toxicogenomics. Used as a predictive tool, toxicogenomics can impact the productivity of discovery organizations through earlier identification of toxicity. As public and private repository of gene expression profiles are expanding, specific signatures predictive of toxic changes are likely to become available. Ultimately, these novel toxicity biomarkers will need to be validated in prospective, well-controlled studies across multiple institutions. Various efforts have already been initiated in the form of industry consortia. For instance, the Predictive Safety Testing Consortium between the C-Path Institute (www.c-path.org) and several large pharmaceutical companies is a consortium formed to share proprietary markers or laboratory methods to improve the prediction and monitoring of toxicity. When used as a mechanistic tool, toxicogenomics represents an effective approach to rapidly elucidate the mechanism of toxic changes. The objective here is to rapidly generate relevant molecular data that can be used to formulate hypotheses. These hypotheses can then be quickly confirmed or refuted in orthogonal studies. Once mechanisms of toxicity are understood, risks can be better assessed and compounds can be either moved forward or terminated based on more reliable information. Furthermore, this mechanistic information can be used to set up appropriate counterscreens to select back-up compounds unlikely to have similar safety liabilities. Figure 5.5 illustrates the integration of toxicogenomics analysis in an exploratory toxicology testing paradigm. In this chapter, we have focused on a few well-defined applications. It should be understood, however, that toxicogenomics is relevant to many areas of toxicology, such as immunotoxicity, muscle toxicity, or teratology (Foster et al., 2007; Baken et al., 2007, 2008; Kultima et al., 2004). In fact, virtually any aspect of toxicology can be theoretically interrogated at the transcriptomics level. It remains, however, to be seen where the use of gene expression profiling provides enough value to justify its use.

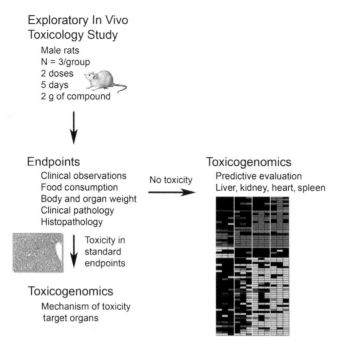

Figure 5.5. Integration of toxicogenomics into an exploratory toxicology program. The small, brief study design minimizes the requirement for compound. Standard toxicological endpoints provide the most economical evaluation of toxicity. In the absence of a toxic signal from standard endpoints, toxicogenomic analysis is performed to predict toxicity after longer duration exposures. Predictive analysis is performed with a trained machine learning algorithm that has already been forward validated. In the presence of a toxic signal from standard endpoints, the toxicogenomic analysis of target tissues is used to generate hypotheses regarding the mechanism of toxicity.

REFERENCES

AbouHaidar, M. G., and Ivanov, I. G. (1999). Non-enzymatic RNA hydrolysis promoted by the combined catalytic activity of buffers and magnesium ions. *Z. Naturforsch. [C]* 54:542–548.

Andrew, A. S., Warren, A. J., Barchowsky, A., Temple, K. A., Klei, L., Soucy, N. V., O'Hara, K. A., and Hamilton, J. W. (2003). Genomic and proteomic profiling of responses to toxic metals in human lung cells. *Environ. Health Perspect.* 111:825–835.

Baken, K. A., Vandebriel, R. J., Pennings, J. L., Kleinjans, J. C., and van Loveren, H. (2007). Toxicogenomics in the assessment of immunotoxicity. *Methods* 41:132–141.

Baken, K. A., Pennings, J. L., Jonker, M. J., Schaap, M. M., de Vries, A., van Steeg, H., Breit, T. M., and van Loveren, H. (2008). Overlapping gene expression profiles of model compounds provide opportunities for immunotoxicity screening. *Toxicol. Appl. Pharmacol.* 226:46–59.

Barash, Y., Dehan, E., Krupsky, M., Franklin, W., Geraci, M., Friedman, N., and Kaminski, N. (2004). Comparative analysis of algorithms for signal quantitation from oligonucleotide microarrays. *Bioinformatics* 20:839–846.

Bell, G. W., and Lewitter, F. (2006). Visualizing networks. *Methods Enzymol.* 411: 408–421.

Bishop, C. M. (1995). *Neural Networks for Pattern Recognition.* New York: Oxford University Press, p. 116.

Blaauboer, B. J. (2001). Toxicodynamic modelling and the interpretation of in vitro toxicity data. *Toxicol. Lett.* 120:111–123.

Boess, F., Kamber, M., Romer, S., Gasser, R., Muller, D., Albertini, S., and Suter, L. (2003). Gene expression in two hepatic cell lines, cultured primary hepatocytes, and liver slices compared to the in vivo liver gene expression in rats: Possible implications for toxicogenomics use of in vitro systems. *Toxicol. Sci.* 73:386–402.

Brazma, A., Hingamp, P., Quackenbush, J., Sherlock, G., Spellman, P., Stoeckert, C., Aach, J., Ansorge, W., Ball, C. A., Causton, H. C., Gaasterland, T., Glenisson, P., Holstege, F. C., Kim, I. F., Markowitz, V., Matese, J. C., Parkinson, H., Robinson, A., Sarkans, U., Schulze-Kremer, S., Stewart, J., Taylor, R., Vilo, J., and Vingron, M. (2001). Minimum information about a microarray experiment (MIAME)-toward standards for microarray data. *Nat. Genet.* 29:365–371.

Brown, C. S., Goodwin, P. C., and Sorger, P. K. (2001). Image metrics in the statistical analysis of DNA microarray data. *Proc. Natl. Acad. Sci. U. S. A.* 98:8944–8949.

Bushel, P. R., Hamadeh, H. K., Bennett, L., Green, J., Ableson, A., Misener, S., Afshari, C. A., and Paules, R. S. (2002). Computational selection of distinct class- and subclass-specific gene expression signatures. *J. Biomed. Inform.* 35:160–170.

Calza, S., Raffelsberger, W., Ploner, A., Sahel, J., Leveillard, T., and Pawitan, Y. (2007). Filtering genes to improve sensitivity in oligonucleotide microarray data analysis. *Nucleic Acids Res.* 35:e102.

Chou, C. C., Chen, C. H., Lee, T. T., and Peck, K. (2004). Optimization of probe length and the number of probes per gene for optimal microarray analysis of gene expression. *Nucleic Acids Res.* 32:e99.

Churchill, G. A. (2002). Fundamentals of experimental design for cDNA microarrays. *Nat. Genet.* 32(Suppl):490–495.

Copois, V., Bibeau, F., Bascoul-Mollevi, C., Salvetat, N., Chalbos, P., Bareil, C., Candeil, L., Fraslon, C., Conseiller, E., Granci, V., Maziere, P., Kramar, A., Ychou, M., Pau, B., Martineau, P., Molina, F., and Del Rio, M. (2007). Impact of RNA degradation on gene expression profiles: Assessment of different methods to reliably determine RNA quality. *J. Biotechnol.* 127:549–559.

de Longueville, F., Atienzar, F. A., Marcq, L., Dufrane, S., Evrard, S., Wouters, L., Leroux, F., Bertholet, V., Gerin, B., Whomsley, R., Arnould, T., Remacle, J., and Canning, M. (2003). Use of a low-density microarray for studying gene expression patterns induced by hepatotoxicants on primary cultures of rat hepatocytes. *Toxicol. Sci.* 75: 378–392.

Duda, R. O., Hart, P. E., and Stork, D. G. (2001a). Maximum-likelihood and Bayesian parameter estimation. In *Pattern Classification*, 2nd ed., Wiley, New York, pp. 84–160.

Duda, R. O., Hart, P. E., and Stork, D. G. (2001b). Linear discriminant functions. In *Pattern Classification*, 2nd ed., Wiley, New York, pp. 215–281.

Dudley, A. M., Aach, J., Steffen, M. A., and Church, G. M. (2002). Measuring absolute expression with microarrays with a calibrated reference sample and an extended signal intensity range. *Proc. Natl. Acad. Sci. U. S. A.* 99:7554–7559.

Dufva, M. (2005). Fabrication of high quality microarrays. *Biomol. Eng.* 22:173–184.

Fan, J., and Niu, Y. (2007). Selection and validation of normalization methods for c-DNA microarrays using within-array replications. *Bioinformatics* 23:2391–2398.

Farcomeni, A. (2008). A review of modern multiple hypothesis testing, with particular attention to the false discovery proportion. *Stat. Methods Med.* 17:347–388.

Farkas, D., and Tannenbaum, S. R. (2005). In vitro methods to study chemically-induced hepatotoxicity: A literature review. *Curr. Drug Metab.* 6:111–125.

Fielden, M. R., Eynon, B. P., Natsoulis, G., Jarnagin, K., Banas, D., and Kolaja, K. L. (2005). A gene expression signature that predicts the future onset of drug-induced renal tubular toxicity. *Toxicol. Pathol.* 33:675–683.

Fielden, M. R., Brennan, R., and Gollub, J. (2007). A gene expression biomarker provides early prediction and mechanistic assessment of hepatic tumor induction by nongenotoxic chemicals. *Toxicol. Sci.* 99:90–100.

Foster, W. R., Chen, S. J., He, A., Truong, A., Bhaskaran, V., Nelson, D. M., Dambach, D. M., Lehman-McKeeman, L. D., and Car, B. D. (2007). A retrospective analysis of toxicogenomics in the safety assessment of drug candidates. *Toxicol. Pathol.* 35:621–635.

Fuller, A. P., Palmer-Toy, D., Erlander, M. G., and Sgroi, D. C. (2003). Laser capture microdissection and advanced molecular analysis of human breast cancer. *J. Mammary Gland Biol. Neoplasia* 8:335–345.

Ganter, B., Tugendreich, S., Pearson, C. I., Ayanoglu, E., Baumhueter, S., Bostian, K. A., Brady, L., Browne, L. J., Calvin, J. T., Day, G. J., Breckenridge, N., Dunlea, S., Eynon, B. P., Furness, L. M., Ferng, J., Fielden, M. R., Fujimoto, S. Y., Gong, L., Hu, C., Idury, R., Judo, M. S., Kolaja, K. L., Lee, M. D., McSorley, C., Minor, J. M., Nair, R. V., Natsoulis, G., Nguyen, P., Nicholson, S. M., Pham, H., Roter, A. H., Sun, D., Tan, S., Thode, S., Tolley, A. M., Vladimirova, A., Yang, J., Zhou, Z., and Jarnagin, K. (2005). Development of a large-scale chemogenomics database to improve drug candidate selection and to understand mechanisms of chemical toxicity and action. *J. Biotechnol.* 119:219–244.

Gay, C. G., Zuerner, R., Bannantine, J. P., Lillehoj, H. S., Zhu, J. J., Green, R., and Pastoret, P. P. (2007). Genomics and vaccine development. *Rev. Sci. Tech.* 26:49–67.

George, R. A. (2006). The printing process: Tips on tips. *Methods Enzymol.* 410:121–135.

Glasbey, C. A., and Ghazal, P. (2003). Combinatorial image analysis of DNA microarray features. *Bioinformatics* 19:194–203.

Gollub, J., and Sherlock, G. (2006). Clustering microarray data. *Methods Enzymol.* 411:194–213.

Gunderson, K. L., Kruglyak, S., Graige, M. S., Garcia, F., Kermani, B. G., Zhao, C., Che, D., Dickinson, T., Wickham, E., Bierle, J., Doucet, D., Milewski, M., Yang, R., Siegmund, C., Haas, J., Zhou, L., Oliphant, A., Fan, J. B., Barnard, S., and Chee, M. S. (2004). Decoding randomly ordered DNA arrays. *Genome Res.* 14:870–877.

Han, T., Melvin, C. D., Shi, L., Branham, W. S., Moland, C. L., Pine, P. S., Thompson, K. L., and Fuscoe, J. C. (2006). Improvement in the reproducibility and accuracy of DNA microarray quantification by optimizing hybridization conditions. *BMC Bioinformatics* 7 (Suppl 2):S17.

Harries, H. M., Fletcher, S. T., Duggan, C. M., and Baker, V. A. (2001). The use of genomics technology to investigate gene expression changes in cultured human liver cells. *Toxicol. In Vitro* 15:399–405.

Harrison, A. P., Johnston, C. E., and Orengo, C. A. (2007). Establishing a major cause of discrepancy in the calibration of Affymetrix GeneChips. *BMC Bioinformatics* 8:195.

Hays, T., Rusyn, I., Burns, A. M., Kennett, M. J., Ward, J. M., Gonzalez, F. J., and Peters, J. M. (2005). Role of peroxisome proliferator-activated receptor-alpha (PPARalpha) in bezafibrate-induced hepatocarcinogenesis and cholestasis. *Carcinogenesis* 26:219–227.

Hegde, P., Qi, R., Abernathy, K., Gay, C., Dharap, S., Gaspard, R., Hughes, J. E., Snesrud, E., Lee, N., and Quackenbush, J. (2000). A concise guide to cDNA microarray analysis. *Biotechniques* 29:548–550, 552–544, 556.

Heller, M. J. (2002). DNA microarray technology: Devices, systems, and applications. *Annu. Rev. Biomed. Eng.* 4:129–153.

Hesterberg, T., Moore, D. S., Monaghan, S., Clipson, A., and Epstein, R. (2006). Bootstrap methods and permutation tests. In *Introduction to the Practice of Statistics*, 5th ed. W H Freeman, New York.

Irwin, R. D., Parker, J. S., Lobenhofer, E. K., Burka, L. T., Blackshear, P. E., Vallant, M. K., Lebetkin, E. H., Gerken, D. F., and Boorman, G. A. (2005). Transcriptional profiling of the left and median liver lobes of male f344/n rats following exposure to acetaminophen. *Toxicol. Pathol.* 33:111–117.

Jeffery, I. B., Higgins, D. G., and Culhane, A. C. (2006). Comparison and evaluation of methods for generating differentially expressed gene lists from microarray data. *BMC Bioinformatics* 7:359.

Jessen, B. A., Mullins, J. S., De Peyster, A., and Stevens, G. J. (2003). Assessment of hepatocytes and liver slices as in vitro test systems to predict in vivo gene expression. *Toxicol. Sci.* 75:208–222.

Kadota, K., Miki, R., Bono, H., Shimizu, K., Okazaki, Y., and Hayashizaki, Y. (2001). Preprocessing implementation for microarray (PRIM): An efficient method for processing cDNA microarray data. *Physiol. Genomics* 4:183–188.

Karakach, T. K., and Wentzell, P. D. (2007). Methods for estimating and mitigating errors in spotted, dual-color DNA microarrays. *Omics* 11:186–199.

Kerr, M. K., and Churchill, G. A. (2001). Experimental design for gene expression microarrays. *Biostatistics* 2:183–201.

Khondoker, M. R., Glasbey, C. A., and Worton, B. J. (2007). A comparison of parametric and nonparametric methods for normalising cDNA microarray data. *Biom. J.* 49:815–823.

Kreil, D. P., Russell, R. R., and Russell, S. (2006). Microarray oligonucleotide probes. *Methods Enzymol.* 410:73–98.

Kroll, T. C., and Wolfl, S. (2002). Ranking: A closer look on globalisation methods for normalisation of gene expression arrays. *Nucleic Acids Res.* 30:e50.

Kuhn, K., Baker, S. C., Chudin, E., Lieu, M. H., Oeser, S., Bennett, H., Rigault, P., Barker, D., McDaniel, T. K., and Chee, M. S. (2004). A novel, high-performance random array platform for quantitative gene expression profiling. *Genome Res.* 14:2347–2356.

Kultima, K., Nystrom, A. M., Scholz, B., Gustafson, A. L., Dencker, L., and Stigson, M. (2004). Valproic acid teratogenicity: A toxicogenomics approach. *Environ. Health Perspect.* 112:1225–1235.

Lausted, C. G., Warren, C. B., Hood, L. E., and Lasky, S. R. (2006). Printing your own inkjet microarrays. *Methods Enzymol.* 410:168–189.

Leighton, J. K., DeGeorge, J., Jacobson-Kram, D., MacGregor, J., Mendrick, D., and Worobec, A. (2004). Pharmacogenomic data submissions to the FDA: Non-clinical case studies. *Pharmacogenomics* 5:507–511.

Lesko, L. J., Salerno, R. A., Spear, B. B., Anderson, D. C., Anderson, T., Brazell, C., Collins, J., Dorner, A., Essayan, D., Gomez-Mancilla, B., Hackett, J., Huang, S. M., Ide, S., Killinger, J., Leighton, J., Mansfield, E., Meyer, R., Ryan, S. G., Schmith, V., Shaw, P., Sistare, F., Watson, M., and Worobec, A. (2003). Pharmacogenetics and pharmacogenomics in drug development and regulatory decision making: Report of the first FDA-PWG-PhRMA-DruSafe Workshop. *J. Clin. Pharmacol.* 43:342–358.

Liguori, M. J., Blomme, E. A., and Waring, J. F. (2007). Trovafloxacin-induced gene expression changes in liver-derived in vitro systems: Comparison of primary human hepatocytes to HepG2 cells. *Drug Metab. Dispos.* 36:223–233.

Lio, P. (2003). Wavelets in bioinformatics and computational biology: State of art and perspectives. *Bioinformatics* 19:2–9.

Liu, W. M., Li, R., Sun, J. Z., Wang, J., Tsai, J., Wen, W., Kohlmann, A., and Williams, P. M. (2006). PQN and DQN: Algorithms for expression microarrays. *J. Theor. Biol.* 243:273–278.

Olsavsky, K. M., Page, J. L., Johnson, M. C., Zarbl, H., Strom, S. C., and Omiecinski, C. J. (2007). Gene expression profiling and differentiation assessment in primary human hepatocyte cultures, established hepatoma cell lines, and human liver tissues. *Toxicol. Appl. Pharmacol.* 222:42–56.

Olson, H., Betton, G., Robinson, D., Thomas, K., Monro, A., Kolaja, G., Lilly, P., Sanders, J., Sipes, G., Bracken, W., Dorato, M., Van Deun, K., Smith, P., Berger, B., and Heller, A. (2000). Concordance of the toxicity of pharmaceuticals in humans and in animals. *Regul. Toxicol. Pharmacol.* 32:56–67.

Orr, M. S., Goodsaid, F., Amur, S., Rudman, A., and Frueh, F. W. (2007). The experience with voluntary genomic data submissions at the FDA and a vision for the future of the voluntary data submission program. *Clin. Pharmacol. Ther.* 81:294–297.

Page, G. P., Edwards, J. W., Gadbury, G. L., Yelisetti, P., Wang, J., Trivedi, P., and Allison, D. B. (2006). The PowerAtlas: A power and sample size atlas for microarray experimental design and research. *BMC Bioinformatics* 7:84.

Peirson, S. N., and Butler, J. N. (2007). RNA extraction from mammalian tissues. *Methods Mol. Biol.* 362:315–327.

Quackenbush, J. (2002). Microarray data normalization and transformation. *Nat. Genet.* 32(Suppl):496–501.

Rockett, J. C., Burczynski, M. E., Fornace, A. J., Herrmann, P. C., Krawetz, S. A., and Dix, D. J. (2004). Surrogate tissue analysis: Monitoring toxicant exposure and health status of inaccessible tissues through the analysis of accessible tissues and cells. *Toxicol. Appl. Pharmacol.* 194:189–199.

Rouse, R., and Hardiman, G. (2003). Microarray technology—an intellectual property retrospective. *Pharmacogenomics* 4:623–632.

Salerno, R. A., and Lesko, L. J. (2004a). Pharmacogenomic data: FDA voluntary and required submission guidance. *Pharmacogenomics* 5:503–505.

Salerno, R. A., and Lesko, L. J. (2004b). Pharmacogenomics in drug development and regulatory decision-making: The genomic data submission (GDS) proposal. *Pharmacogenomics* 5:25–30.

Schena, M., Shalon, D., Davis, R. W., and Brown, P. O. (1995). Quantitative monitoring of gene expression patterns with a complementary DNA microarray. *Science* 270:467–470.

Schroeder, A., Mueller, O., Stocker, S., Salowsky, R., Leiber, M., Gassmann, M., Lightfoot, S., Menzel, W., Granzow, M., and Ragg, T. (2006). The RIN: An RNA integrity number for assigning integrity values to RNA measurements. *BMC Mol. Biol.* 7:3.

Seo, J., and Hoffman, E. P. (2006). Probe set algorithms: Is there a rational best bet? *BMC Bioinformatics* 7:395.

Shi, L., Tong, W., Goodsaid, F., Frueh, F. W., Fang, H., Han, T., Fuscoe, J. C., and Casciano, D. A. (2004). QA/QC: Challenges and pitfalls facing the microarray community and regulatory agencies. *Expert Rev. Mol. Diagn.* 4:761–777.

Shi, L., Tong, W., Fang, H., Scherf, U., Han, J., Puri, R. K., Frueh, F. W., Goodsaid, F. M., Guo, L., Su, Z., Han, T., Fuscoe, J. C., Xu, Z. A., Patterson, T. A., Hong, H., Xie, Q., Perkins, R. G., Chen, J. J., and Casciano, D. A. (2005a). Cross-platform comparability of microarray technology: Intra-platform consistency and appropriate data analysis procedures are essential. *BMC Bioinformatics* 6(Suppl 2):S12.

Shi, L., Tong, W., Su, Z., Han, T., Han, J., Puri, R. K., Fang, H., Frueh, F. W., Goodsaid, F. M., Guo, L., Branham, W. S., Chen, J. J., Xu, Z. A., Harris, S. C., Hong, H., Xie, Q., Perkins, R. G., and Fuscoe, J. C. (2005b). Microarray scanner calibration curves: Characteristics and implications. *BMC Bioinformatics* 6(Suppl 2):S11.

Shi, L., Reid, L. H., Jones, W. D., Shippy, R., Warrington, J. A., Baker, S. C., Collins, P. J., de Longueville, F., Kawasaki, E. S., Lee, K. Y., Luo, Y., Sun, Y. A., Willey, J. C., Setterquist, R. A., Fischer, G. M., Tong, W., Dragan, Y. P., Dix, D. J., Frueh, F. W., Goodsaid, F. M., Herman, D., Jensen, R. V., Johnson, C. D., Lobenhofer, E. K., Puri, R. K., Schrf, U., Thierry-Mieg, J., Wang, C., Wilson, M., Wolber, P. K., Zhang, L., Amur, S., Bao, W., Barbacioru, C. C., Lucas, A. B., Bertholet, V., Boysen, C., Bromley, B., Brown, D., Brunner, A., Canales, R., Cao, X. M., Cebula, T. A., Chen, J. J., Cheng, J., Chu, T. M., Chudin, E., Corson, J., Corton, J. C., Croner, L. J., Davies, C., Davison, T. S., Delenstarr, G., Deng, X., Dorris, D., Eklund, A. C., Fan, X. H., Fang, H., Fulmer-Smentek, S., Fuscoe, J. C., Gallagher, K., Ge, W., Guo, L., Guo, X., Hager, J., Haje, P. K., Han, J., Han, T., Harbottle, H. C., Harris, S. C., Hatchwell, E., Hauser, C. A., Hester, S., Hong, H., Hurban, P., Jackson, S. A., Ji, H., Knight, C. R., Kuo, W. P., LeClerc, J. E., Levy, S., Li, Q. Z., Liu, C., Liu, Y., Lombardi, M. J., Ma, Y., Magnuson, S. R., Maqsodi, B., McDaniel, T., Mei, N., Myklebost, O., Ning, B., Novoradovskaya, N., Orr, M. S., Osborn, T. W., Papallo, A., Patterson, T. A., Perkins, R. G., Peters, E. H., Peterson, R., et al. (2006). The MicroArray Quality Control (MAQC) project shows inter- and intraplatform reproducibility of gene expression measurements. *Nat. Biotechnol.* 24:1151–1161.

Simon, R. (2003). Diagnostic and prognostic prediction using gene expression profiles in high-dimensional microarray data. *Br. J. Cancer* 89:1599–1604.

Strand, C., Enell, J., Hedenfalk, I., and Ferno, M. (2007). RNA quality in frozen breast cancer samples and the influence on gene expression analysis—a comparison of three evaluation methods using microcapillary electrophoresis traces. *BMC Mol. Biol.* 8:38.

Tan, P. K., Downey, T. J., Spitznagel, E. L., Jr., Xu, P., Fu, D., Dimitrov, D. S., Lempicki, R. A., Raaka, B. M., and Cam, M. C. (2003). Evaluation of gene expression measurements from commercial microarray platforms. *Nucleic Acids Res.* 31:5676–5684.

Takahashi, Y., Nishida, Y., Ishii, Y., Ishikawa, K., and Asai, S. (2005). Monitoring expression of cytochrome P450 genes during postischemic rat liver reperfusion using DNA microarrays. *J. Pharmacol. Sci.* 97:153–156.

Thomas, D. C. (2001). Introduction: Bayesian models and Markov chain Monte Carlo methods. *Genet. Epidemiol.* 21(Suppl 1):S660–661.

Thum, T., and Borlak, J. (2007). Detection of early signals of hepatotoxicity by gene expression profiling studies with cultures of metabolically competent human hepatocytes. *Arch. Toxicol.* 82:89–101.

Tong, W., Lucas, A. B., Shippy, R., Fan, X., Fang, H., Hong, H., Orr, M. S., Chu, T. M., Guo, X., Collins, P. J., Sun, Y. A., Wang, S. J., Bao, W., Wolfinger, R. D., Shchegrova, S., Guo, L., Warrington, J. A., and Shi, L. (2006). Evaluation of external RNA controls for the assessment of microarray performance. *Nat. Biotechnol.* 24:1132–1139.

Trepicchio, W. L., Williams, G. A., Essayan, D., Hall, S. T., Harty, L. C., Shaw, P. M., Spear, B. B., Wang, S. J., and Watson, M. L. (2004). Pharmacogenomic data submissions to the FDA: Clinical case studies. *Pharmacogenomics* 5:519–524.

Tusher, V. G., Tibshirani, R., and Chu, G. (2001). Significance analysis of microarrays applied to the ionizing radiation response. *Proc. Natl. Acad. Sci. U. S. A.* 98:5116–5121.

Viale, A., Li, J., Tiesman, J., Hester, S., Massimi, A., Griffin, C., Grills, G., Khitrov, G., Lilley, K., Knudtson, K., Ward, B., Kornacker, K., Chu, C. Y., Auer, H., and Brooks, A. I. (2007). Big results from small samples: Evaluation of amplification protocols for gene expression profiling. *J. Biomol. Tech.* 18:150–161.

Vinciotti, V., Khanin, R., D'Alimonte, D., Liu, X., Cattini, N., Hotchkiss, G., Bucca, G., de Jesus, O., Rasaiyaah, J., Smith, C. P., Kellam, P., and Wit, E. (2005). An experimental evaluation of a loop versus a reference design for two-channel microarrays. *Bioinformatics* 21:492–501.

Waring, J. F., Liguori, M. J., Luyendyk, J. P., Maddox, J. F., Ganey, P. E., Stachlewitz, R. F., North, C., Blomme, E. A., and Roth, R. A. (2006). Microarray analysis of lipopolysaccharide potentiation of trovafloxacin-induced liver injury in rats suggests a role for proinflammatory chemokines and neutrophils. *J. Pharmacol. Exp. Ther.* 316: 1080–1087.

Wilfinger, W. W., Mackey, K., and Chomczynski, P. (1997). Effect of pH and ionic strength on the spectrophotometric assessment of nucleic acid purity. *Biotechniques* 22:474–476, 478–481.

Wu, M. J., Lai, L. W., and Lien, Y. H. (2004). Effect of calbindin-D28K on cyclosporine toxicity in cultured renal proximal tubular cells. *J. Cell Physiol.* 200:395–399.

Yang, Y. H., and Speed, T. (2002). Design issues for cDNA microarray experiments. *Nat. Rev. Genet.* 3:579–588.

Yang, Y., Abel, S. J., Ciurlionis, R., and Waring, J. F. (2006). Development of a toxicogenomics in vitro assay for the efficient characterization of compounds. *Pharmacogenomics* 7:177–186.

Yue, L., and Reisdorf, W. C. (2005). Pathway and ontology analysis: Emerging approaches connecting transcriptome data and clinical endpoints. *Curr. Mol. Med.* 5:11–21.

6

MOLECULAR PATHOLOGY AS A WAY TO FIND THE RIGHT DOSE FOR A DRUG

F. Rojo, A. Rovira, S. Serrano, and J. Albanell

6.1. INTRODUCTION

Anticancer drug discovery and development are currently undergoing a period of rapid and unprecedented transformation. Advances in molecular biology and genomic approaches lead to an increasingly detailed understanding of the genetic abnormalities of malignancies, and extensive progress has been achieved in the knowledge of cancer and malignant phenotype. This emerging identification of cancer-causing genes and the cellular pathways that their encoded proteins control supports a basis for drug discovery, development, and clinical testing to identify the target population. At the same time, drug development is being accelerated by numerous innovative technologies, particularly high-throughput methodologies for genomics, screening, structural biology, pharmacokinetics, and combinatorial chemistry. The nature of the drugs emerging from these new approaches is also changing. The previous generation of anticancer agents was dominated by cytotoxic agents, whose precise molecular mechanisms of action were not clear during their preclinical and early clinical development. The new generation of molecular therapies, called targeted therapies, is now entering in cancer treatment. These targeted therapies are directed against modulators of proliferative signal transduction, telomere regulation, cell cycle progression,

Molecular Pathology in Drug Discovery and Development, Edited by J. Suso Platero
Copyright © 2009 John Wiley & Sons, Inc.

apoptosis and survival, invasion, angiogenesis, and metastasis. Clinical development of such agents is still in the early stages, but the promise of this approach has already been shown through the regulatory approval of trastuzumab, a humanized monoclonal antibody for Human Epidermal Growth Factor Receptor 2 (*HER2*)-positive breast cancer; imatinib mesilate, a Breakpoint Cluster Region-Abelson Leukemia (*Bcr-Abl*) and *c-Kit* (CD117) inhibitor in chronic myelocytic leukemia and gastrointestinal stromal tumors (GIST); and the epidermal growth factor receptor inhibitors and the monoclonal antibody bevacizumab, which acts on the vascular endothelial growth factor receptor ligand, VEGF-A.

Traditionally, cytotoxic drugs have been developed through dose selection based on maximum tolerable toxicity (MTD) in phase I trials and screening for efficacy based on clinical response in phase II trials. This selection has been based on preclinical studies that correlated doses and observed antitumor effects and safety profiles. Application of these procedures to targeted therapies may be problematic because neither toxicity nor tumor shrinkage is useful surrogate for dose selection or activity, and the dose that inhibits a specific target may not necessarily be one that induces toxicity.

Indeed, measurement of molecular effects and identification of the appropriate biomarkers in clinical and preclinical development of targeted therapies is important to provide demonstration of proof of concept for molecular and biologic mechanisms of action, to evaluate the desired biological effect, to select the adequate population to be treated, to identify the optimal dose and schedule, to help the interpretation of clinical data, to evaluate the clinical response, and to contribute to decisions for final approval by authorities. In phase I clinical trials, it is no longer sufficient only to define the nature of the dose-limiting toxicity, the maximum tolerated dose, and the recommended dose for phase II trial. Phase I trials are increasingly extensions of the preclinical mechanistic drug development process, and extensive studies incorporating pharmacokinetic and pharmacodynamic endpoints have been conducted. Pharmacokinetics explores the effects of the organism on the drug in terms of absorption, distribution, metabolism, and excretion, including the concentration–time relationship and its dependence on dose, whereas pharmacodynamics is centered on the molecular, biochemical, and physiological effects of the drug on the organism, analyzing how the drug binds and modulates the target, initiates the mechanism of action, produces a therapeutic effect, and finally develops toxic side effects.

Throughout the process of preclinical and clinical drug development, pharmacodynamic endpoints determine and quantify the biological activity of a determined drug on its therapeutic target or targets when administered and are used to define the optimal biological dose (OBD) in vivo. Pharmacodynamics is based on the study of sequential samples from patients at different time points, ideally the target tissue. A wide range of invasive and minimally invasive procedures are now being tested in early clinical trials. Increasingly, clinical studies involve dose escalations to define the OBD and to catalog the toxic side effects. The collection of serial tumor biopsies for correlative purposes has several disadvantages such as invasiveness, electiveness—because not every patient is suitable for biopsy—and sampling error. A potential solution to this problem is represented by the use of normal tissue, skin biopsies, or peripheral blood cells. Moreover, these studies permit to analyze not only the biological effects produced by the drug on the target or the downstream signaling pathways but also try to identify the biomarkers that would permit to predict the individual response of each patient against a concrete drug. These biomarkers should be identified during preclinical studies carried out on in vitro cellular models or in vivo animal models, generally using high-throughput techniques that generate a large number of potential or candidate biomarkers. Afterward, these candidates must be evaluated and validated in order to determine its real utility to select patients or to define OBD in clinical trials using protein or messenger ribonucleic acid (mRNA) methods that may include immunohistochemistry, enzyme-linked immunosorbent assay (ELISA), reverse transcription–polymerase chain reaction (RT-PCR), gene expression profiling, western blotting, protein lysate arrays, or proteomic mass spectrometry. In addition to molecular and tissue-based techniques, advances in novel imaging technologies also have profound implications for drug development. These molecular and functional imaging platforms include technologies to assess cellular metabolism using 18F-fluorodeoxyglucose positron emission tomography (PET), cell proliferation and apoptosis using 18F-fluoro-L-thymidine and 99mTc-annexin imaging, and resistance to chemotherapy using 99mTc-sestamibi imaging and vascular dynamic contrast-enhanced computed tomography and magnetic resonance imaging. Other technical advances include simultaneous combined modality imaging, as PET/computed tomography or PET/magnetic resonance imaging, which offers great promise in integrating functional and anatomical information.

This chapter will discuss the most relevant pharmacodynamic studies in oncology, using molecular pathology, and their contribution to the development of targeted therapies.

6.2. ANTI-EGFR-TARGETED THERAPIES: THE PHARMACODYNAMIC EXPERIENCE

Epidermal growth factor receptor (EGFR) is a member of ErbB membrane receptor family. The family is composed by four receptors: ErbB1/EGFR, ErbB2/HER2, ErbB3/HER3, and ErbB4/HER4. EGFR is activated by specific ligands such as epidermal growth factor (EGF) or transforming growth factor alpha (TGF-α) that bind to the extracelullar domain of the receptor and induce dimerization, leading to a conformational modification and the activation of the intracellular kinase domain by phosphorylation. This activation initiates a downstream cascade of intracellular signals to the nucleus that regulates proliferation, cell growth, differentiation, mobility, adhesion, and cell survival by preventing apoptosis. It is well documented that EGFR is expressed in a broad spectrum of normal tissues, including epidermis or gastrointestinal mucosa. Interestingly, EGFR expression is increased or overexpressed in a large number of solid tumors, such as non-small-cell lung cancer (NSCLC), colorectal cancer, ovary tumors, and squamous cell head and neck carcinomas (SCHNC). Moreover, the EGFR overexpression has been related to poor prognosis and chemoresistance (Mendelsohn and Baselga, 2003). For these reasons, EGFR is an attractive target in cancer therapy. EGFR is targeted using two different strategies: use of monoclonal antibodies against the extracellular domain of the receptor and use of small molecules that inhibit the intracellular tyrosine kinase domain Among all these agents, best characterized are the tyrosine kinase inhibitors (TKIs) gefitinib (ZD1839, Iressa, AstraZeneca) and erlotinib (OSI-774, Tarceva, Roche), and the monoclonal antibody cetuximab (IMC-225, Erbitux, ImClone, Merck, and Bristol-Myers Squibb). These compounds have demonstrated antitumor activity, although identification of sensitive population to EGFR therapies is now one of the most crucial priorities in oncology. Indeed, clinical development of EGFR inhibitors has permitted the first demonstration of the biological activity of targeted therapies directly on samples from treated patients by phamacodynamic (PD) assays. Molecular endpoints in PD assays with EGFR inhibitors are based in the in vitro knowledge of the biology of the receptor and its downstream effects (Baselga and Albanell, 2002) (Fig. 6.1). This biology could be broken into the following steps:

1. *EGFR activation:* Binding of ligand to EGFR leads to intracellular domain phosphorylation and activation as a first event of the intracellular signaling pathway. This activation could be demonstrated by the use of antibodies that specifically recognize the phosphorylated form of EGFR and tested on tissues by immunohistochemistry (IHC).

2. *Signaling transduction:* Two major signaling pathways are involved in the response to Epidermal Growth factor (EGF), ras-raf-Mitogen-Activated Protein Kinase (Ras-Raf-MAPK) and Phosphoinositide 3 Kinase–Protein Kinase B (PI3K-AKT) cascades. They control a myriad of molecular downstream targets as cyclin, c-fos, p21 or p27. Studying the activity of

---

Figure 6.1. (A) Ras-Raf-ERK1/2 signaling pathway. Following ligand binding, growth factor receptor tyrosine kinases become activated. This induces the binding of adaptor proteins and then activates Ras. In GTP form, Ras activates the kinase activity of Raf and its downstream cascade. Raf phosphorylates the mitogen-activated protein kinase (MAPK) kinase (MEK). After that, MAPK (ERK1/2) are phosphorylated and activates several subsequent kinases, which induce transcriptional factors, resulting changes in gene regulation affect cell cycle progression and/or cell motility in a cell-dependent manner. (B) Overview of the PI3K-AKT signaling pathway. The pathway is activated either by the p85 PI3K regulatory subunit binding to an activated tyrosine residue on the activated membrane receptor or by the p110 PI3K subunit binding to activate Ras. Both result in membrane localization of PI3K and the phosphorylate AKT. Phosphatases that inhibit activity are PTEN and SHIP. AKT activation has been implicated in cell survival by apoptosis inhibition, inducing phosphorylation and inactivation of the pro-apoptotic Bad protein, in control of cell cycle progression by blocking FOX, increasing p27[KIP1], Chk-1, c-Fos, and cyclin D1 transcription, in cell growth by mTOR activation and neoplastic transformation.

(A)

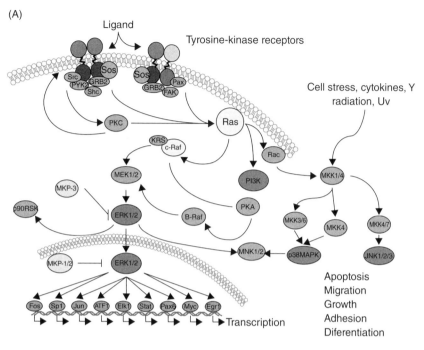

(B)

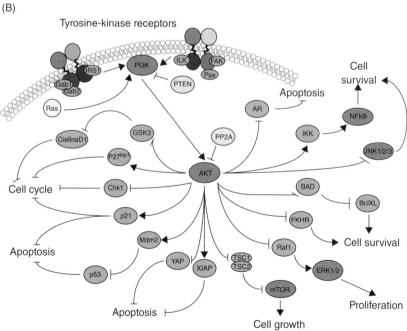

these signaling pathways and their targets, correlations with receptor inhibition induced by the therapies may be established.

3. *Phenotype:* EGFR activation in cells induces proliferation, cell survival, promotes angiogenesis, and stimulates metastasis. Analysis of the effects of target inhibition on differentiation, proliferation, and apoptosis allows studying the biological EGFR dependency of tumors.

Epidermal growth factor receptor activation might be the more appropriate and direct pharmacodynamic endpoint. However, studies in vitro have provided a better understanding of the role of EGFR in human cancer. Gefitinib and cetuximab in cell lines have demonstrated that drug concentrations induced a maximum proliferation inhibition, blocked EGFR activation, and also ERK1/2 signaling (Albanell et al., 2001). These findings have confirmed the relevance of signaling molecules as surrogate biomarkers for the definition of the biological activity and the OBD. The relevance of these biomarkers has been emphasised in studies in vivo using breast cancer models treated with gefinitib (Rojo et al., 2002). In this model, gefinitib was able to induce in tumors from treated animals a maximum inhibition of epidermal growth factor receptor (EGFR) and extracellular signal-regulated kinase (ERK1/2) and a partial inhibition of AKT (Protein Kinases B, PKB). This suggested that AKT in this model might play a role in the tumor as a resistance factor to EGFR inhibitors. Additional studies using other EGFR inhibitors provided new evidence for alternative markers to EGFR, such as AKT, p27, p63, cyclin D1, PAK1 or c-Src (Wakeling et al., 2002; Busse et al., 2000; Moasser et al., 2001; Shien et al., 2004; Matheny et al., 2003; Yang et al., 2004). In retrospect, series of human tumors, such as head and neck squamous carcinoma, gastric carcinoma, breast cancer, colorectal, or NSCL, that show significant correlation between EGFR and ERK1/2 expression in tumor cells has been described. However, other molecular EGFR-independent mechanisms have been reported as activators of ERK1/2: insulinlike growth factor receptor (IGF1R), estrogen receptor (ER), protease receptor type 2 (PAR2), and activating mutations of Ras or other kinases. Moreover, overexpression of *EGFR* in different tumor types did not correlate with high activation of the ERK1/2 pathway but induced an increased signaling by Janus kinase/signal transducers and activators of transcription (JAK/STAT) or PI3K/AKT. In summary, the enormous complexity should be considered for selecting best candidates for EGFR inhibitor therapy and should enforce the incorporation of new massive data analysis methods, including transcriptional and proteomic profiles.

6.3. MOLECULAR PATHOLOGY WITH SMALL MOLECULES GEFITINIB AND ERLOTINIB

The first reported pharmacodynamic studies with gefitinib were performed in two phase I clinical trials, one in the United States and another in Europe, Australia, and Asia (Herbst et al., 2002; Baselga et al., 2002). These trials included patients with advanced solid tumors treated at increasing orally daily doses of gefinitib

(150 to 1000 mg). A PD clinical study was assayed using sequential skin biopsies from 41 patients, obtained before and after 28 days of treatment. The idea was to demonstrate the inhibition of *EGFR* and of the events downstream the receptor by using a molecular pathology assay (Albanell et al., 2002). The skin assay was justified by accessibility to obtain sequential biopsies and the documented biological EGFR dependence of epidermis. This study demonstrated that most patients showed an inhibition of the EGFR activity in vivo after gefitinib treatment, pointing out that an orally administered dose could reach and inhibit the target in skin cells. However, minimal levels of EGFR activity persisted in a subset of patients, independent of the dose and gefitinib plasma levels. The biological basis of this uncompleted inhibition is still unknown. During the treatment with gefitinib, ERK1/2 activity was also inhibited, although not completely. This fact suggests that other signaling mechanism, not EGFR dependent, or receptor activity that persisted above the detection threshold might also activate ERK in skin keratinocytes. In addition to EGFR and ERK1/2 inhibition, proliferation of keratinocytes was reduced and the expression of cyclin-dependent kinase (CDK) inhibitor, $p27^{KIP1}$, was up-regulated (Fig. 6.2). Definitivly, these molecular pathology assays in vivo proved that gefitinib could carry out a great variety of biological effects associated with an effective EGFR inhibition using skin tissue from treated patients as a model. However, no correlation between PD effects, gefitinib doses,

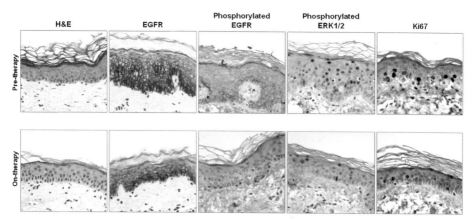

Figure 6.2. Pharmacodynamic effects on sequential skin biopsies—baseline and after 28 days of therapy—from a patient treated with gefitinib at 250 mg/day. Baseline (upper panel) and on-therapy (lower panel) for hematoxylin-eosin (H&E), and EGFR, phosphorylated EGFR, phosphorylated ERK1/2, and Ki67 immunohistochemistry assays. On-therapy, the stratum corneum was thinner and apoptotic cells increased in the H&E examination. Activated EGFR in baseline keratinocytes was abolished after treatment. Inhibition of ERK1/2 at on-therapy epidermis was observed. Reduced Ki67 in keratinocytes was also detected. The immunohistochemistry assay is performed on formalin-fixed paraffin-embedded tissues using appropriate specific antibodies against molecular targets, including phosphorylated or activated forms of the proteins and based on a peroxidase reaction used as detection method.

plasma levels, or skin rash was observed. This observation could be explained by the fact that even in the initial dose of 150 mg/day, EGFR was already inhibited. Moreover, this should be supported by the observation that clinical benefit and antitumoral response in patients were reached at all dose level (Herbst et al., 2002; Baselga et al., 2002). It is important to emphasize that the MTD was not reached until 1000 mg/day, when unacceptable gastrointestinal toxicity appeared. Since all the molecular effects related to the target inhibition were observed at lower doses than the MTD, these results support the use of PD assays to select the MTD and to define the efficacy and safety of these drugs (Lorusso et al., 2003).

After these results, additional PD assays with gefitinib were performed in patients treated at doses of 250 and 500 mg/day, which demonstrated EGFR inhibition, therapeutic effect, and minimal adverse events, supporting the Optimal Biological Dose (OBD) previously defined (Cella, 2003; Herbst, 2003). Further studies carried out in Non Small Cell Lung Cancer (NSCLC) patients demonstrated that gefitinib administered 250 mg/day showed similar antitumoral effect as 500 mg/day dose but with lower incidence of skin rash. These findings might suggest that in some tumor types, a 250-mg/day dose could be therapeutically superior to higher doses.

In addition to PD studies on skin biopsies, other pharmacodynamic markers have been applied to studies with gefitinib using molecular pathology assays in sequential tumor biopsies from colorectal tumors, breast cancer, and gastric cancer (Fig. 6.3). In colorectal cancer, the study with escalating doses of gefitinib demonstrated that therapy induced a decrease in the activation of EGFR, ERK1/2, and AKT in tumor cells (Goss et al., 2005). Similarly, a multicentric phase II study performed in advanced breast cancer patients treated with

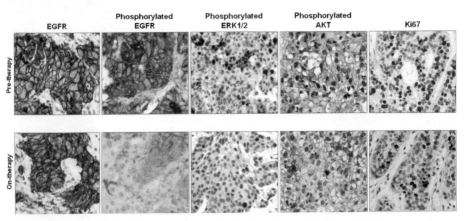

Figure 6.3. Pharmacodynamic effects on sequential tumor biopsies—baseline and after 28 days of therapy—from a patient treated with gefitinib at 250 mg/day. Baseline (upper panel) and on-therapy (lower panel) for EGFR, phosphorylated EGFR, phosphorylated ERK1/2, phosphorylated AKT, and Ki67 immunohistochemistry assays in a gastric carcinoma. On-therapy, inhibition of p-EGFR, p-ERK1/2 was detected, whereas only a reduction of p-AKT and proliferation was observed. No changes in total EGFR expression were present in tumor cells. See insert for color representation of this figure.

500 mg/day of gefinitib in monotherapy compared the biological effects in tumor and skin biopsies (Baselga et al., 2005a). Although clinical benefit was modest and responses were not observed, in agreement with previous trials with EGFR TKIs in breast cancer (Robertson et al., 2003; Albain et al., 2002; Tan et al., 2004), gefitinib inhibited EGFR and ERK1/2 phosphorylation both in skin and tumor biopsies of treated patients, corroborating the biological activity of the drug. However, downstream effects of the receptor inhibition were different in tumor than in skin: p27^{KIP1} expression and proliferation were modified only in skin but not in tumors. Supporting these findings, gefitinib did not inhibit AKT in tumor, pointing a potential resistance mechanism in breast cancer to EGFR TKI therapies. In conclusion, clinical resistance to gefitinib might not be attributed to a lack of biological activity of the drug but to the fact that EGFR inhibition is not enough to obtain a relevant clinical benefit in breast cancer.

Similar findings have been reported in a phase II trial in patients with ovarian carcinoma treated at 500 mg/day of gefitinib (Posadas et al., 2007). In the PD study, a proteomic approach using protein lysate arrays was used on sequential tumor samples. Inhibition of EGFR activation and a decrease in the total amount of this protein after 4 weeks of gefitinib treatment was demonstrated. However, ERK1/2 and AKT signaling pathways were not blocked. In this tumor, EGFR inhibition could not be related with clinical response either. Another study from a phase II trial in gastric cancer patients treated with 250 or 500 mg/day of gefitinib also demonstrated a complete inhibition of EGFR in tumor cells at both doses but not inhibition of ERK1/2 or AKT signaling pathways (Rojo et al., 2006). Interestingly, patients who showed an inhibition of AKT activation after therapy presented with an increased rate of apoptosis reached in the tumor that correlated with plasma levels of the drug.

Similar PD assays have been reported in clinical trials with NSCLC patients treated with erlotinib. Erlotinib has demonstrated a significant therapeutic benefit measured in terms of overall survival and disease-free survival. Molecular effects of the drug were analyzed in phase I trials with PD and pharmacokinetic (PK) studies carried out in patients with different solid tumor types (Malik et al., 2003; Hidalgo et al., 2001). The MTD was defined at 150 mg/day, and this dose was selected for phase II trials. However, this dose reached plasma drug concentrations higher than biological levels necessary to inhibit completely EGFR, as previously defined according to preclinical studies carried out in animal models (Hidalgo et al., 2001). To resolve that, a PD study was designed in a phase I/II trial with increasing doses of erlotinib. Interim data analysis showed an inhibition of EGFR, ERK1/2, and AKT in more than 50% of the patients, and a p27^{KIP1} dose-dependent up-regulation in epidermal keratinocytes (Malik et al., 2003). Similar results were described in a PD phase I/II clinical trial in which tumor samples obtained from patients with metastatic or relapsed head and neck tumors and treated with erlotinib and cisplatin (Agulnik et al., 2007). This study demonstrated that EGFR and nuclear factor kappa B (NFkB) inhibition induced by the treatment significantly correlated with an increase of survival.

Recently, a second generation of EGFR TKI is emerging in oncology. EKB-569 (Wyeth) is an orally administered irreversible EGFR TKI that inhibits the growth of EGFR-overexpressing tumor cell lines. A recently published phase I study with EKB-569 monotherapy established the MTD at 75 mg/day, the dose-limiting toxicity (DLT) being diarrhea. In this study, two heavily pretreated patients with metastatic colorectal carcinoma achieved prolonged tumor stabilization (Erlichman et al., 2006). Because of the known synergistic clinical effect of anti-EGFR agents in combination with irinotecan, a PK/PD phase I trial of EKB-569 in combination with FOLFIRI (irinotecan/5-fluorouracil [5-FU]/leucovorin [LV]) in patients with metastatic colorectal carcinoma (mCRC) was conducted. To assess the optimal recommended dose of this combination, the safety profile and the molecular PD effects in sequential skin and tumor biopsies of FOLFIRI alone and EKB-569 in combination with FOLFIRI were assessed (Casado et al., 2004). The recommended dose was 25 mg EKB-569 plus full-dose FOLFIRI, which resulted in complete inhibition of activated EGFR and downstream receptor signaling in skin and tumor samples. Interestingly, FOLFIRI alone did not affect EGFR but inhibited epidermal proliferation and activated MAPK and induced p27 expression. It was noted that activated Akt was not inhibited in the tumors after administration of FOLFIRI and EKB-569, speculating that activation of PI3K/Akt is mediated via other growth factor receptors, or that loss of activity of the tumor suppressor gene PTEN, or presence of PI3K mutations results in enhanced PI3K/Akt activity. An important contribution of this study was to analyze the effects on PD markers induced by chemotherapy alone prior to the introduction of EKB-569. The implication of these findings was that chemotherapy alone may interfere, probably through a variety of nonspecific mechanisms, with the activation status of some of the PD markers that are frequently analyzed in clinical trials with targeted agents directed at signal transduction pathways. Therefore, caution should be introduced with the interpretation of PD studies of targeted agents when given in combination with chemotherapy.

Globally, these PD studies of EGFR TKIs have contributed to the knowledge of the mechanism of action of the drugs in vivo and their biological effects in tissues and provided useful information for the optimization of treatment schedules. The differences in the effects and the efficacy of different drugs against the same target could be explained by the differences in the specificity or sensitivity of the assays, statistical analysis, treated population or the different affinity of the drugs to the receptor. In fact, the definition of OBD is extremely attractive, but still it does not exist as a prospective clinical validation to demonstrate its superiority to MTD.

6.4. MOLECULAR PATHOLOGY WITH CETUXIMAB AND OTHER MONOCLONAL ANTIBODIES TO EGFR

Initial phase I studies with the monoclonal antibody against the extracellular domain of EGFR, cetuximab, defined the OBD and the weekly administration at doses 200 to 400 mg/m^2 provided an appropriate PK plasma clearance and receptor saturation (Baselga et al., 2000). Although the MTD was not reached in this study, the therapeutic doses were higher than concentrations that inhibited cell growth in EGFR-dependent tumors in vitro. Aiming to complete the cetuximab activity knowledge, a phase Ib PD study was designed combining cetuximab and cisplatin in squamous head and neck cell carcinoma (SCHNC) patients (Shin et al., 2001). Sequential tumor biopsies were obtained in 12 patients treated with a loading dose of 100, 400, or $500\,mg/m^2$ and maintenance doses of 100, 400, or $500\,mg/m^2$, combined with $100\text{-}mg/m^2$ doses of cisplatin every 3 weeks. The EGFR saturation was analyzed in tumor cells. Results revealed that higher inhibition of the tyrosine kinase activity of the receptor and presence of EGFR/Cetuximab complexes, after the treatment, were observed at $100\,mg/m^2$ than higher doses. Following these studies, a loading dose of $400\,mg/m^2$ and subsequent doses of $250\,mg/m^2$ were selected as schedule of cetuximab treatment for phase II and III trials. Supporting this schedule, a phase I PD-PK trial in patients with advanced solid tumors treated with cetuximab at doses of 50, 100, 250, 400, and $500\,mg/m^2$ was conducted (Fracasso et al., 2007). Sequential tumor and skin biopsies were obtained. EGFR and downstream signaling pathway inhibition were achieved in a dose-dependent manner, reaching a maximum biological effect at $250\,mg/m^2$ (Fig. 6.4). At this dose, cetuximab

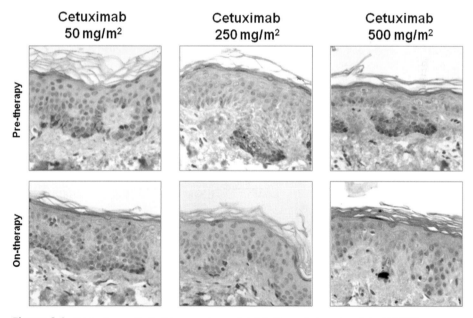

Figure 6.4. Dose-dependent pharmacodynamic inhibition of phosphorylated EGFR in sequential skin biopsies from patients treated with cetuximab at 50, 250, and $500\,mg/m^2$. Samples were obtained baseline and after 28 days of therapy. Baseline expression is mainly detected in basal keratinocytes by immunohistochemistry and reduced in a dose-dependent manner after treatment. See insert for color representation of this figure.

inhibited ERK1/2 activation and cellular proliferation in keratinocytes (Albanell et al., 2001b), showing clinical activity in colorectal cancer (Saltz et al., 2004). Different administration schedules have been also explored as PD endpoints. A phase II study in patients with colorectal cancer, inhibition of EGFR, ERK1/2, AKT, proliferation and up-regulation of p27^{KIP1} were demonstrated at protein and RNA levels (Cervantes et al., 2007). This study compared a weekly 250-mg/m^2 cetuximab administration with 400- to 700-mg/m^2 doses administered every 2 weeks. The biological effects and the PK of the drug were similar, becoming an attractive scheduling alternative.

The biological effects of combination of two different treatments against EGFR have also been explored in vivo. The combined treatment with cetuximab and gefitinib has been studied in animal models, showing a synergistic effect on cell proliferation and a superior inhibition of EGFR-dependent signaling and induction of apoptosis (Matar et al., 2004). The single-agent gefitinib or cetuximab resulted in transient complete tumor remission only at the highest doses. In contrast, suboptimal doses of gefitinib and cetuximab given in combination resulted in a complete and permanent regression of large tumors. In the combination-treated tumors, there was a superior inhibition of EGFR, ERK1/2, and AKT, as well as greater inhibition of cell proliferation, vascularization, and enhanced apoptosis. Using complementary DNA (cDNA) arrays, genes were found to be differentially regulated, including genes related to cell proliferation and differentiation, transcription, DNA synthesis and repair, angiogenesis, signaling molecules, cytoskeleton organization, and tumor invasion and metastasis. These findings were applied on a phase I PD clinical trial in patients with *EGFR* biologically dependent tumors, including NSCLC, colorectal cancer, and SCHNC (Baselga et al., 2006). Encouraging clinical activity in advanced colorectal and SCHNC patients in combination therapy was observed. In addition, the PD studies confirmed a synergistic effect of gefitinib and cetuximab compared with monotherapies, reporting a profound inhibition in tumor, not only in receptor activation but also in ERK1/2, AKT, and proliferation. In addition, extensive tumor apoptosis was observed in patients at the combinatory group (Naret et al., 2006). Gene expression analysis was also performed in treated patients. Results obtained demonstrated that the combination was able to down-regulate differentially the expression of pivotal genes implied in cell survival and proliferation; ligands related to the ErbB receptor network and cell motility and invasion factors, as proangiogenic matrix proteases.

On top of the large experience with cetuximab, new monoclonal antibodies against EGFR are being incorporated in clinics. In this respect, a new monoclonal antibody in clinical development is the humanized monoclonal antibody h-R3, which presents different PK properties than others. In preclinical studies, h-R3 has demonstrated important antiproliferative, proapoptotic, and antiangiogenic activity. In a phase I clinical trial in SCHNC patients treated with h-R3 combined with radiation, increased overall survival was observed at highest doses. The PD study in tumor correlated antitumoral response with antiproliferative and antiangiogenic effects (Crombet et al., 2004). Mathematical models were developed to relate EGFR antigen expression in tissues and h-R3 doses, antibody–antigen affinity, and PK profile, aimed to compare the antibody distribution in normal and tumor tissues of patients.

Matuzumab (EMD72000, Merck KGaA) is another antibody against EGFR. It is a humanized murine antibody with high affinity to EGFR, with antitumoral activity in animal models, and prolonged half-life. Phase I studies reported that matuzumab was well tolerated at doses between 400 and 1600 mg and demonstrated antitumor activity in several tumor types, including esophagus, ovary, lung, and colorectal carcinoma (Socinski, 2007). Diverse pharmacodynamic assays in sequential tumor and skin biopsies have showed a dose-dependent inhibition of EGFR and ERK1/2 in keratynocytes and tumor cells. The OBD was defined at 1200 mg, which achieved a maximum biological effect on target and downstream proteins, with similar activity comparing different administration schedules, weekly, every 2 or 3 weeks (Vanhoefer et al., 2004; Salazar et al., 2004).

6.5. PROTEASOME INHIBITORS: PHARMACODYNAMICS ON BLOOD SAMPLES

The proteasome is a multicatalytic protease present in all eukaryotic cells, and its main function is to degrade intracellular proteins. Relevant proteins implicated in the regulation of basic cell processes, proliferation, cell growth, and survival are degraded by proteasome, such as p21, p27, p53, c-myc, Ikb, and others. This mechanism is essential for cell homeostasis, and its inhibition leads in a stop of proliferation and apoptosis (Ciechanover, 1998). This observation and the feature that malignant cells are more sensitive to cell cycle inhibition and survival signals than normal cells provide a rationale for proteasome inhibition as a new strategy for cancer treatment.

Bortezomib (PS-341, Velcade, Millenium) is a reversible proteasome inhibitor that has already demonstrated preclinical and clinical antitumor activity (Albanell and Adams, 2002; Adams, 2002a). Bortezomib works on an innovative mechanism of action, with a wide antitumoral and cytotoxic activity, by sensitizing tumor cells to chemotherapy. Multiple molecular effects have been described induced by bortezomib: intracellular signaling interference, cell death by apoptosis, CDK stabilization, angiogenesis inhibition, and functional inhibition of NFkB. In cellular in vitro models, bortezomib has been combined with different antineoplastic agents. The proteasome inhibition blocked the NFkB activation induced by chemotherapy, increased apoptosis, and resulted in antitumoral effects (Adams, 2002b).

Clinical studies have reported that bortezomib has been well tolerated at doses that showed biological activity. A phase I study incorporated a PD assay ex vivo aimed to analyze the kinetics of inhibition by a direct measurement of proteasome activity in blood or tissues (Lightcap et al., 2000). This bioassay was crucial in initial bortezomib clinical studies because 90% of the drug is eliminated in the first 15 minutes from the plasma compartment after administration. Due to this effect, PK studies have not been developed, but the bioassay demonstrated inhibitory proteasome activity in a dose and administration-time-dependent manner (Papandreou et al., 2004). However, bortezomib schedule and administration doses are nowadays well established in the clinical practice, making the bioassay not necessary anymore. Reported toxicity was diarrhea and neurotoxicity, but any hematological limiting toxicity was not observed; following these results, recommended dose has been established at $1.56 \, \text{mg/m}^2$. Additional phase I PD studies in patients with refractory malignant hematological disease treated with increasing doses of bortezomib confirmed limiting toxicity as thrombocytopenia, hyponatremia, hypokalemia, and asthenia, establishing a new recommended dose at $1.04 \, \text{mg/m}^2$. Antitumoral effect was observed in non-Hodgkin's lymphoma and multiple myeloma (Aghajanian et al., 2002; Orlowski et al., 2002). Interestingly, a clinical trial using bortezomib administered every week for 4 or 5 weeks in patients with advanced solid tumors showed a maximum PD effect, observed as a reversible proteasome inhibition, one hour after administration, and a recovery of activity at 48 to 72 hours later (Nix et al., 2001). Relating to proteasome inhibition, a decrease in blood levels of interleukin 6 (IL-6) was observed, suggesting that bortezomib inhibited Nuclear Factor kappa-light-chain-ENHANCER of Activated B (NFkB) pathway (Papandreou et al., 2004).

Furthermore, bortezomib has demonstrated antitumoral activity in phase II and III studies in different tumors, which include myeloid and lymphoproliferative disorders, malignant melanoma, prostate, kidney, head and neck, and lung cancer, as monotherapy or in combination with anticancer agents (Adams, 2002a; Mitchell, 2003; Richardson et al., 2003; Montagut et al., 2005). Combination with docetaxel in breast cancer has been well tolerated at all doses and schedules analyzed, showing a promising activity level (Albanell et al., 2003).

6.6. PHARMACODYNAMICS WITH RAPAMYCIN ANALOGS

The mTOR (mammalian target of rapamycin) kinase plays a pivotal role as controller of cell growth and, indirectly, proliferation. At a transcriptional level, mTOR is responsible for induction of RNA polymerase activity by the stimulation of the transcriptional activator STAT, and at translational level mTOR activates p70S6 kinase and 4E-BP1 factor. The p70S6 kinase recruits ribosomal subunit 40S in the translational active polysomes, and 4EBP1 allows liberation and activation of the translation initiator factor eIF-4E, which incorporates mRNA into ribosome. The mTOR is activated by growth factors, including insulin or Platelet-Derived Growth Factor (PDGF), through PI3K-AKT signaling pathway or by cellular stress. The presence of mTOR has been described in all mammalian cells, and overexpression has been frequently described in cancer, correlating with poor outcome, becoming an attractive therapeutic target for cancer treatment (Hay, 2005; Rojo et al., 2007).

Rapamycin (sirolimus), and its analogs, inhibit mTOR by irreversible binding to FKBP-12, a factor necessary for mTOR activation. Nowadays, three rapamycin analogs are in clinical development: Temsirolimus (CCI-779, Wyeth Ayest), Everolimus (RAD001, Novartis) and Amplimexon (AP23573, Ariad) (Vignot et al., 2005). In vitro models have showed that mTOR inhibition reduces transcriptional and translational functions and decreases protein synthesis and mRNA translation. Ribosomal proteins and other components that are implied in cell growth by controlling cell cycle are down-regulated by mTOR activation such as IGF-II (insulin growth factor-II), c-myc, or cyclin D1 (Vignot et al., 2005). Moreover, mTOR has effects controlling apoptosis, regulating proteins such as p53, Bad, Bcl-2, or c-myc.

Phase I and II clinical studies with Temsirolimus have demonstrated well-tolerated administration and antitumoral activity in kidney and breast cancers (Raymond et al., 2004; Atkins et al., 2004). Controversially, antitumoral activity occurred in a wide range of doses and different administration schedules. Moreover, the toxicity of the drug did not correlate with doses, restricting the selection of appropriate administration. Aiming to establish the dose with a maximum biological effect against mTOR, a PD assay was conducted in a phase II study with different doses of Temsirolimus, ranging from 25 to 250 mg (Atkins et al., 2004; Peralba et al., 2003). The PD study quantified the p70S6 kinase activity in peripheral blood mononuclear cells (PBMC), as a marker of mTOR inhibition, demonstrating that the activity decreased linearly 2, 4, and 8 days after treatment. No correlation with dose was observed, suggesting that Temsirolimus achieved maximal biological activity at doses lower or equal to 25 mg (Peralba et al., 2003). Moreover, the results obtained in a phase II PD study performed in 111 patients showed no correlation between efficacy, toxicity, or administered dose. However, a linear relation between p70S6 kinase inhibition and progression disease period was reported. Two phase I PD studies with Everolimus have described a complete biological mTOR inhibition (Tabernero et al., 2005; Lerut et al., 2005). Treatment with Everolimus, even daily or weekly, showed p70S6 kinase inhibition, and a reduction in the phosphorylation of 4EB-P1, eIF-4G, and ribosomal protein S6, which translates to a decrease in cell proliferation in tumor and normal tissues (Fig. 6.5). Moreover, these effects were dose dependent, reflecting a good bioavailability of the drug, although no clinical response was achieved in patients. However, the mTOR inhibitory drug rapamycin up-regulates insulin receptor substrate-1 (IRS-1) protein levels and induces AKT phosphorylation, protein kinase activity, and downstream signaling in a variety of cell lines and in clinical samples from patients treated with Everolimus (O'Reilly et al., 2006). Preclinical models have reported that tumor cells with activated mTOR displayed a phenotype functionally equivalent to insulin-resistant diabetes with an exaggerated down-regulation of upstream signaling molecules such as IRS-1. An increase in IRS-1 adapter protein levels may induce AKT activity by augmenting IGF-IR signaling to PI3K/AKT. These results also suggested a new model for the development of combinatorial anticancer therapy. Combined inhibition of constitutively activated oncoproteins and of normal pathways that are down-regulated

(A)

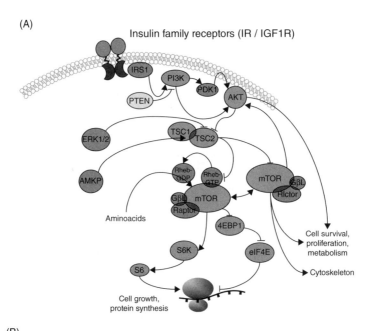

(B)

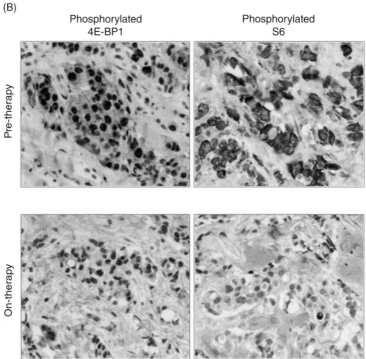

by oncoprotein inhibition may be much more effective than either alone. For the rapamycin analogs, these findings provide a rationale for tailored combination therapy with an mTOR inhibitor and an inhibitor of the growth factor receptor, such as insulin-like growth factor 1 receptor (IGF-IR), which normally drives PI3K activity in that tumor.

6.7. SECOND GENERATION OF TARGETED THERAPIES: MULTITARGET AGENTS

Evidence from previously discussed PD studies suggested that the inhibition of more than one target should increase the antitumor effects and the efficacy of the therapy. Thus, a growing development of multitarget agents in cancer is entering clinical trials. The new generation of compounds with activity against receptors of the family erbB includes lapatinib (Tykerb, GlaxoSmithKline). Lapatinib is a reversible tyrosine kinase inhibitor of EGFR and HER2. A phase I clinical trial in patients with advanced solid tumors with EGFR expression and/or HER2 overexpression used lapatinib as a single agent, and revealed a clinical benefit of 30%, including breast cancer patients refractory to trastuzumab (Burris et al., 2005; Spector et al., 2005). A PD study incorporating molecular pathology techniques on sequential tumor biopsies from those patients demonstrated an inhibition of activation of the targets EGFR and HER2, downstream proteins ERK1/2, AKT, and a reduction of expression of cyclin D1 and TGF-α. Interestingly, the inhibition correlated with clinical response. Moreover, patients with clinical benefit showed high baseline expression of HER2, phosphorylated HER2, ERK1/2, activated ERK1/2, IGFR-1, p70S6 kinase, and TGF-α, achieving superior tumor apoptosis after therapy. However, PK profile or therapeutical doses did not correlate with the PD effects.

Biomarkers to predict the sensitivity population to lapatinib come from in vitro models. In breast cancer, the presence in tumor cells of a truncated form of

---

Figure 6.5. (A) Regulation of mTOR activity by growth factors is mediated by the PI3K/AKT signaling pathway, leading to phophorylation and inhibition of tuberin (TSC2) by AKT and to the subsequent activation of Rheb, which activates mTOR. The mTOR also receives nutrient input signals. The Raptor/mTOR complex mediates the phosphorylation of eukaryotic initiation factor 4E (eIF-4E) binding protein (4E-BP1) and ribosomal protein S6 kinase (p70S6K1). 4EB-P1 and p70S6K1 are mTOR downstream effector molecules that function as regulators of ribosome biogenesis and protein translation. (B) Pharmacodynamic effects on sequential tumor biopsies—baseline and after 28 days of therapy—from a patient treated with a rapamycin-analog mTOR inhibitor. Baseline (upper panel) and on-therapy (lower panel) for phosphorylated 4E-BP1 (p-4E-BP1) and phosphorylated S6 (p-S6) immunohistochemistry assays in a breast carcinoma. On-therapy, inhibition of p-4E-BP1 and p-S6 was detected in tumor cells. See insert for color representation of this figure.

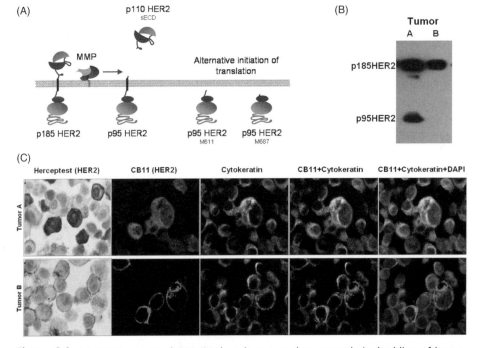

Figure 6.6. (A) HER2 receptor (p185HER2) undergoes a slow proteolytic shedding of its ectodomain that is detected in the serum of patients with advanced breast cancer. The shedding generates an NH2 terminally truncated fragment (p95HER2) that is membrane associated and has kinase activity. Membrane p95HER2 forms are largely synthesized by alternative initiation of translation from methionines 611 and 687, located before and after transmembrane region. The expression of truncated p95HER2 in breast cancer, detected by immunofluorescence assays, has been correlated with poor prognosis and resistance to trastuzumab. (B) Two infiltrating ductal breast carcinomas were subjected to Western blot analysis using an anti-HER2 antibody against intracellular domain of the receptor. Tumor A expresses both HER2 full-length receptor (p185) and truncated form receptor (p95). Tumor B expresses only the p185 HER2 receptor. (C) Two serial sections from tumors in (B) were assayed by immunofluorescence using an antibody to the extracellular domain of the receptor (ECD) and to the intracellular domain of HER2 (ICD), in red. Staining of cytoplasmic compartment was performed with an antibody anticytokeratin (green) and nuclei were stained with DAPI (blue). Tumor A shows membrane staining with the ECD but combined membrane and cytoplasmic staining with the ICD antibody, which co-localized with the anticytokeratin antibody (yellow). Tumor B shows only membrane staining with both antibodies. See insert for color representation of this figure.

HER2 could be a potential resistance mechanism to trastuzumab and, conversely, define sensitivity population to lapatinib (Scaltriti et al., 2007). This truncated form, named p95HER2, correlates with poor prognosis in breast cancer patients and lacks the extracellular domain. Double-fluorescence confocal-based methods have been reported as screening test for routine tissue samples (Fig. 6.6).

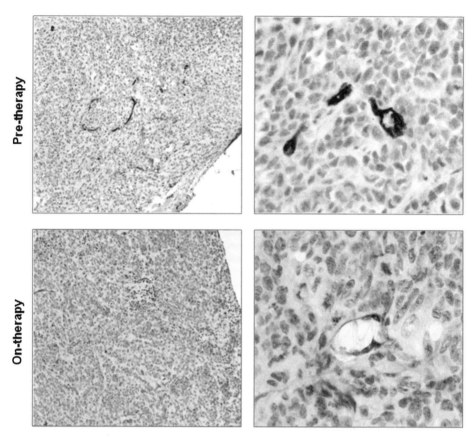

Figure 6.7. Pharmacodynamic inhibition of phosphorylated KDR (p-KDR) in a breast cancer, studied by immunohistochemistry. Baseline (upper panel) and on-therapy (lower panel) expression for p-KDR at ×100 (left panel) and ×400 magnification (right panel). On-therapy p-KDR detection was reduced in endothelial cells into tumor stroma.

Other multitarget agents have demonstrated activity on growth receptors and angiogenesis. In humans, angiogenesis is present in adults in the ovary cycle, endometrial development, and reparative processes but is necessary for the growth, progression, and dissemination of malignancies, and most of neoplasias show an important angiogenesis component (Fig. 6.7). Antiangiogenic agents are effective against tumors with high proliferation rate and, consequently, high requirements of nutrients and oxygen. These antiangiogenic agents would be more efficient than standard therapies because they target endothelial cells only inside the tumor, which are more genetically stable and tend to be more resistant to pharmacological agents. Angiogenesis is a complex and dynamic process regulated by a myriad of pro- and antiangiogenic factors (Carmeliet and Jain, 2000). Some proangiogenic factors are the vascular endothelial cell growth factor (VEGF), its specific receptors vascular endothelial growth factor receptor 1–3 (VEGFR 1–3), the platelet-derived growth factor (PDGF), and its receptors PDGFR-α and PDGFR-β.

Sutent (SU11248, sunitinib malate, Pfizer) is a potent mutitarget agent with high activity against the tyrosine kinase domains of both PDGFR and VEGFR, but also against c-Kit, FLT-3, y RET. Biochemical in vitro studies have revealed that Sutent is able to inhibit the ligand-dependent phosphorylation of receptors at nanomolar range. In animal models, Sutent demonstrated regression or stabilization in colorectal (Colo205) and glial (C6) tumors (Mendel et al., 2003). Aimed to define biomarkers to monitor the biological activity of Sutent, gene expression studies were performed using microarrays (Morimoto et al., 2004). Sutent therapy up-regulated, in animal models, mRNA and protein expression of cadherin-11. This finding was corroborated in tumor biopsies from patients included in clinical trials. Sutent showed antitumoral activity in phase II and III trials including patients with imatinib-resistant gastrointestinal stromal tumors (GIST) and patients with cytokines-resistant renal carcinoma. Additional phase II studies in neuroendocrine tumors also demonstrated clinical activity as monotherapy.

Another promising multitarget agent is AEE788 (Novartis), a TKI with activity against EGFR, HER2, and KDR (VEGFR2, Flk-1). In a phase I PD clinical trial, patients were treated with increasing daily doses of AEE788 ranging from 25 to 550 mg (Baselga et al., 2005b). The PD study included tumor, skin, and wound assessments in order to measure the anti-erbB and antiangiogenic activity. One of the goals of wound assessments is to explore potential antiangiogenic effects of therapies in skin as a surrogate tissue. Adult endothelial cells in nontumoral situations are in a nonproliferative state. To overcome this situation, a wound tissue assay on skin has been developed. This wound assay explores a skin granulation tissue, composed by young blood vessels with proliferating endothelial cells, active fibroblasts, inflammatory cells, and a reparative epidermis. To induce a baseline wound tissue sample, a skin biopsy from a normal area is performed, and this area is re biopsied 7 days later. Antiangiogenic activity must be measured in endothelial cells at protein expression level. In skin keratinocytes, AEE788 administration for 4 weeks inhibited in a dose-dependent manner the phosphorylation of EGFR, ERK1/2, and proliferation and up-regulated p27^{KIP1}, achieving a maximum effect at doses higher than 150 to 200 mg. Interestingly, the antiangiogenic effect on endothelial cells in skin wound tissue was observed at doses ≥300 mg. These results corroborated the biochemical in vitro assays that reported anti-KDR activity at higher doses (twofold) of AEE788 compared to doses that achieved EGFR target inhibitory effect (Traxler et al., 2004). Correlation of PD findings on skin and wound tissue with PK profiles demonstrated a relationship between molecular effects and plasma levels of AEE788 and its active metabolites with exposures to the drug. These PD findings defined an OBD on skin and wound tissue at 300 mg. Conversely, PD changes in tumor revealed a profound inhibition of EGFR, HER2, ERK1/2, AKT, and proliferation, as well as KDR down-regulation, regardless of AEE788 dose levels or tumor type. Drug accumulation and different bioavailability in tumor tissue could explain the differences with the skin results. Compiling all these results, phase II and III clinical studies have been developed using 350-mg doses of AEE788 that demonstrated molecular activity in vivo against EGFR, HER2, and KDR in normal and tumor tissues.

Vandetanib (Zactima, ZD6474, AstraZeneca) is an orally bioavailable, small-molecule TKI of Vascular Endothelial Growth Factor Receptor 2 (VEGFR2), EGFR, and RET (Rearranged During Transfection). Preclinical studies have showed that dual blockade of VEGFR2 and EGFR produces additive or synergistic antitumor effects (Hanrahan and Heymach, 2007). Early clinical results also suggested that dual targeting of these pathways may have activity greater than blocking either pathway alone. In a phase I/II trial assessing the safety and efficacy of bevacizumab—a monoclonal antibody against VEGF-A—and erlotinib in patients with metastatic NSCLC, an objective response rate of 20% was observed. Vandetanib was initially evaluated at 100- to 300-mg doses in two phase I clinical trials among patients with advanced solid tumors refractory to standard therapy. In these trials, a PD study was conducted on sequential skin samples, including wound assay to measure the antiangiogenic activity of the drug (Baselga et al., 2005c). Vandetanib partially inhibited EGFR activation in keratinocytes after 4 weeks of therapy. In addition, abrogation of activated Kinase Insert Domain Receptor (KDR) and VEGFR2 in endothelial cells was observed in a dose-dependent manner, in parallel to reduction of downstream ERK1/2 and proliferation in reparative tissue.

6.8. CONCLUSIONS AND PERSPECTIVES: PHASE 0 CLINICAL TRIALS

Because of our increasingly detailed understanding of the genomics and molecular biology of cancer, enormous expectations are being placed on the development of new molecular therapies that exploit this growing knowledge. The identification of pharmacokinetic and pharmacodynamic endpoints provides a powerful mechanism for improving the quality of drug development and accelerating their regulatory approval. Pharmacodynamics must be considered as an essential part in the development of anticancer agents and has the potential to make drug development more rational, thereby optimizing preclinical and clinical drug development and ultimately delivering timely benefits to patients. In fact, cancer research is incorporating molecular assays at initial steps in clinical development. The relevance of this discipline is demonstrated as a concept in phase 0 clinical trials, aimed to investigate the biology of the target, to evaluate biomarkers, and to provide PK data directly in human samples. It is expected that phase 0 trials will help us to identify and validate therapeutical targets, to screen and to optimize candidate-targeted therapies, to provide demonstration of proof of concept for agents and models, to enhance mechanistic understanding of drug or drug combination effects, to identify sensitive target population, to predict response, resistance, and toxicity, and, in definitive ways, to accelerate the development of targeted therapies.

REFERENCES

Adams, J. (2002a). Proteasome inhibition: A novel approach to cancer therapy. *Trends Mol. Med.* 8(4 Suppl):S49–54.

Adams, J. (2002b). Preclinical and clinical evaluation of proteasome inhibitor PS-341 for the treatment of cancer. *Curr. Opin. Chem. Biol.* 6(4):493–500.

Aghajanian, C., et al. (2002). A phase I trial of the novel proteasome inhibitor PS341 in advanced solid tumor malignancies. *Clin. Cancer Res.* 8(8):2505–2511.

Agulnik, M., et al. (2007). Predictive and pharmacodynamic biomarker studies in tumor and skin tissue samples of patients with recurrent or metastatic squamous cell carcinoma of the head and neck treated with erlotinib. *J. Clin. Oncol.* 25(16):2184–2190.

Albain, K., et al. (2002). Open-label, phase II, multicenter trial of ZD1839 (Iressa) in patients with advanced breast cancer. *Breast Cancer Res. Treat.* 76(S33):Suppl 1; Abstr. 20.

Albanell, J., and Adams, J. (2002). Bortezomib, a proteasome inhibitor for cancer therapy: From concept to clinic. *Drugs Future* 27:1–14.

Albanell, J., Rojo, F., and Baselga, J. (2001a). Pharmacodynamic studies with the epidermal growth factor receptor tyrosine kinase inhibitor ZD1839. *Semin. Oncol.* 28(5 Suppl 16):56–66.

Albanell, J., et al. (2001b). Activated extracellular signal-regulated kinases: Association with epidermal growth factor receptor/transforming growth factor alpha expression in head and neck squamous carcinoma and inhibition by anti-epidermal growth factor receptor treatments. *Cancer Res.* 61(17):6500–6510.

Albanell, J., et al. (2002). Pharmacodynamic studies of the epidermal growth factor receptor inhibitor ZD1839 in skin from cancer patients: Histopathologic and molecular consequences of receptor inhibition. *J. Clin. Oncol.* 20(1):110–124.

Albanell, J., et al. (2003). Phase I study of bortezomib in combination with docetaxel in antracycline-pretreated advanced breast cancer. *Proc. ASCO* 22(Abst. 63).

Atkins, M. B., et al. (2004). Randomized phase II study of multiple dose levels of CCI-779, a novel mammalian target of rapamycin kinase inhibitor, in patients with advanced refractory renal cell carcinoma. *J. Clin. Oncol.* 22(5):909–918.

Baselga, J., and Albanell, J. (2002). Targeting epidermal growth factor receptor in lung cancer. *Curr. Oncol. Rep.* 4(4):317–324.

Baselga, J., et al. (2000). Phase I studies of anti-epidermal growth factor receptor chimeric antibody C225 alone and in combination with cisplatin. *J. Clin. Oncol.* 18(4):904–914.

Baselga, J., et al. (2002). Phase I safety, pharmacokinetic, and pharmacodynamic trial of ZD1839, a selective oral epidermal growth factor receptor tyrosine kinase inhibitor, in patients with five selected solid tumor types. *J. Clin. Oncol.* 20(21):4292–4302.

Baselga, J., et al. (2005a). Phase II and tumor pharmacodynamic study of gefitinib in patients with advanced breast cancer. *J. Clin. Oncol.* 23(23):5323–5333.

Baselga, J., et al. (2005b). Phase I study of AEE788, a novel multitargeted inhibitor of ErbB and VEGF receptor family tyrosine kinases: A pharmacokinetic-pharmacodynamic study to identify the optimal therapeutic dose regimen. *J. Clin. Oncol. ASCO Annual Meeting Proceedings*, 23(16S), Part I of II (June 1 Suppl): 3028, 2005.

Baselga, J., et al. (2005c). Pharmacodynamic assessment of ZD6474 (ZACTIMA™) in the skin of patients with previously treated metastatic breast cancer. 17th NCI-EORTC-AACR Symposium on New Drugs in Cancer Therapy, Abs. 165, November.

Baselga, J., et al. (2006). A phase I pharmacokinetic and molecular pharmacodynamic study of the combination of two anti-EGFR therapies, the monoclonal antibody cetuximab and the tyrosine kinase inhibitor gefitinib, in patients with advanced colorectal, head and neck and non-small cell lung cancer. *J. Clin. Oncol.* 2006 ASCO Annual Meeting Proceedings, Part I, 24(18S) (June 20 Suppl): 3006, 2006.

Burris, H. A., 3rd, et al. (2005). Phase I safety, pharmacokinetics, and clinical activity study of lapatinib (GW572016), a reversible dual inhibitor of epidermal growth factor receptor tyrosine kinases, in heavily pretreated patients with metastatic carcinomas. *J. Clin. Oncol.* 23(23):5305–5313.

Busse, D., et al. (2000). Reversible G(1) arrest induced by inhibition of the epidermal growth factor receptor tyrosine kinase requires up-regulation of p27(KIP1) independent of MAPK activity. *J. Biol. Chem.* 275(10):6987–6995.

Carmeliet, P., and Jain, R. K. (2000). Angiogenesis in cancer and other diseases. *Nature* 407(6801):249–257.

Casado, E., et al. (2004). Phase I pharmacokinetic/pharmacodynamic study of EKB-569—an irreversible inhibitor of the epidermal growth factor receptor (EGFR) tyrosine kinase—in combination with irinotecan, 5-fluorouracil and leucovorin (FOLFIRI) in first-line treatment of patients with metastatic colorectal cancer. *J. Clin. Oncol.* ASCO Annual Meeting Proceedings (Post-Meeting Edition), 22(14S):3543.

Cella, D. (2003). Impact of ZD1839 on non-small cell lung cancer-related symptoms as measured by the functional assessment of cancer therapy-lung scale. *Semin. Oncol.* 30(1 Suppl 1):39–48.

Cervantes, A., Rivera, F., Rojo, F., Casado, E., Rodriguez-Braun, E., Martinelli, E., Kisker, O., Baselga, B., and Tabernero, J. (2007). Optimal dose of cetuximab administered every 2 weeks (q2w): A phase I safety, pharmacokinetics and pharmacodynamics study of weekly (q1w) and q2w schedules in patients with metastatic colorectal cancer. In American Association for Cancer Research Annual Meeting: Proceedings, Los Angeles, CA. Philadelphia (PA): AACR. Abstract nr LB-352.

Ciechanover, A. (1998). The ubiquitin-proteasome pathway: On protein death and cell life. *Embo J.*, 17(24):7151–7160.

Crombet, T., et al. (2004). Use of the humanized anti-epidermal growth factor receptor monoclonal antibody h-R3 in combination with radiotherapy in the treatment of locally advanced head and neck cancer patients. *J. Clin. Oncol.* 22(9):1646–1654.

Erlichman, C., Hidalgo, M., and Boni, J. P. (2006). Phase I study of EKB-569, an irreversible inhibitor of the epidermal growth factor receptor, in patients with advanced solid tumors. *J. Clin. Oncol.* 24:2252–2260.

Fracasso, P. M., et al. (2007). A phase 1 escalating single-dose and weekly fixed-dose study of cetuximab: Pharmacokinetic and pharmacodynamic rationale for dosing. *Clin. Cancer Res.* 13(3):986–993.

Goss, G., et al. (2005). A phase I study of oral ZD 1839 given daily in patients with solid tumors: IND.122, a study of the Investigational New Drug Program of the National Cancer Institute of Canada Clinical Trials Group. *Invest. New Drugs* 23(2):147 155.

Hanrahan, E. O., and Heymach, J. V. (2007). Vascular endothelial growth factor receptor tyrosine kinasa inhibitors vandetanib (ZD6474) and AZD2171 in lung cancer. *Clin. Cancer Res.* 13(15 Suppl):4617–4622.

Hay, N. (2005). The Akt-mTOR tango and its relevance to cancer. *Cancer Cell* 8(3): 179–183.

Herbst, R. S. (2003). Dose-comparative monotherapy trials of ZD1839 in previously treated non-small cell lung cancer patients. *Semin. Oncol.* 30(1 Suppl 1):30–38.

Herbst, R. S., et al. (2002). Selective oral epidermal growth factor receptor tyrosine kinase inhibitor ZD1839 is generally well-tolerated and has activity in non-small-cell lung cancer and other solid tumors: results of a phase I trial. *J. Clin. Oncol.* 20(18): 3815–3825.

Hidalgo, M., et al. (2001). Phase I and pharmacologic study of OSI-774, an epidermal growth factor receptor tyrosine kinase inhibitor, in patients with advanced solid malignancies. *J. Clin. Oncol.* 19(13):3267–3279.

Lerut, E., et al. (2005). Molecular pharmacodynamic evaluation of dose and schedule of RAD001 (everolimus) in patients with operable prostate carcinoma. *J. Clin. Oncol.* 2005 ASCO Annual Meeting Proceedings, 23(16S), Part I of II (June 1 Suppl): 3071, 2005.

Lightcap, E. S., et al. (2000). Proteasome inhibition measurements: Clinical application. *Clin. Chem.* 46(5):673–683.

Lorusso, P. M. (2003). Phase I studies of ZD1839 in patients with common solid tumors. *Semin. Oncol.* 30(1 Suppl 1):21–29.

Malik, S. N., et al. (2003). Pharmacodynamic evaluation of the epidermal growth factor receptor inhibitor OSI-774 in human epidermis of cancer patients. *Clin. Cancer Res.* 9(7):2478–2486.

Matar, P., et al. (2004). Combined epidermal growth factor receptor targeting with the tyrosine kinase inhibitor gefitinib (ZD1839) and the monoclonal antibody cetuximab (IMC-C225): Superiority over single-agent receptor targeting. *Clin. Cancer Res.* 10(19):6487–6501.

Matheny, K. E., et al. (2003). Inhibition of epidermal growth factor receptor signaling decreases p63 expression in head and neck squamous carcinoma cells. *Laryngoscope* 113(6):936–939.

Mendel, D. B., et al. (2003). In vivo antitumor activity of SU11248, a novel tyrosine kinase inhibitor targeting vascular endothelial growth factor and platelet-derived growth factor receptors: Determination of a pharmacokinetic/pharmacodynamic relationship. *Clin. Cancer Res.* 9(1):327–337.

Mendelsohn, J., and Baselga, J. (2003). Status of epidermal growth factor receptor antagonists in the biology and treatment of cancer. *J. Clin. Oncol.* 21(14):2787–2799.

Mitchell, B. S., (2003). The proteasome—an emerging therapeutic target in cancer. *N. Engl. J. Med.* 348(26):2597–2598.

Moasser, M. M., et al. (2001). The tyrosine kinase inhibitor ZD1839 ("Iressa") inhibits HER2-driven signaling and suppresses the growth of HER2-overexpressing tumor cells. *Cancer Res.* 61(19):7184–7188.

Montagut, C., et al. (2005). Preclinical ans clinical development of the proteasome inhibitor bortezomib in cancer treatment. *Drugs Today* 41(5):299–315.

Morimoto, A. M., et al. (2004). Gene expression profiling of human colon xenograft tumors following treatment with SU11248, a multitargeted tyrosine kinase inhibitor. *Oncogene* 23(8):1618–1626.

Naret, C. L., Beattie, L., Mayfield, S. D., Lu, H., Langer, C., and Belani, C. P. (2006). Total blockade of the epidermal growth factor receptor with the combination of cetuximab and gefitinib: A phase I study for patients with recurrent non-small cell lung cancer.

J. Clin. Oncol. 2006 ASCO Annual Meeting Proceedings Part I, 24(18S) (June 20 Suppl): 17045.

Nix, D., et al. (2001). Clinical development of a proteasome inhibitor, PS341, for the treatment of cancer. *Proc. Am. Soc. Clin. Oncol.* 20(Abstr. 86).

O'Reilly, K. E., et al. (2006). mTOR inhibition induces upstream receptor tyrosine kinase signaling and activates Akt. *Cancer Res.* 66(3):1500–1508.

Orlowski, R. Z., et al. (2002). Phase I trial of the proteasome inhibitor PS-341 in patients with refractory hematologic malignancies. *J. Clin. Oncol.* 20(22):4420–4427.

Papandreou, C. N., et al. (2004). Phase I trial of the proteasome inhibitor bortezomib in patients with advanced solid tumors with observations in androgen-independent prostate cancer. *J. Clin. Oncol.* 22(11):2108–2121.

Peralba, J. M., et al. (2003). Pharmacodynamic evaluation of CCI-779, an inhibitor of mTOR, in cancer patients. *Clin. Cancer Res.* 9(8):2887–2892.

Posadas, E. M., et al. (2007). A phase II and pharmacodynamic study of gefitinib in patients with refractory or recurrent epithelial ovarian cancer. *Cancer* 109(7):1323–1330.

Raymond, E., et al. (2004). Safety and pharmacokinetics of escalated doses of weekly intravenous infusion of CCI-779, a novel mTOR inhibitor, in patients with cancer. *J. Clin. Oncol.* 22(12):2336–2347.

Richardson, P. G., et al. (2003). A phase 2 study of bortezomib in relapsed, refractory myeloma. *N. Engl. J. Med.* 348(26):2609–2617.

Robertson, J., et al. (2003). Gefitinib (ZD 1839) is active in acquired tamoxifen (TAM)-resistant oestrogen receptor (ER)-positive and ER-negative breast cancer: Results from a phase II study. *Proc. Am. Soc. Clin. Oncol.* 22(7):Abstr. 23.

Rojo, F., et al. (2002). Dose dependent pharmacodynamic effects of ZD1839 correlate with tumor growth inhibition in BT-474 breast cancer xenografts. *Proc. Am. Assoc. Cancer Res.* 43:705(Abstr. 3893).

Rojo, F., et al. (2006). Pharmacodynamic studies of gefitinib in tumor biopsy specimens from patients with advanced gastric carcinoma. *J. Clin. Oncol.* 24(26):4309–4316.

Rojo, F., et al. (2007). 4E-binding protein 1, a cell signaling hallmark in breast cancer that correlates with pathologic grade and prognosis. *Clin. Cancer Res.* 13(1):81–89.

Salazar, R., et al. (2004). Dose-dependent inhibition of the EGFR and signaling pathways with the anti-EGFR monoclonal antibody EMD 72000 administered every three weeks. A phase I pharmacokinetic/pharmacodynamic study to define the optimal biological dose. *J. Clin. Oncol.* 2004 ASCO Annual Meeting Proceedings (Post-Meeting Edition), 22(14S) (July 15 Suppl): 2002.

Saltz, L. B., et al. (2004). Phase II trial of cetuximab in patients with refractory colorectal cancer that expresses the epidermal growth factor receptor. *J. Clin. Oncol.* 22(7): 1201–1208.

Scaltriti, M., et al. (2007). Expression of p95HER2, a truncated form of the HER2 receptor, and response to anti-HER2 therapies in breast cancer. *J. Natl. Cancer Inst.* 99(8):628–638.

Shien, T., et al. (2004). PLC and PI3K pathways are important in the inhibition of EGF-induced cell migration by gefitinib ("Iressa", ZD1839). *Breast Cancer* 11(4):367–373.

Shin, D. M., et al. (2001). Epidermal growth factor receptor-targeted therapy with C225 and cisplatin in patients with head and neck cancer. *Clin. Cancer Res.* 7(5):1204–1213.

Socinski, M. A. (2007). Antibodies to the epidermal growth factor receptor in non small cell lung cancer: Current status of matuzumab and panitumumab. *Clin. Cancer Res.* 13(15):4597s–4601s.

Spector, N. L., et al. (2005). Study of the biologic effects of lapatinib, a reversible inhibitor of ErbB1 and ErbB2 tyrosine kinases, on tumor growth and survival pathways in patients with advanced malignancies. *J. Clin. Oncol.* 23(11):2502–2512.

Tabernero, J., et al. (2005). A phase I study with tumor molecular pharmacodynamic evaluation of dose and schedule of the oral mTOR-inhibitor Everolimus (RAD001) in patients with advanced solid tumors. *J. Clin. Oncol.* 2005 ASCO Annual Meeting Proceedings, 23(16S), Part I of II (June 1 Suppl): 3007.

Tan, A. R., et al. (2004). Evaluation of biologic end points and pharmacokinetics in patients with metastatic breast cancer after treatment with erlotinib, an epidermal growth factor receptor tyrosine kinase inhibitor. *J. Clin. Oncol.* 22(15):3080–3090.

Traxler, P., et al. (2004). AEE788: A dual family epidermal growth factor receptor/ErbB2 and vascular endothelial growth factor receptor tyrosine kinase inhibitor with antitumor and antiangiogenic activity. *Cancer Res.* 64(14):4931–4941.

Vanhoefer, U., et al. (2004). Phase I study of the humanized antiepidermal growth factor receptor monoclonal antibody EMD72000 in patients with advanced solid tumors that express the epidermal growth factor receptor. *J. Clin. Oncol.* 22(1):175–184.

Vignot, S., et al. (2005). mTOR-targeted therapy of cancer with rapamycin derivatives. *Ann. Oncol.* 16(4):525–537.

Wakeling, A. E., et al. (2002). ZD1839 (Iressa): An orally active inhibitor of epidermal growth factor signaling with potential for cancer therapy. *Cancer Res.* 62(20): 5749–5754.

Yang, Z., et al. (2004). The epidermal growth factor receptor tyrosine kinase inhibitor ZD1839 (Iressa) suppresses c-Src and Pak1 pathways and invasiveness of human cancer cells. *Clin. Cancer Res.* 10(2):658–667.

MOLECULAR PATHOLOGY IN LIFE-CYCLE MANAGEMENT IN DRUG DEVELOPMENT

Martha Quezado, Carlos A. Torres-Cabala, and David Berman

7.1. INTRODUCTION

Since at least the mid nineteenth century, the diagnosis, therapy, and prognosis of tumors have primarily been derived from clinicopathological analysis of the tumor. This approach was practical since chemotherapeutic options have historically been limited. With the introduction of anti-cancer-targeted agents, research has turned to biological markers (biomarkers) that predict sensitivity to the drug. Biomarkers are also fragmenting tumors into new biologically and clinically relevant tumor subclasses—previously diagnostically indistinguishable—and providing important prognostic information (Bertucci et al., 2003). The use of biomarkers is no longer limited to academic labs but is gaining widespread acceptance in general pathology practice (Netto and Saad, 2006). This chapter will review the fundamentals of the most practical molecular pathology techniques and provide clinical examples likely to be experienced in a routine pathology laboratory.

7.2. MOLECULAR PATHOLOGY TECHNIQUES

Until the 1970s, molecular analysis of tumors simply referred to descriptive karyotypic analysis, the resolution limited to the entire chromosome. In 1970, the field of cancer cytogenetics was revolutionized with the introduction of

Molecular Pathology in Drug Discovery and Development, Edited by J. Suso Platero
Copyright © 2009 John Wiley & Sons, Inc.

chromosomal banding, wherein the resolution of cytogenetics was extended to regions (or bands) of the chromosome (Roylance, 2002). The most famous clinical application was the demonstration of a reciprocal translocation t (9; 22) (q34; q11), the Philadelphia chromosome, in patients with chronic myelogenous leukemia. Until recently, cytogenetic analysis required obtaining fresh tumor or blood and culturing the cells with inhibitors of cell division to trap the cells in metaphase or interphase, which is amenable to cytogenetic analysis. The most widely used technique is fluorescence in situ hybridization (FISH), which uses a fluorescently labeled probe for the visualization of DNA sequences on metaphase spreads or interphase nuclei (Roylance, 2002). Current molecular cytogenetic techniques can routinely identify numerical and structural chromosomal aberrations on a range of pathology specimens, including archival material. FISH probes include whole-chromosome, arm-specific, centromere-specific, gene-sequence-specific, and low copy sequence probes (Crocker, 2002). The classic example of FISH in archived tumor tissue is the detection of *HER2* amplification in breast cancer, a negative prognostic biomarker and a predictor of antitumor response to trastuzumab (Herceptin). The next generation of FISH is exploring the ability to detect amplifications from minute number of cells such as touch imprints of breast cancer core biopsies (Kaneko et al., 2002).

Traditional FISH used a single probe to interrogate the degree of amplification of a single chromosome region. Multiplex FISH, also called spectral karyotype imaging, or SKY, employs 24 chromosome probes each labeled with a different combination of fluorochromes, which, with appropriate filters, cameras, and software, can uniquely discriminate numerous loci. This technique permits the analysis of extremely complex karyotyping that is impossible to resolve with classical cytogenetics (Going and Gusterson, 1999). One clinically relevant application of SKY is in the evaluation of acute lymphoblastic leukemia (ALL). The ALL karyotype is an independent prognostic and can provide additional information in more than 50% of cases of ALL on otherwise undetectable chromosomal rearrangements (Nordgren, 2003). FISH requires special microscope filters and imaging equipment, not always available in routine pathology laboratories. The recent development of the chromogenic in situ hybridization (CISH), a variant of FISH, has permitted the utilization of bright-field microscopy for interpretation of cytogenetic studies. CISH allows detection of a labeled DNA probe with peroxidase-labeled polymerized antibodies and can be performed in routine pathology laboratories. CISH has been used to demonstrate HER2 gene amplification in breast carcinoma (Li-Ning et al., 2005; Bilous et al., 2006) and epidermal growth factor receptor (*EGFR*) status in primary glioblastoma multiforme (GBM) (Quezado et al., 2005). FISH/CISH analysis of non-small-cell lung cancer biopsies is currently being studied to identify patients with *EGFR* gene amplification, a biomarker of sensitivity to EGFR inhibitors (Daniele et al., 2007).

Comparative genomic hybridization (CGH) compares the chromosomal copy number of tumor DNA relative to normal DNA. Two labeled DNA samples—usually from normal and tumor tissues—are hybridized to normal metaphase chromosome spreads. The quantitative ratio of the two different fluorescent molecules allows the determination of DNA sequence copy number across the whole genome. CGH has became an important tool in the discovery of novel deletions, amplifications, and polysomies in tumors (Going and Gusterson, 1999). DNA is a remarkably physicochemically stable molecule compared to ribonucleic acid (RNA) and extraction does not pose major technical difficulties. Polymerase chain reaction (PCR) is frequently used to amplify small amounts of DNA. Quantitative real-time PCR (Q-PCR) permits the real-time quantification of PCR products and can be used to assess minimal residual disease following targeted therapy. Q-PCR permits the evaluation of residual myelogenous leukemia cells carrying the target translocation following administration of *BCR-ABL* tyrosine kinase inhibitors dasatinib and imatinib and following bone marrow transplantation (Netto and Saad, 2006). PCR-based gene rearrangement studies may be used to differentiate benign lymphoid proliferations (polyclonal) from lymphoma (monoclonal).

Current technology for purification of RNA from archived tissue is more limited to that of DNA. However, RNA can be purified from fresh or frozen tissue. Reverse transcriptase PCR (RT-PCR) allows the amplification of messenger RNA (mRNA) gene product from oncogenic fusion genes. RT-PCR is used in pathology for the detection of the oncogenic gene products of *EWS/FLI1*, *EWS/WT1*, and *SYT/SSX* fusion genes in the diagnosis of peripheral neuroectodermal tumor/Ewing sarcoma, desmoplastic small round cell tumor, and synovial sarcoma, respectively.

Analysis of microsatellites—DNA segments arranged in repetitive units— by PCR has been of tremendous importance in the discovery of pathogenic mechanisms of hereditary and nonhereditary conditions. Mutations that occur in microsatellites are referred to as microsatellite instability (MSI), which characterizes conditions such as hereditary nonpolyposis colorectal cancer (HNPCC). Therefore, detection of MSI in a particular clinical setting is determinant for diagnosis, prognosis, genetic counseling, and therapy. Since microsatellites are located in several important gene loci, assessment of specific microsatellites is widely used for evaluation of allelic imbalance or loss of heterozygosity (LOH) of various genes (Naidoo and Chetty, 1998). Identification of LOH of specific genes may suggest a role for them in the development and progression of cancer and a potential use of these genes as molecular therapeutic targets (Cacev et al., 2005). LOH can also be applied on the investigation of clonality of tumors.

DNA sequencing of a gene of interest is probably the ultimate goal of the molecular pathologist (Crocker, 2002). Most mutation detection methods use a PCR-based sequencing approach. Large population-based studies of mutations of the *KIT* gene in gastrointestinal stromal tumors (GISTs) have demonstrated that mutational analysis of *KIT* and its relative platelet-derived growth factor receptor α (*PDGFRα*) is of significance for treatment with tyrosine kinase inhibitors such as imatinib mesylate (Gleevec) (Steigen et al., 2007).

DNA microarray-based gene expression profiling has emerged as a powerful tool for prognosis and prediction to drug therapy (Mazumder and Wang, 2006). High-throughput DNA microarray technology allows for the simultaneous measurement of the expression level of thousands of genes (Bertucci et al., 2003). Each array consists of a solid support (usually a glass slide) in which complementary DNA (cDNA) or oligonucleotides are spotted in a known pattern (Mocellin et al., 2005). The gene expression signatures have been demonstrated to be important for the prediction of aggressiveness, chance of relapse of tumors, and survival (Vasselli et al., 2003; Mazumder and Wang, 2006). Besides providing researchers with novel molecular targets, DNA microarray technology is expected to foster in an unprecedented way the development of patient-tailored antiblastic therapy since preclinical trials have demonstrated that the gene signature can predict tumor sensitivity to chemotherapeutic drugs (Mocellin et al., 2005).

Until recently, molecular pathology has been limited to studies of DNA in paraffin-embedded tissue since RNA is rapidly degraded. However, recent improvements in technology have used labeled probes to detect RNA transcripts. For example, probes for the Epstein–Barr virus encoded RNA (EBER) are able to detect the presence of viral RNA in paraffin-embedded tissue. A recent technology called the Nucleic Acid Index, (NAI) is able to calculate the ratio of cellular RNA to DNA from paraffin-embedded tissue that can then be correlated with the aggressiveness of the tumor (Berman et al., 2005). The current generation of molecular pathology is broadening analysis to RNA expression, circulating tumor cells, and functional analysis of tumor. For example, RNA expression from diffuse large B-cell lymphoma can be analyzed to form a multivariate predictor of survival after chemotherapy (Staudt, 2003). However, RNA expression analysis requires fresh tissue and specialized technology not yet available in standard pathology laboratories. Circulating tumor cells are more accessible than the tumor tissue; although this technology is still in its infancy. Finally, a return to standard immunohistochemistry is being used to characterize the functional status of tumors with the goal of directing therapy. For example, the presence of *ERCC1* in non-small-lung cancer indicates good DNA repair activity and predicted poor response to platinum agents (Reed, 2006).

Pathological changes within an organ might be reflected in protein patterns (Jain, 2004). The proteomics approach has been used to identify novel biomarkers, even in cytology specimens (Torres-Cabala et al., 2006) or serum (Petricoin et al., 2002). Since cancer is a very heterogeneous disease, a new approach of personalized management of cancer based on proteomic patterns may improve responses to therapy. Proteomic technologies combined with protein microarray assays represent a new tool for detecting disease and monitoring response to therapy (Jain, 2004).

7.3. PRACTICAL APPLICATIONS OF MOLECULAR PATHOLOGY BIOMARKERS

7.3.1. Selection of Methylating Chemotherapeutic Regimen

Oligodendrogliomas represent about 10 to 15% of all gliomas. These tumors are more frequent in young adults who may present with a seizure episode after a long, asymptomatic latent period (Burger, 2002). Radiologic features include calcifications of a curvilinear/gyriform distribution best seen on computed tomography (CT) scan, and by magnetic resonance imagining (MRI); these are T2 or Flair bright lesions with or without enhancement, and variable degrees of mass effect. The pathological diagnosis is based on Hematoxylin and Eosin (H&E) morphology of an infiltrating neoplasm with a monomorphic cell population with round nuclei, perinuclear halos (an artifact of formalin fixation), delicate, branching vessels, the so-called chicken-wire vasculature, and calcifications. As per the World Health Organization (WHO) classification, oligodendrogliomas are classified as well-differentiated (WHO grade II) and frankly malignant/anaplastic (WHO grade III) (Reifenberger, 2007). Grade III oligodendrogliomas are characterized by greater cellularity, atypia, and mitotic activity.

Historically, the diagnosis, prognosis, and selection of therapy of brain tumors have relied on histopathology. There is intersubject variability as there is for all histological diagnosis, with tumors being interpreted, based solely on their morphology, as astrocytic, oligodendroglial, or even mixed astrocytic/oligodendroglial in nature. To compound this issue, there are no immunohistochemical markers specific for oligodendroglial tumors. Myelin basic protein, myelin proteolipid protein, and myelin-associated glycoprotein, which are produced by oligodendrocytes, are not highly expressed in oligodendrogliomas (Schwechheimer et al., 1992; Sung et al., 1996). Well-differentiated oligodendroglioma cells are mostly immunonegative for glial fibrillary acidic protein (GFAP), but positive staining can be appreciated in the so-called transitional oligodendroglioma cells, including minigemystocytes and gliofibrillary oligodendrocytes. The basic helix–loop–helix transcription factor OLIG2 is specifically expressed in human oligodendrocytes (Marie et al., 2001; Yokoo et al., 2004) but is also expressed in various diffuse gliomas, limiting their specificity (Ligon et al., 2004; Rousseau et al., 2006). Potential, novel markers of oligodendroglial tumor cells include the transcription factors ASCL1 and NKX2-2 (Rousseau et al., 2006).

In the last two decades, anaplastic oligodendrogliomas were observed to respond more favorably to a chemotherapy regimen of procarbazine, lomustine/CCNU, and vincristine (PCV) than do astrocytic brain tumors (Cairncross and Macdonald, 1988; Cairncross et al., 1992, 1994, 1998, 2006; Bauman et al., 2000; Chahlavi et al., 2003; Hoang-Xuan et al., 2004; van den Bent et al., 2006). This observation necessitated the development of better molecular biomarkers to diagnose anaplastic oligodendrogliomas since chemotherapy would be added to patient therapy. In 1998, Cairncross and collaborators (1998) reported that oligodendrogliomas with the combined 1p/19q deletion had improved therapeutic response and longer survival. The combined 1p/19q deletion was demonstrated to be specific for oligodendroglial tumors and is reported in 50 to 80% of such cases (Bello et al., 1994; Reifenberger et al., 1994; Kros et al., 1999; Nigro et al., 2001; Hatanpaa et al., 2003; Felsberg et al., 2004; Fuller and Perry, 2005). This pattern of deletion appears to be associated with methylation of the *MGMT* promoter (Hegi et al., 2005; Mollemann et al., 2005), which may explain the better response to alkylating chemotherapeutic agents. *TP53* mutations, loss of

10q, loss of 9q, and amplification of the *EGFR* are inversely associated with 1p/19q deletions (Hoang-Xuan et al., 2001; Ino et al., 2001; Sasaki et al., 2001; Reifenberger and Louis, 2003; Huang et al., 2004; Jeon et al., 2007). Absence of 1p/19q deletion and aberrant expression of *p53* or loss of *p16* are poor prognostic biomarkers (Jeon et al., 2007).

Various molecular techniques may be used to detect these genetic alterations including loss of heterozygosity (LOH), comparative genomic hybrization (CGH), quantitative microsatellite analysis, chromogenic in situ hybridization (CISH), and fluorescence in situ hybridization (FISH). Recent literature suggests that combined 1p/19q deletions are associated with a balanced translocation between chromosomes 1 and 19 forming two derivative chromosomes, followed by loss of der(1:19)(p10:q10) and retention of der(1:19)(q10:p10) (Griffin et al., 2006; Jenkins et al., 2006).

The genomic signature can also be used in the diagnosis, prognosis, and selection of chemotherapy regimen for other brain tumors. As described above, loss of 1p/19q and the silencing of *MGMT* are genetic predictors of response to methylating chemotherapeutic agents. Other examples of genetic signatures used to differentiate brain tumors include infiltrating astrocytoma (most with 1p/19q intact; *p53* mutations, GFAP positivity), small-cell variants of anaplastic astrocytoma and glioblastoma multiforme (GBM, chromosome 10 loss, *EGFR* amplification), and dysembryoplastic neuroepithelial tumor (DNET; occurs in children; 1p/19q intact). As delineated above, today it is well accepted that patients with classical oligodendroglioma histology and combined loss of 1p/19q are more likely to respond to various chemotherapy and/or radiation therapy and have a more favorable outcome, which supports the role of 1p/19q status as a predictive and prognostic marker. It is yet unclear if this has to do with the signature genetic alterations they carry, or it has to do with their more indolent biological behavior. Nevertheless, it is clear that the loss of 1p/19q and the silencing of *MGMT* are genetic predictors of response and that they are used for guiding conventional therapy. Knowledge of the molecular characteristics of brain tumors will hopefully help in the development of additional, effective molecularly targeted therapy.

In the case example described below, the 1p/19q status revealed a deletion, supporting the use of chemotherapy and suggesting a better prognosis than patients with similar grade astrocytic tumors.

Case 1. Patient is a 23-year-old female who presents to the ER after a seizure episode. CT/MRI scans reveal a superficially situated, well-delineated tumor mass with curvilinear intracortical calcifications. A stereotactic brain biopsy is performed. Microscopic evaluation reveals an infiltrating glioma with monotonous bland cells with perinuclear halo, round nuclei, chicken-wire type vasculature, and focal calcifications. GFAP stain is negative, which helps exclude an astrocytic neoplasm. OLIG2 expression is prominent. MIB-1 index is low (less than 2%). A diagnosis of well-differentiated oligodendroglioma (WHO grade II) is rendered (Fig. 7.1). The clinician requests evaluation of chromosome 1p/19q status, which reveals the deletion (Fig. 7.2).

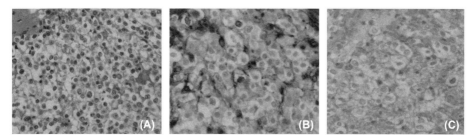

Figure 7.1. Oligodendroglioma. (A) Distinctive feature of oligodendrogliomas, perinuclear halos (a fixation artifact) highlight the uniform, perfectly round nuclei. (B) Occasional tumor cells with eosinophilic cytoplasm can be immunoreactive with GFAP. Most tumor cells are GFAP negative. (C) Low-grade oligodendrogliomas usually have very few MIB-1 immunopositive nuclei. See insert for color representation of this figure.

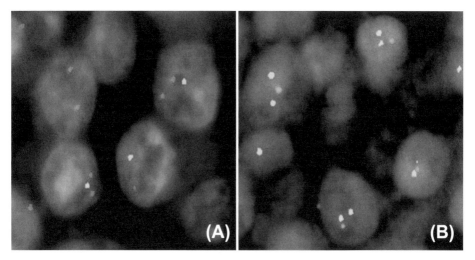

Figure 7.2. Representative FISH images. (A) and (B) are FISH images from an oligodendroglioma tumor. (A) 1p deletion is represented (the green signal is 1p32 and red is 1q42; mostly 1 green, 2 red signal pattern). (B) 19q deletion is represented (the green is 19p13 and red is 19q13.4 (mostly 2 green, 1 red pattern). (Courtesy of Dr. Arie Perry, St. Louis, Missouri.) See insert for color representation of this figure. [39]

7.3.2. Epidermal Growth Factor Receptor Expression Is Important Biomarker in Many Tumors

Glioblastoma multiforme (GBM, WHO grade IV) is a devastating disease, being the most common malignant glioma in adults, and it has a dismal prognosis (case 2). Two GBM subtypes are well recognized, the primary and secondary GBM (Kleihues and Ohgaki, 1999; Ohgaki and Kleihues, 2007). Primary or de novo GBM (likely diagnosis for the patient described below; case 2) is characterized by a short clinical history, with no clinicoradiological or histological evidence of a prior less malignant neoplasm. Secondary GBM develops as a progression from astrocytic tumors WHO grade II or III. Morover, these disease subtypes are also genetically distinct.

Primary GBM is characterized by overexpression and/or amplification of the *EGFR* gene, coupled with additional genetic alterations including deletion or mutation of the phosphatase and tensin homolog deleted from chromosome 10 (*PTEN*), homozygous deletions of *CDKN2A* (*p16*) gene, and murine double minute 2 gene (*MDM2*) amplification. Secondary GBM is associated with *P53* gene mutation, mainly involving codons 248 and 273 at CpG sites, and over-expression of platelet-derived growth factor (PDGF) ligand and receptors. *EGFR* amplification and/or overexpression and P53 mutations appear to be exclusive. Differences in pattern of promoter methylation, RNA, and protein levels are also distinct among primary and secondary GBM subtypes.

Colorectal carcinoma (CRC) is a common malignancy, and metastatic CRC is the second leading cause of cancer-related death in the United States. Surgery is potentially a curative treatment, but many patients develop metastatic CRC following radical surgery. In recent years, the standard first-line regimen for metastatic CRC includes a combination of 5FU-irinotecan or 5FU-oxaliplatin (Braun et al., 2004). Nevertheless, overall treatment results remain less than optimal. In the last few decades, molecular-targeted strategies for the treatment of patients who fail traditional therapy has brought hope to the oncology field. In solid tumors, the use of *EGFR* inhibitor agents singly or in association with other agents are being assessed in multiple phases I to III trials. *EGFR* inhibitors target either the extracellular domain (e.g., monoclonal antibodies such as cetux-imab) and against tyrosine kinase domain (e.g., tyrosine kinase inhibitors such as erlonitib). In contrast to *HER2*, the value of *EGFR* status as a predictive marker of response to therapy and prognostic indicator of disease progression is still being elucidated.

The ErbB receptor tyrosine kinase superfamily is composed of four related transmembrane proteins ErbB1 (EGFR), ErbB2 (HER2), ErbB3 (HER3), and ErbB4 (HER4). The *EGFR* is a 170-kDa glycoprotein composed of an extracel-lular ligand binding domain, a hydrophobic transmembrane region, and a cyto-plasmic domain containing both a tyrosine kinase domain as well as receptor regulatory motifs. Upon ligand binding, *EGFR* homo or heterodimerization occurs followed by tyrosine autophosphorylation. These phosphorylated tyro-sines serve as sites for activation of numerous signal transducers and adaptor molecules that, when activated, trigger a wide array of downstream signaling pathways, including the ras-raf-mitogen activated protein kinase (MAPK) pathway and the phosphatidylinositol 3-kinase (P13K)/Akt pathway (Salomon et al., 1995; Blume-Jensen and Hunter, 2001; Yarden and Sliwkowski, 2001; Baselga and Arteaga, 2005; Normanno et al., 2006; Scaltriti and Baselga, 2006). While the activation of *EGFR* in normal cells is under tight control, supra-physiologic activation of *EGFR* may occur in certain epithelial tumors. Unregulated activation may occur as a result of various pathways including mutations, gene amplification/overexpression, and structural rearrangements. The pathophysiologic result of such dysregulation includes oncogenic activities such as proliferation, migration, angiogenesis, stromal invasion, and resistance to apoptosis signals.

Epidermal growth factor receptor is known to be overexpressed in a variety of human cancers including head and neck carcinomas, non-small-cell lung carcinomas (NSCLC), pancreatic adenocarcinomas, brain gliomas, and colon carcinoma (Ozanne et al., 1986; Gullick, 1991; Arteaga, 2001; Adjei and Rowinsky, 2003; Syed and Rowinsky, 2003). Mutations of the *EGFR* gene may occur in NSCLC where they are reported to confer increased sensitivity to tyrosine kinase inhibitors. EGFR overexpression/activation is reportedly associated with advanced disease and poor prognosis (Mendelsohn and Baselga, 2000; Brabender et al., 2001; Cooke et al., 2001; Nicholson et al., 2001; Earp et al., 2003), and the presence of *EGFRvIII* mutant gene confers poor prognosis (Feldkamp et al., 1999). In brain tumors, *EGFR* is overexpressed in 24 to 95% of GBMs and amplified in 27 to 62% of the *EGFR*-overexpressing tumors, establishing a good correlation between amplification and overexpression in these tumors, especially in the small-cell GBM variant (Haas-Kogan et al., 2005; Quan et al., 2005; Quezado et al., 2005). The mutant *EGFRvIII* (which results from a large deletion involving exons 2 to 7) is observed in up to 70% of *EGFR*-overexpressing GBMs (Nishikawa et al., 2004). *EGFR* overexpression is appreciated in a high percentage of colorectal carcinomas (Salomon et al., 1995; Meropol, 2005; Ferrara et al., 2007) and has been found to correlate with progression and development of metastasis (Hayashi et al., 1994; Radinsky et al., 1995; Galizia et al., 2006).

Preliminary data suggest that some *EGFR* tyrosine kinase inhibitors may induce response in patients with tumors that had *EGFR* amplification/overexpression and low levels of phosphorylated PKB/Akt (Haas-Kogan et al., 2005b) and in tumors with co-expression of *EGFRvIII* and *PTEN* (Mellinghoff et al., 2005). However, a definitive correlation between drug sensitivity and *EGFR* status has not yet been proven (Lassman et al., 2005).

Cetuximab, a chimeric monoclonal antibody directed against *EGFR*, has shown efficacy in the treatment of patients with refractory CRC. Initial colorectal carcinoma clinical trials required *EGFR* positivity by immunohistochemistry (IHC) as an entry criterion (Cunningham et al., 2004; Saltz et al., 2004), which was based on the logical assumption that a target needs to be present for the drug to inhibit. *EGFR* expression was included in the drug label, since current Food and Drug Administration (FDA)-approved indication limits therapy to mCRC patients who overexpress *EGFR*. However, recent evidence indicates that EGFR expression irrespective of intensity and percentage of cells stained may not predict response to treatment since both *EGFR* expressors and nonexpressor tumors showed similar response rates to cetuximab therapy (Chung et al., 2005; Meropol, 2005; Dei Tos, 2007). *EGFR* expression may occur at different frequencies in the primary and metastatic disease from the same patient, suggesting that *EGFR* detection by current methodology may be inadequate to evaluate response in patients with metastatic disease (Scartozzi et al.,

2004). Moreover, current immunohistochemical methods of EGFR status detection may be inadequate. This is due to many reasons, including availability of multiple immunohistochemistry kits, and lack of standard criteria for reporting of results.

The utility of *EGFR* expression, amplification, and or mutation status as predictive versus prognostic biomarkers has not been fully resolved. Gene mutation and amplification status can be studied in formalin-fixed tissue; however, this is typically done only in academic centers or by companies. To detect amplification, FISH and CISH methodologies have been utilized and have shown to be effective in fresh, frozen, and formalin-fixed, paraffin-embedded tissues. The use of IHC to evaluate *EGFR* expression is common but also not considered standard pathology practice. As for other IHC stains, similar problems of subjective interpretation and variability in detection kits hinder interpretation. Nevertheless, the practicing pathologist in the near future will undoubtedly require robust knowledge of signal transduction pathways and the awareness of ever evolving technologies. Specifically, pathologists should become familiar with patterns of *EGFR* overexpression/amplification in tumor samples as detected by immunohistochemistry or more sophisticated methods such as CISH and FISH. Further studies should include the development of more predictive assays to evaluate for sensitivity for therapy.

The cases below are examples of potential utility of anti-EGFR-targeted therapy to human cancers.

Case 2. The patient is a 42-year-old male who presented to the ER after fainting at his daughter's soccer game. CT/MRI images revealed a large, contrast-enhancing, ring-shaped mass situated in the left frontal lobe and surrounded by area of cerebral edema. Microscopic evaluation revealed an infiltrating malignant neoplasm composed of monotonous, small, hyperchromatic undifferentiated cells, with areas of pseudopalisading necrosis, increased mitotic activity, and vascular proliferation. GFAP immunostaining was positive. Immunostaining for leukocyte common antigen (CD45) was negative. MIB-1 index was high (more than 40%). *P53* stains were negative. The most important differential diagnosis to consider would be primary or secondary malignant lymphoma. The presence of glial filaments within tumor cells was established by positivity reaction with GFAP staining, a marker of astrocytic differentiation. Immunostaining for CD45 was negative, helping to rule out the diagnosis of lymphoma. A diagnosis of glioblastoma mutiforme (WHO grade IV astrocytoma), small-cell variant was rendered (Fig. 7.3).

The patient underwent multimodality therapy including surgical debulking, radiation, and chemotherapy but progressed. The neurooncologist requested evaluation of *EGFR* status in original tumor represented on the formalin-fixed, paraffin-embedded tissue blocks. *EGFR* staining by IHC was 3+ (3/3), and true amplification was detected by CISH (Fig. 7.4). He was offered experimental treatment with anti-EGFR agent erlotinib (tyrosine kinase inhibitor) but had disease progression. The patient died one year after initial diagnosis.

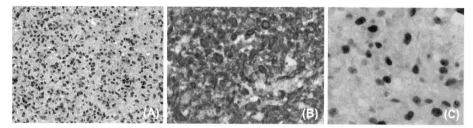

Figure 7.3. Small-cell GBM. (A) H&E morphology chracterized by monotonous population of bland, round cells. (B) Glial nature of the tumor established by strong GFAP positivity. (C) MIB-1 (Ki-67) labeling index is markedly elevated.

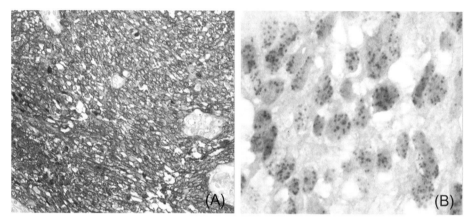

Figure 7.4. EGFR immunohistochemistry and CISH evaluation. (A) GBM, small-cell variant showing strong EGFR immunostaining (3+). (B) EGFR amplification detected by CISH.

Case 3. The patient is a 75-year-old female who presented with rectal bleeding. Colonoscopy revealed a fungating tumor in the left colon. Biopsy showed an invasive colonic adenocarcinoma, positive for cytokeratin 20 and negative for cytokeratin 7 (Fig. 7.5). This diagnosis is supported by the morphology in conjunction with the typical immunohistochemical profile of CK20 positivity/CK7 negativity, which is highly characteristic of colorectal cancer (Tot, 1999; Kummar et al., 2002; Park et al., 2002) and has been correlated with histologic grade and location (Park et al., 2002). CT scans during staging procedures detected multiple metastases to the liver. The patient was treated with an approved first-line treatment of FOLFOX but progressed. The original tumor and metastatic disease to liver were subsequently stained for *EGFR* and found to be positive (Fig. 7.5). The patient was then treated with cetuximab (anti-EGFR monoclonal antibody). One year later, the patient died from tumor progression.

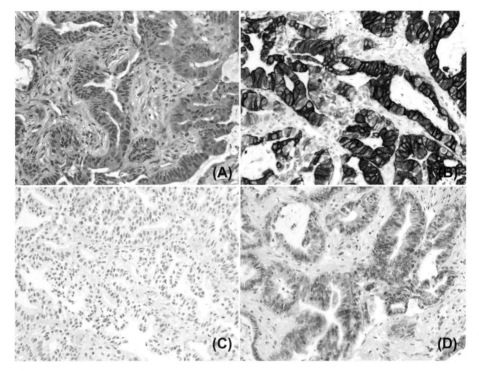

<u>Figure 7.5.</u> Colorectal adenocarcinoma. (A) Invasive moderately differentiated adenocarcinoma with a desmoplastic background. (B, C) Typical CD20+ (B)/CD7-(C) immunohistochemical profile. (D) Positive membranous/cytoplasmic EGFR staining. See insert for color representation of this figure.

7.3.3. Gastrointestinal Stromal Tumor and KIT Evaluation

Mesenchymal tumors of the gastrointestinal tract are not rare and include lesions similar to their soft-tissue counterparts as well as a heterogeneous group of tumors referred to as gastrointestinal stromal tumors (GISTs). GISTs are the most common mesenchymal tumors of the GI tract, accounting for 80% of such tumors (Miettinen and Lasota, 2001). Since the discovery of activating *KIT* or *PDGFRα* gene mutations in GISTs and their dramatic response to tyrosine kinase inhibitors, the accurate diagnosis of these tumors has become crucial. In 1998, these tumors were discovered to originate from the interstitial cells of Cajal (Hirota et al., 1998; Kindblom et al., 1998). Transgenic mouse models demonstrated that constitutional activation of *KIT* by mutations induces proliferation of Cajal cells and forms GISTs (Sommer et al., 2003; Rubin et al., 2005).

The *KIT* gene is located at chromosome 4q12 adjacent to a highly homologous *PDGFRα* gene. The c-KIT protein is a 145-kDa transmembrane protein belonging to the type III subfamily of the receptor tyrosine kinase and contains an extracellular and intracellular tyrosine kinase domain (Stenman et al., 1989; Pawson, 2002). Mutually exclusive mutations of two receptor tyrosine kinase proteins encoding genes, *KIT* and *PDGFRα*, are frequently encountered in GISTs, 80 to 85% of GISTs have *KIT* mutations, 5 to 10% harbor *PDGFRα* mutations, and the remaining 10% are wild type (Rubin, 2006).

Given the substantial morphologic variability within GIST tumors, immuno-phenotyping is often used to confirm the diagnosis. GIST tumors express CD117 (KIT; >95%), CD34 (60 to 70%), h-caldesmon (85%), SMA (30 to 40%), Desmin (1 to 2%), S100 (5%), and Keratin (1 to 2%) (Sarlomo-Rikala et al., 1998; Miettinen et al., 1999; Fletcher et al., 2002; Miettinen and Lasota, 2006; Rubin et al., 2007). Until recently, *KIT* expression was recognized as an absolute requirement for their diagnosis and implied an association to *KIT* mutations. In 2003, it became clear that some mesenchymal tumors with highly characteristic H&E morphology of GIST remained *KIT* immunonegative and *c-KIT* wild type. Of these *KIT* immunonegative GISTS, molecular evaluation demonstrated the presence of *PDGFRα* or *KIT* mutations in many (Heinrich et al., 2003b; Debiec-Rychter et al., 2004; Emile et al., 2004; Tzen and Mau, 2005). Evaluation of *PDGFRα* expression is currently limited by the absence of commercially useful antibodies for formalin-fixed, paraffin-embedded tissues (Hornick and Fletcher, 2007). KIT-negative IHC tumors that contain *KIT/PDGFRα* mutations may be imanitib sensitive (Corless et al., 2005; Weisberg et al., 2006). Recent clinical studies report that the presence and location of *KIT* and *PDGFRα* mutations correlate with response to imanitib therapy (Heinrich et al., 2003b; Debiec-Rychter et al., 2004a) and in the selection of the optimal dose of imanitib (Debiec-Rychter et al., 2006). Specifically, patients with tumor mutation in the most common c-KIT juxtamembrane domain in the proximal part of exon 11 (codons 550 to 562) are expected to be excellent responders to imanitib therapy, while patients with tumor mutation in the *PDGFRα* exon 18 (D842V) or with no *KIT* mutation are less likely to have favorable responses to imanitib treatment. Unfortunately, the majority of patients eventually develop progressive disease associated with the development of new *KIT/PDGFRα* imanitib-resistant muta-tions (Wakai et al., 2004; Antonescu et al., 2005; Chen et al., 2005).

As described above, the pathologist needs to be aware that KIT positivity is not a requirement for diagnosis but is frequently seen in GISTs. On the other hand, KIT positivity is also seen in other tumors and a broad immunohistochemi-cal panel may be necessary to establish the correct diagnosis. Lack of or weak KIT expression does not seem to correlate with type of *KIT* mutation or likeli-hood of response to tyrosine kinase inhibitor therapy. At this moment, KIT nega-tivity in tissue specimens should not discard the diagnosis of GIST and should not be grounds for denial for Tyrosine Kinase Inhibitors (TKI) drug therapy. While it is tempting to consider mutational analysis as a means to predict response to therapy, this is not feasible currently. Nevertheless, pathologists should be able to triage cases that despite KIT immunonegative are still best classified as GISTs. Patients with such tumors can benefit from targeted therapy.

Case 4. A 63-year-old male presents to his family doctor complaining of vague stomach pain, fullness, and a recent episode of hematemesis. Gastrointestinal

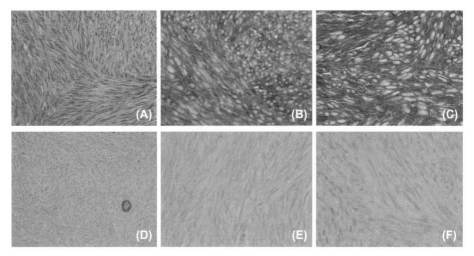

Figure 7.6. Gastrointestinal stromal tumor H&E and immunohistochemical phenotype. (A) Spindle cell neoplasm with moderate cellularity. (B) Strong membranous KIT positivity. (C) Extensive CD34 positivity. (D, E, F) Negative staining for SMA, desmin and S100, repectively. See insert for color representation of this figure.

workup detects a large gastric mass (estimated 15 cm in largest dimension) possibly extending to the pancreas. A biopsy is obtained and shows a cellular spindle cell neoplasm positive for CD117 (CKIT), CD34, negative for alpha smooth muscle actin (SMA), and for S100 and desmin (Fig. 7.6). MIB1 staining shows a high proliferative index (>10%). A diagnosis of GIST was rendered. Since the mass was deemed unresectable, with possible pancreatic involvement, the patient was placed on KIT/PDGFR tyrosine kinase inhibitor, imatinib. After 6 months on therapy, the mass was amenable to surgical resection.

7.3.4. Chronic Myeloid Leukemia and BCR-ABL Protooncogene

Chronic myeloid leukemia (CML) is a rare disease with an annual incidence of 1.6 cases/100,000 adults (Jemal et al., 2006). The median patient age at diagnosis is 65 years and about 90% of patients are diagnosed at chronic phase with little or no symptoms, followed by an accelerated phase, and the terminal blastic phase (Faderl et al., 1999a, 1999b; Mughal and Goldman, 2006; Quintas-Cardama and Cortes, 2006). Elevated white blood cell count with basophilia, decreased neutrophil alkaline phosphatase, and the presence of the Philadelphia chromosome, as observed in the case described below, are characteristic of CML.

The oncogene that causes CML is the *BCR-ABL* oncogene, the product of Philadelphia chromosome (Ph)22q (Bartram et al., 1983; Barnes and Melo, 2002). This protooncogene derives from a reciprocal translocation involving the *BCR* gene on chromosome 22q11 and the *ABL* protooncogene on chromosome 9q34 (t[9;22][q34;q11]). It encodes for the 210-kDa BCR-ABL oncoprotein, an abnormal, non-membrane-bound protein expressed in about 95% of patients with CML. The BCR-ABL oncoprotein has a constitutively activated ABL tyrosine kinase activity that activates numerous signal transduction pathways including Ras/Raf/mitogen-activated protein kinase (MAPK), phosphatidylinositol 3 kinase P13K, STAT5/Janus kinase, and Myc. Deregulation of these pathways is associated with cell proliferation, decreased apoptosis, and consequent expansion of malignant pluripotent stem cells in the bone marrow. Additional molecular alterations, including involvement of the Src family kinases, may be implicated in the progression of chronic to blastic CML phases (Lionberger et al., 2000; Donato et al., 2003).

Chronic myeloid leukemia patients with the *BCR-ABL* oncogene have benefited tremendously by the development of drugs targeting the BCR-ABL tyrosine kinase, including imatinib and dasatinib. The current standard of care for first-line treatment for CML is targeted therapy with imatinib mesylate, a small-molecule tyrosine kinase inhibitor. Most patients receive a trial of imatinib before being considered for allogeneic hematopoietic cell transplantation (Giralt et al., 2007). Patients with the best response include those in chronic phase, but not acute or blastic phase, and remission is characterized by normalization or near normalization of bone marrow in most cases. Imatinib therapy is associated with hematological response rates of more than 90% and complete cytogenetic response rates of 50% (Giralt et al., 1993; Druker et al., 2001). The phase III International Randomized Study of Interferon and ST1571 trial has demonstrated the efficacy of imanitib, which reports the superiority of imanitib in comparison to Interferon α (IFN-α)-based treatment in regards to hematologic response, cytogenetic response, molecular response, and progression-free survival. While the success rate with this drug has revolutionized the treatment and prognosis of patients with CML, primary and secondary resistance to imanitib is well documented and a significant treatment hurdle. Various mechanisms contribute to imanitib resistance, including mutations in several areas of the BCR-ABL molecule (Hochhaus et al., 2002; Branford et al., 2003; Lahaye et al., 2005; Martinelli et al., 2005). Mutations in the ATP-binding site (P-loop) have been reportedly associated with a poor prognosis (Branford et al., 2003). In order to overcome imanitib resistance, both imanitib dose escalation and development of new targeted therapies have been clinically accepted.

Dasatinib (also known as Sprycel), one of the newest, extremely potent tyrosine kinase inhibitor binds both the active and inactive conformations of the BCR-ABL protein and blocks multiple different oncogenic proteins including Scr family kinase, Kit, PDGFR, and ephrin A receptor kinase (Nam et al., 2005; Schittenhelm et al., 2006). It appears to "counteract" all imanitib-resistant kinase domain mutations but one. Dasatinib has been demonstrated to induce hematologic and cytogenetic response in all phases of CML and in patients with imanitib resistance or intolerance (Talpaz et al., 2006; Cortes et al., 2007). As a result of these very encouraging findings, dasatinib has been recently FDA approved for CML patients of all phases who present with resistance/intolerance to prior treatments.

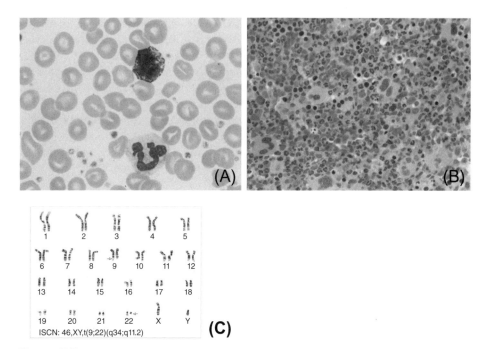

ISCN: 46,XY,t(9;22)(q34;q11.2)

Figure 7.7. Chronic myelogenous leukemia. (A) CML, peripheral blood. (B) CML, bone marrow aspirate. (A,B Courtesy of Dr. Irina Maric, HEMATOLOGY, CC/NIH) (C) G-banded karyotype of a bone marrow metaphase cell from a patient with CML showing a single Philadelphia chromosome (Ph) arising from the common 9;22 translocation. (Courtesy of Dr. Diane Arthur, LP/NCI/NIH)

Case 5. A 65-year-old male presents to his internist for his annual routine physical evaluation. He complains of fatigue but is otherwise asymptomatic. Upon physical exam, splenomegaly is detected. Blood examination reveals an unexpected elevated white blood cell count with numerous basophils. Bone marrow sections are hypercellular with increased granulocytes and megakaryocytes. Myeloblasts in blood and marrow smears are less than 5%. The diagnosis of CML, chronic phase, is rendered. Cytogenetics/molecular analysis illustrated the presence of Philadelphia chromosome (Fig. 7.7). The patient was placed on imatinib therapy but failed to show complete hematological remission. He was then placed on dasatinib therapy.

7.4. CONCLUSION

The era of targeted therapy has arrived and demands molecular pathology to guide treatment and provide prognostic and diagnostic support. This rapidly changing environment requires pathologists to extend their understanding of disease pathology beyond that of bright-field microscopy. Molecular pathology in the past was primarily of diagnostic and prognostic value. Today, molecular pathology is also being used to predict those patients likely to respond to chemotherapeutic and targeted anticancer agents.

REFERENCES

Adjei, A. A., and Rowinsky, E. K. (2003). Novel anticancer agents in clinical development. *Cancer Biol. Ther.* 2(4 Suppl 1):S5–15.

Antonescu, C. R., Besmer, P., et al. (2005). Acquired resistance to imatinib in gastrointestinal stromal tumor occurs through secondary gene mutation. *Clin. Cancer Res.* 11(11):4182–4190.

Arteaga, C. L. (2001). The epidermal growth factor receptor: From mutant oncogene in nonhuman cancers to therapeutic target in human neoplasia. *J. Clin. Oncol.* 19(18 Suppl):32S–40S.

Barnes, D. J., and Melo, J. V. (2002). Cytogenetic and molecular genetic aspects of chronic myeloid leukaemia. *Acta Haematol.* 108(4):180–202.

Bartram, C. R., de Klein, A., et al. (1983). Translocation of c-abl oncogene correlates with the presence of a Philadelphia chromosome in chronic myelocytic leukaemia. *Nature* 306(5940):277–280.

Baselga, J., and Arteaga, C. L. (2005). Critical update and emerging trends in epidermal growth factor receptor targeting in cancer. *J. Clin. Oncol.* 23(11):2445–2459.

Bauman, G. S., Ino, Y., et al. (2000). Allelic loss of chromosome 1p and radiotherapy plus chemotherapy in patients with oligodendrogliomas. *Int. J. Radiat. Oncol. Biol. Phys.* 48(3):825–830.

Bello, M. J., Vaquero, J., et al. (1994). Molecular analysis of chromosome 1 abnormalities in human gliomas reveals frequent loss of 1p in oligodendroglial tumors. *Int. J. Cancer* 57(2):172–175.

Berman, D. M., Wincovitch, S., et al. (2005). Grading melanocytic dysplasia in paraffin wax embedded tissue by the nucleic acid index. *J. Clin. Pathol.* 58(11):1206–1210.

Bertucci, F., Viens, P., et al. (2003). DNA arrays in clinical oncology: Promises and challenges. *Lab. Invest.* 83(3):305–316.

Bilous, M., Morey, A., et al. (2006). Chromogenic in situ hybridisation testing for HER2 gene amplification in breast cancer produces highly reproducible results concordant with fluorescence in situ hybridisation and immunohistochemistry. *Pathology* 38(2): 120–124.

Blume-Jensen, P., and Hunter, T. (2001). Oncogenic kinase signalling. *Nature* 411(6835): 355–365.

Brabender, J., Danenberg, K. D., et al. (2001). Epidermal growth factor receptor and HER2-neu mRNA expression in non-small cell lung cancer Is correlated with survival. *Clin. Cancer Res.* 7(7):1850–1855.

Branford, S., Rudzki, Z., et al. (2003). Detection of BCR-ABL mutations in patients with CML treated with imatinib is virtually always accompanied by clinical resistance, and mutations in the ATP phosphate-binding loop (P-loop) are associated with a poor prognosis. *Blood* 102(1):276–283.

Braun, A. H., Achterrath, W., et al. (2004). New systemic frontline treatment for metastatic colorectal carcinoma. *Cancer* 100(8):1558–1577.

Burger, P. C., Scheithauer, B. W., and Vogel, F. S. (2002). The brain: Tumors. In *Oligodendroglioma and Mixed Glioma (Oligoastrocytoma). Surgical Pathology of the Nervous System and Its Coverings.* Burger, P. C., Scheithauer B. W., and Vogel, F. S. (Eds.). Elsevier, Amsterdam, pp. 223–241.

Cacev, T., Radosevic, S., et al. (2005). NF1 gene loss of heterozygosity and expression analysis in sporadic colon cancer. *Gut* 54(8):1129–1135.

Cairncross, J. G., and Macdonald, D. R. (1988). Successful chemotherapy for recurrent malignant oligodendroglioma. *Ann. Neurol.* 23(4):360–364.

Cairncross, J. G., Macdonald, D. R., et al. (1992). Aggressive oligodendroglioma: A chemosensitive tumor. *Neurosurgery* 31(1):78–82.

Cairncross, G., Macdonald, D., et al. (1994). Chemotherapy for anaplastic oligodendroglioma. National Cancer Institute of Canada Clinical Trials Group. *J. Clin. Oncol.* 12(10):2013–2021.

Cairncross, J. G., Ueki, K., et al. (1998). Specific genetic predictors of chemotherapeutic response and survival in patients with anaplastic oligodendrogliomas. *J. Natl. Cancer Inst.* 90(19):1473–1479.

Cairncross, G., Berkey, B., et al. (2006). Phase III trial of chemotherapy plus radiotherapy compared with radiotherapy alone for pure and mixed anaplastic oligodendroglioma: Intergroup Radiation Therapy Oncology Group Trial 9402. *J. Clin. Oncol.* 24(18):2707–2714.

Chahlavi, A., Kanner, A., et al. (2003). Impact of chromosome 1p status in response of oligodendroglioma to temozolomide: Preliminary results. *J. Neurooncol.* 61(3):267–273.

Chen, L. L., Sabripour, M., et al. (2005). Imatinib resistance in gastrointestinal stromal tumors. *Curr. Oncol. Rep.* 7(4):293–299.

Chung, K. Y., Shia, J., et al. (2005). Cetuximab shows activity in colorectal cancer patients with tumors that do not express the epidermal growth factor receptor by immunohistochemistry. *J. Clin. Oncol.* 23(9):1803–1810.

Cooke, T., Reeves, J., et al. (2001). The value of the human epidermal growth factor receptor-2 (HER2) as a prognostic marker. *Eur. J. Cancer* 37(Suppl 1):3–10.

Corless, C. L., Schroeder, A., et al. (2005). PDGFRA mutations in gastrointestinal stromal tumors: Frequency, spectrum and in vitro sensitivity to imatinib. *J. Clin. Oncol.* 23(23): 5357–5364.

Cortes, J., Rousselot, P., et al. (2007). Dasatinib induces complete hematologic and cytogenetic responses in patients with imatinib-resistant or -intolerant chronic myeloid leukemia in blast crisis. *Blood* 109(8):3207–3213.

Crocker, J. (2002). Demystified ... Molecular pathology in oncology. *Mol. Pathol.* 55(6): 337–347.

Cunningham, D., Humblet, Y., et al. (2004). Cetuximab monotherapy and cetuximab plus irinotecan in irinotecan-refractory metastatic colorectal cancer. *N. Engl. J. Med.* 351(4): 337–345.

Daniele, L., Macri, L., et al. (2007). Predicting gefitinib responsiveness in lung cancer by fluorescence in situ hybridization/chromogenic in situ hybridization analysis of EGFR and HER2 in biopsy and cytology specimens. *Mol. Cancer Ther.* 6(4):1223–1229.

Debiec-Rychter, M., Dumez, H., et al. (2004a). Use of c-KIT/PDGFRA mutational analysis to predict the clinical response to imatinib in patients with advanced gastrointestinal stromal tumours entered on phase I and II studies of the EORTC Soft Tissue and Bone Sarcoma Group. *Eur. J. Cancer* 40(5):689–695.

Debiec-Rychter, M., Wasag, B., et al. (2004b). Gastrointestinal stromal tumours (GISTs) negative for KIT (CD117 antigen) immunoreactivity. *J. Pathol.* 202(4):430–438.

Debiec-Rychter, M., Sciot, R., et al. (2006). KIT mutations and dose selection for imatinib in patients with advanced gastrointestinal stromal tumours. *Eur. J. Cancer* 42(8): 1093–1103.

Dei Tos, A. P. (2007). The biology of epidermal growth factor receptor and its value as a prognostic/predictive factor. *Int. J. Biol. Markers* 22(1 Suppl 4):S3–9.

Donato, N. J., Wu, J. Y., et al. (2003). BCR-ABL independence and LYN kinase overexpression in chronic myelogenous leukemia cells selected for resistance to STI571. *Blood* 101(2):690–698.

Druker, B. J., Sawyers, C. L., et al. (2001). Activity of a specific inhibitor of the BCR-ABL tyrosine kinase in the blast crisis of chronic myeloid leukemia and acute lymphoblastic leukemia with the Philadelphia chromosome. *N. Engl. J. Med.* 344(14):1038–1042.

Earp, H. S., 3rd, Calvo, B. F., et al. (2003). The EGF receptor family—multiple roles in proliferation, differentiation, and neoplasia with an emphasis on HER4. *Trans. Am. Clin. Climatol. Assoc.* 114:315–333; discussion 333–334.

Emile, J. F., Theou, N., et al. (2004). Clinicopathologic, phenotypic, and genotypic characteristics of gastrointestinal mesenchymal tumors. *Clin. Gastroenterol. Hepatol.* 2(7):597–605.

Faderl, S., Kantarjian, H. M., et al. (1999a). Chronic myelogenous leukemia: Update on biology and treatment. *Oncol. (Williston Park)* 13(2):169–180; discussion 181, 184.

Faderl, S., Talpaz, M., et al. (1999b). Chronic myelogenous leukemia: Biology and therapy. *Ann. Intern. Med.* 131(3):207–219.

Feldkamp, M. M., Lala, P., et al. (1999). Expression of activated epidermal growth factor receptors, Ras-guanosine triphosphate, and mitogen-activated protein kinase in human glioblastoma multiforme specimens. *Neurosurgery* 45(6):1442–1453.

Felsberg, J., Erkwoh, A., et al. (2004). Oligodendroglial tumors: Refinement of candidate regions on chromosome arm 1p and correlation of 1p/19q status with survival. *Brain Pathol.* 14(2):121–130.

Ferrara, G., Palombi, N., et al. (2007). Epidermal growth factor receptor and prognosis in colon cancer: A crack in the wall? *Ann. Surg. Oncol.* 14(7):2169–2170.

Fletcher, C. D., Berman, J. J., et al. (2002). Diagnosis of gastrointestinal stromal tumors: A consensus approach. *Hum. Pathol.* 33(5):459–465.

Fuller, C. E., and Perry, A. (2005). Molecular diagnostics in central nervous system tumors. *Adv. Anat. Pathol.* 12(4):180–194.

Galizia, G., Lieto, E., et al. (2006). Prognostic significance of epidermal growth factor receptor expression in colon cancer patients undergoing curative surgery. *Ann. Surg. Oncol.* 13(6):823–835.

Giralt, S. A., Kantarjian, H. M., et al. (1993). Effect of prior interferon alfa therapy on the outcome of allogeneic bone marrow transplantation for chronic myelogenous leukemia. *J. Clin. Oncol.* 11(6):1055–1061.

Giralt, S. A., Arora, M., et al. (2007). Impact of imatinib therapy on the use of allogeneic haematopoietic progenitor cell transplantation for the treatment of chronic myeloid leukaemia. *Br. J. Haematol.* 137(5):461–467.

Going, J. J., and Gusterson, B. A. (1999). Molecular pathology and future developments. *Eur. J. Cancer* 35(14):1895–1904.

Griffin, C. A., Burger, P., et al. (2006). Identification of der(1;19)(q10;p10) in five oligodendrogliomas suggests mechanism of concurrent 1p and 19q loss. *J. Neuropathol. Exp. Neurol.* 65(10):988–994.

Gullick, W. J. (1991). Prevalence of aberrant expression of the epidermal growth factor receptor in human cancers. *Br. Med. Bull.* 47(1):87–98.

Haas-Kogan, D. A., Prados, M. D., et al. (2005a). Biomarkers to predict response to epidermal growth factor receptor inhibitors. *Cell Cycle* 4(10):1369–1372.

Haas-Kogan, D. A., Prados, M. D., et al. (2005b). Epidermal growth factor receptor, protein kinase B/Akt, and glioma response to erlotinib. *J. Natl. Cancer Inst.* 97(12):880–887.

Hatanpaa, K. J., Burger, P. C., et al. (2003). Molecular diagnosis of oligodendroglioma in paraffin sections. *Lab. Invest.* 83(3):419–428.

Hayashi, Y., Widjono, Y. W., et al. (1994). Expression of EGF, EGF-receptor, p53, v-erb B and ras p21 in colorectal neoplasms by immunostaining paraffin-embedded tissues. *Pathol. Int.* 44(2):124–130.

Hegi, M. E., Diserens, A. C., et al. (2005). MGMT gene silencing and benefit from temozolomide in glioblastoma. *N. Engl. J. Med.* 352(10):997–1003.

Heinrich, M. C., Corless, C. L., et al. (2003a). Kinase mutations and imatinib response in patients with metastatic gastrointestinal stromal tumor. *J. Clin. Oncol.* 21(23): 4342–4349.

Heinrich, M. C., Corless, C. L., et al. (2003b). PDGFRA activating mutations in gastrointestinal stromal tumors. *Science* 299(5607):708–710.

Hirota, S., Isozaki, K., et al. (1998). Gain-of-function mutations of c-kit in human gastrointestinal stromal tumors. *Science* 279(5350):577–580.

Hoang-Xuan, K., He, J., et al. (2001). Molecular heterogeneity of oligodendrogliomas suggests alternative pathways in tumor progression. *Neurology* 57(7):1278–1281.

Hoang-Xuan, K., Capelle, L., et al. (2004). Temozolomide as initial treatment for adults with low-grade oligodendrogliomas or oligoastrocytomas and correlation with chromosome 1p deletions. *J. Clin. Oncol.* 22(15):3133–3138.

Hochhaus, A., Kreil, S., et al. (2002). Molecular and chromosomal mechanisms of resistance to imatinib (STI571) therapy. *Leukemia* 16(11):2190–2196.

Hornick, J. L., and Fletcher, C. D. (2007). The role of KIT in the management of patients with gastrointestinal stromal tumors. *Hum. Pathol.* 38(5):679–687.

Huang, H., Okamoto, Y., et al. (2004). Gene expression profiling and subgroup identification of oligodendrogliomas. *Oncogene* 23(35):6012–6022.

Ino, Y., Betensky, R. A., et al. (2001). Molecular subtypes of anaplastic oligodendroglioma: Implications for patient management at diagnosis. *Clin. Cancer Res.* 7(4):839–845.

Jain, K. K. (2004). Role of oncoproteomics in the personalized management of cancer. *Expert. Rev. Proteomics* 1(1):49–55.

Jemal, A., Siegel, R., et al. (2006). Cancer statistics, 2006. *CA Cancer J. Clin.* 56(2): 106–130.

Jenkins, R. B., Blair, H., et al. (2006). A t(1;19)(q10;p10) mediates the combined deletions of 1p and 19q and predicts a better prognosis of patients with oligodendroglioma. *Cancer Res.* 66(20):9852–9861.

Jeon, Y. K., Park, K., et al. (2007). Chromosome 1p and 19q status and p53 and p16 expression patterns as prognostic indicators of oligodendroglial tumors: a clinicopathological study using fluorescence in situ hybridization. *Neuropathology* 27(1):10–20.

Kaneko, S., Gerasimova, T., et al. (2002). The use of FISH on breast core needle samples for the presurgical assessment of HER-2 oncogene status. *Exp. Mol. Pathol.* 73(1): 61–66.

Kindblom, L. G., Remotti, H. E., et al. (1998). Gastrointestinal pacemaker cell tumor (GIPACT): Gastrointestinal stromal tumors show phenotypic characteristics of the interstitial cells of Cajal. *Am. J. Pathol.* 152(5):1259–1269.

Kleihues, P., and Ohgaki, H. (1999). Primary and secondary glioblastomas: From concept to clinical diagnosis. *Neuro. Oncol.* 1(1):44–51.

Kros, J. M., van Run, P. R., et al. (1999). Genetic aberrations in oligodendroglial tumours: An analysis using comparative genomic hybridization (CGH). *J. Pathol.* 188(3):282–288.

Kummar, S., Fogarasi, M., et al. (2002). Cytokeratin 7 and 20 staining for the diagnosis of lung and colorectal adenocarcinoma. *Br. J. Cancer* 86(12):1884–1887.

Lahaye, T., Riehm, B., et al. (2005). Response and resistance in 300 patients with BCR-ABL-positive leukemias treated with imatinib in a single center: A 4.5-year follow-up. *Cancer* 103(8):1659–1669.

Lassman, A. B., Rossi, M. R., et al. (2005). Molecular study of malignant gliomas treated with epidermal growth factor receptor inhibitors: tissue analysis from North American Brain Tumor Consortium Trials 01-03 and 00-01. *Clin. Cancer Res.* 11(21): 7841–7850.

Li-Ning, T. E., Ronchetti, R., et al. (2005). Role of chromogenic in situ hybridization (CISH) in the evaluation of HER2 status in breast carcinoma: Comparison with immunohistochemistry and FISH. *Int. J. Surg. Pathol.* 13(4):343–351.

Ligon, K. L., Alberta, J. A., et al. (2004). The oligodendroglial lineage marker OLIG2 is universally expressed in diffuse gliomas. *J. Neuropathol. Exp. Neurol.* 63(5):499–509.

Lionberger, J. M., Wilson, M. B., et al. (2000). Transformation of myeloid leukemia cells to cytokine independence by Bcr-Abl is suppressed by kinase-defective Hck. *J. Biol. Chem.* 275(24):18581–18585.

Marie, Y., Sanson, M., et al. (2001). OLIG2 as a specific marker of oligodendroglial tumour cells. *Lancet* 358(9278):298–300.

Martinelli, G., Soverini, S., et al. (2005). New tyrosine kinase inhibitors in chronic myeloid leukemia. *Haematologica* 90(4):534–541.

Mazumder, A., and Wang, Y. (2006). Gene-expression signatures in oncology diagnostics. *Pharmacogenomics* 7(8):1167–1173.

Mellinghoff, I. K., Wang, M. Y., et al. (2005). Molecular determinants of the response of glioblastomas to EGFR kinase inhibitors. *N. Engl. J. Med.* 353(19):2012–2024.

Mendelsohn, J., and Baselga, J. (2000). The EGF receptor family as targets for cancer therapy. *Oncogene* 19(56):6550–6565.

Meropol, N. J. (2005). Epidermal growth factor receptor inhibitors in colorectal cancer: it's time to get back on target. *J. Clin. Oncol.* 23(9):1791–1793.

Miettinen, M., and Lasota, J. (2001). Gastrointestinal stromal tumors—definition, clinical, histological, immunohistochemical, and molecular genetic features and differential diagnosis. *Virchows Arch.* 438(1):1–12.

Miettinen, M., and Lasota, J. (2006). Gastrointestinal stromal tumors: Review on morphology, molecular pathology, prognosis, and differential diagnosis. *Arch. Pathol. Lab. Med.* 130(10):1466–1478.

Miettinen, M. M., Sarlomo-Rikala, M., et al. (1999). Calponin and h-caldesmon in soft tissue tumors: Consistent h-caldesmon immunoreactivity in gastrointestinal stromal tumors indicates traits of smooth muscle differentiation. *Mod. Pathol.* 12(8):756–762.

Mocellin, S., Provenzano, M., et al. (2005). DNA array-based gene profiling: From surgical specimen to the molecular portrait of cancer. *Ann. Surg.* 241(1):16–26.

Mollemann, M., Wolter, M., et al. (2005). Frequent promoter hypermethylation and low expression of the MGMT gene in oligodendroglial tumors. *Int. J. Cancer* 113(3):379–385.

Mughal, T. I., and Goldman, J. M. (2006). Chronic myeloid leukemia: Why does it evolve from chronic phase to blast transformation? *Front. Biosci.* 11:198–208.

Naidoo, R., and Chetty, R. (1998). The application of microsatellites in molecular pathology. *Pathol. Oncol. Res.* 4(4):310–315.

Nam, S., Kim, D., et al. (2005). Action of the Src family kinase inhibitor, dasatinib (BMS-354825), on human prostate cancer cells. *Cancer Res.* 65(20):9185–9189.

Netto, G. J., and Saad, R. D. (2006). Diagnostic molecular pathology: An increasingly indispensable tool for the practicing pathologist. *Arch. Pathol. Lab. Med.* 130(9): 1339–1348.

Nicholson, R. I., Gee, J. M., et al. (2001). EGFR and cancer prognosis. *Eur. J. Cancer* 37(Suppl 4):S9–15.

Nigro, J. M., Takahashi, M. A., et al. (2001). Detection of 1p and 19q loss in oligodendroglioma by quantitative microsatellite analysis, a real-time quantitative polymerase chain reaction assay. *Am. J. Pathol.* 158(4):1253–1262.

Nishikawa, R., Sugiyama, T., et al. (2004). Immunohistochemical analysis of the mutant epidermal growth factor, deltaEGFR, in glioblastoma. *Brain Tumor Pathol.* 21(2): 53–56.

Nordgren, A. (2003). Hidden aberrations diagnosed by interphase fluorescence in situ hybridisation and spectral karyotyping in childhood acute lymphoblastic leukaemia. *Leuk. Lymphoma* 44(12):2039–2053.

Normanno, N., De Luca, A., et al. (2006). Epidermal growth factor receptor (EGFR) signaling in cancer. *Gene* 366(1):2–16.

Ohgaki, H., and Kleihues, P. (2007). Genetic pathways to primary and secondary glioblastoma. *Am. J. Pathol.* 170(5):1445–1453.

Ozanne, B., Richards, C. S., et al. (1986). Over-expression of the EGF receptor is a hallmark of squamous cell carcinomas. *J. Pathol.* 149(1):9–14.

Park, S. Y., Kim, H. S., et al. (2002). Expression of cytokeratins 7 and 20 in primary carcinomas of the stomach and colorectum and their value in the differential diagnosis of metastatic carcinomas to the ovary. *Hum. Pathol.* 33(11):1078–1085.

Pawson, T. (2002). Regulation and targets of receptor tyrosine kinases. *Eur. J. Cancer* 38(Suppl 5):S3–10.

Petricoin, E. F., Ardekani, A. M., et al. (2002). Use of proteomic patterns in serum to identify ovarian cancer. *Lancet* 359(9306):572–577.

Quan, A. L., Barnett, G. H., et al. (2005). Epidermal growth factor receptor amplification does not have prognostic significance in patients with glioblastoma multiforme. *Int. J. Radiat. Oncol. Biol. Phys.* 63(3):695–703.

Quezado, M., Ronchetti, R., et al. (2005). Chromogenic in situ hybridization accurately identifies EGFR amplification in small cell glioblastoma multiforme, a common subtype of primary GBM. *Clin. Neuropathol.* 24(4):163–169.

Quintas-Cardama, A., and Cortes, J. E. (2006). Chronic myeloid leukemia: Diagnosis and treatment. *Mayo Clin. Proc.* 81(7):973–988.

Radinsky, R., Risin, S., et al. (1995). Level and function of epidermal growth factor receptor predict the metastatic potential of human colon carcinoma cells. *Clin. Cancer Res.* 1(1):19–31.

Reed, E. (2006). ERCC1 measurements in clinical oncology. *N. Engl. J. Med.* 355(10): 1054–1055.

Reifenberger, G., and Louis, D. N. (2003). Oligodendroglioma: Toward molecular definitions in diagnostic neuro-oncology. *J. Neuropathol. Exp. Neurol.* 62(2):111–126.

Reifenberger, J., Reifenberger, G., et al. (1994). Molecular genetic analysis of oligodendroglial tumors shows preferential allelic deletions on 19q and 1p. *Am. J. Pathol.* 145(5):1175–1190.

Reifenberger, G., Kros, J. M., Louis, D. N., and Collins, V. P. (2007). Oligodendroglial tumors. In *WHO Classification of Tumours of the Central Nervous System.* Louis, D. N., Ohgaki, H., Wiestler, O. D., and Cavenee, W. K. (Eds.). WHO, Geneva, pp. 53–68.

Rousseau, A., Nutt, C. L., et al. (2006). Expression of oligodendroglial and astrocytic lineage markers in diffuse gliomas: Use of YKL-40, ApoE, ASCL1, and NKX2-2. *J. Neuropathol. Exp. Neurol.* 65(12):1149–1156.

Roylance, R. (2002). Methods of molecular analysis: Assessing losses and gains in tumours. *Mol. Pathol.* 55(1):25–28.

Rubin, B. P. (2006). Gastrointestinal stromal tumours: An update. *Histopathology* 48(1):83–96.

Rubin, B. P., Antonescu, C. R., et al. (2005). A knock-in mouse model of gastrointestinal stromal tumor harboring kit K641E. *Cancer Res.* 65(15):6631–6639.

Rubin, B. P., Heinrich, M. C., et al. (2007). Gastrointestinal stromal tumour. *Lancet* 369(9574):1731–1741.

Salomon, D. S., Brandt, R., et al. (1995). Epidermal growth factor-related peptides and their receptors in human malignancies. *Crit. Rev. Oncol. Hematol.* 19(3):183–232.

Saltz, L. B., Meropol, N. J., et al. (2004). Phase II trial of cetuximab in patients with refractory colorectal cancer that expresses the epidermal growth factor receptor. *J. Clin. Oncol.* 22(7):1201–1208.

Sarlomo-Rikala, M., Kovatich, A. J., et al. (1998). CD117: A sensitive marker for gastrointestinal stromal tumors that is more specific than CD34. *Mod. Pathol.* 11(8): 728–734.

Sasaki, H., Zlatescu, M. C., et al. (2001). PTEN is a target of chromosome 10q loss in anaplastic oligodendrogliomas and PTEN alterations are associated with poor prognosis. *Am. J. Pathol.* 159(1):359–367.

Scaltriti, M., and Baselga, J. (2006). The epidermal growth factor receptor pathway: A model for targeted therapy. *Clin. Cancer Res.* 12(18):5268–5272.

Scartozzi, M., Bearzi, I., et al. (2004). Epidermal growth factor receptor (EGFR) status in primary colorectal tumors does not correlate with EGFR expression in related metastatic sites: Implications for treatment with EGFR-targeted monoclonal antibodies. *J. Clin. Oncol.* 22(23):4772–4778.

Schittenhelm, M. M., Shiraga, S., et al. (2006). Dasatinib (BMS-354825), a dual SRC/ABL kinase inhibitor, inhibits the kinase activity of wild-type, juxtamembrane, and activation loop mutant KIT isoforms associated with human malignancies. *Cancer Res.* 66(1): 473–481.

Schwechheimer, K., Gass, P., et al. (1992). Expression of oligodendroglia and Schwann cell markers in human nervous system tumors. An immunomorphological study and western blot analysis. *Acta Neuropathol. (Berl.)* 83(3):283–291.

Sommer, G., Agosti, V., et al. (2003). Gastrointestinal stromal tumors in a mouse model by targeted mutation of the Kit receptor tyrosine kinase. *Proc. Natl. Acad. Sci. U.S.A.* 100(11):6706–6711.

Staudt, L. M. (2003). Molecular diagnosis of the hematologic cancers. *N. Engl. J. Med.* 348(18):1777–1785.

Steigen, S. E., Eide, T. J., et al. (2007). Mutations in gastrointestinal stromal tumors—a population-based study from Northern Norway. *Apmis* 115(4):289–298.

Stenman, G., Eriksson, A., et al. (1989). Human PDGFA receptor gene maps to the same region on chromosome 4 as the KIT oncogene. *Genes Chromosomes Cancer* 1(2):155–158.

Sung, C. C., Collins, R., et al. (1996). Glycolipids and myelin proteins in human oligodendrogliomas. *Glycoconj. J.* 13(3):433–443.

Syed, S., and Rowinsky, E. (2003). The new generation of targeted therapies for breast cancer. *Oncology (Williston Park)* 17(10):1339–1351; discussion 1352, 1355–1356.

Talpaz, M., Shah, N. P., et al. (2006). Dasatinib in imatinib-resistant Philadelphia chromosome-positive leukemias. *N. Engl. J. Med.* 354(24):2531–2541.

Torres-Cabala, C., Bibbo, M., et al. (2006). Proteomic identification of new biomarkers and application in thyroid cytology. *Acta Cytol.* 50(5):518–528.

Tot, T. (1999). Adenocarcinomas metastatic to the liver: The value of cytokeratins 20 and 7 in the search for unknown primary tumors. *Cancer* 85(1):171–177.

Tzen, C. Y., and Mau, B. L. (2005). Analysis of CD117-negative gastrointestinal stromal tumors. *World J. Gastroenterol.* 11(7):1052–1055.

van den Bent, M. J., Carpentier, A. F., et al. (2006). Adjuvant procarbazine, lomustine, and vincristine improves progression-free survival but not overall survival in newly diagnosed anaplastic oligodendrogliomas and oligoastrocytomas: A randomized European Organisation for Research and Treatment of Cancer phase III trial. *J. Clin. Oncol.* 24(18):2715–2722.

Vasselli, J. R., Shih, J. H., et al. (2003). Predicting survival in patients with metastatic kidney cancer by gene-expression profiling in the primary tumor. *Proc. Natl. Acad. Sci. U.S.A.* 100(12):6958–6963.

Wakai, T., Kanda, T., et al. (2004). Late resistance to imatinib therapy in a metastatic gastrointestinal stromal tumour is associated with a second KIT mutation. *Br. J. Cancer* 90(11):2059–2061.

Weisberg, E., Wright, R. D., et al. (2006). Effects of PKC412, nilotinib, and imatinib against GIST-associated PDGFRA mutants with differential imatinib sensitivity. *Gastroenterology* 131(6):1734–1742.

Yarden, Y., and Sliwkowski, M. X. (2001). Untangling the ErbB signalling network. *Nat. Rev. Mol. Cell Biol.* 2(2):127–137.

Yokoo, H., Nobusawa, S., et al. (2004). Anti-human Olig2 antibody as a useful immuno-histochemical marker of normal oligodendrocytes and gliomas. *Am. J. Pathol.* 164(5): 1717–1725.

8

MOLECULAR PATHOLOGY AND MOLECULAR THERAPY

Hewei Li

8.1. INTRODUCTION

Pathology is the study and diagnosis of disease through examination of organs, tissues, bodily fluids, and whole bodies. The first half of twentieth century was characterized by cytopathology enrichment and development phase. In the mid-twentieth century, due to the advent of electronic microscope, ultrastructural pathology developed rapidly. In the last 30 years, advances in cell biology, immunology, genetics, and molecular biology led to the formation of molecular pathology. The emergence of molecular pathology made it possible to investigate the nature of abnormal tissue at the nucleic acid and protein levels by identifying the abnormal molecular events and factors that are responsible for producing the diseased tissue. Nowadays, molecular pathology has been widely applied to molecular diagnosis, prognosis, and therapeutics including molecular therapy of diseases.

Molecular therapy is an approach for correcting defective genes responsible for disease development. With the arrival of recombinant DNA techniques together with viral vectors and other gene transfer methods, cloned genes became available and were used to demonstrate that foreign genes could indeed correct genetic defects and disease phenotypes in vitro and in vivo. Molecular therapy

Molecular Pathology in Drug Discovery and Development, Edited by J. Suso Platero
Copyright © 2009 John Wiley & Sons, Inc.

promises to be an effective and possible curative treatment to human diseases (Anderson, 1984; Friedmann, 1989; Verma, 1990; Anderson, 1992; Miller, 1992; Friedmann, 1992). In the mid-1980s, molecular therapy was focused on treating diseases caused by such single-gene defects as hemophilia, Duchenne's muscular dystrophy, and sickle cell anemia. In the late 1980s and early 1990s, the concept of gene therapy expanded into a number of acquired diseases. By 1989, the first human gene therapy trial was conducted by Rosenberg et al. (1990), and in 1995, public debate led to the consensus that gene therapy has value although many unanswered questions require continued basic research. As the field matured over the last decade, it has caught the attention of the biopharmaceutical industry, which is critical because ultimately this industry will bring gene therapies to large patient populations (Wilson, 1999). This chapter starts with the discussion of six key molecular therapeutic strategies that have been tested, either in animal models or clinical trials. Molecular pathology plays a critical role in assessment of the safety and efficacy of molecular therapeutic agents as detailed in this chapter. Specific examples will be given to illustrate the important role of molecular pathology. The up-to-date status of gene therapy clinical trials worldwide will also be reviewed.

8.2. MOLECULAR THERAPY STRATEGIES

Molecular therapy entails the use of genetic material for therapeutic purposes. Some of the key strategies that are currently developed and applied for human gene therapy are discussed below.

8.2.1. Mutation Compensation

Mutation compensation is an approach by which cancer cells are genetically manipulated to affect the molecular processes contributing to the malignant phenotype. Restoration or inactivation of cellular proliferation controlling genes such as tumor suppressor genes, oncogenes, and other cell cycle control genes proved promising to achieve favorable antitumor effects.

The loss of tumor suppressor gene function is believed to be an important factor in the etiopathogenesis of human cancers (Spitz et al., 1996b; Densmore et al., 2001; Eastham et al., 2000; Clayman et al., 1998; Swisher et al., 1999; Havlik et al., 2002; Ray et al., 1996). Mutation or inactivation of the *p53* tumor suppressor gene is one of the early genetic alterations that may confer a proliferative advantage to cells and is associated with tumor progression (Fults et al., 1992; von Deimling et al., 1992; Sidransky et al., 1992). *p53* is a transcriptional regulator induced by DNA damage. *p53* plays a vital role in cell cycle control and in the cellular response to DNA damage (Ko and Prives, 1996). The mechanism that leads to apoptosis induced by *p53* is still not completely understood. *p53* probably involves the down-regulation of the antiapoptotic protein Bcl-2 (Miyashita et al., 1994) and up-regulation of the proapoptotic protein Bax (Miyashita and Reed,

1995), as well as the death receptors Fas (Muller et al., 1998) and DR5 (Wu et al., 1997). Preclinical studies showed that *p53* overexpression through adenovirus-mediated gene transfer can induce apoptosis and decrease cell proliferation in a wide variety of cancer cell lines irrespective of their endogenous *p53* status (Clayman et al., 1995; Hamada et al., 1996; Gomez-Manzano et al., 1996; Li et al., 1997). In addition, overexpression of wild-type *p53* also increases the radio sensitivity of tumor cells (Pirollo et al., 1997; Spitz et al., 1996a).

Restoration of the nuclear localized Rb protein, a regulator of the cell cycle at the G1 transition point, leads to growth arrest and reduction of tumor growth in xenograft models of bladder, breast, glioblastoma and other cancers (Chatterjee et al., 2004; Bosco et al., 2007; Fueyo et al., 1998). Similarly, adenovirus-mediated gene transfer and overexpression of the tumor suppressor gene *PTEN*, a chromosome 10p gene that is frequently deleted in tumor cells, inhibits prostate cancer cell and glioma cell proliferation in vitro and impairs in vivo tumorigenicity (Anai et al., 2006; Lu et al., 2004). More importantly, alterations in these tumor suppressor molecules are now becoming enticing targets for novel therapeutics.

An example of how molecular pathology can be applied to the adenovirus-mediated *p53* tumor suppressor gene therapy for experimental human glioma has been shown by Li and colleagues (1999). Glioblastoma is the most malignant form of primary cerebral neoplasms. Unlike most other malignant tumors, glioblastoma does not metastasize outside of brain. Its fatal outcome is due to local effects on the intracranial contents. Pathologically, glioblastoma cells spread from the original site(s) through myelinated nerve bundles within the cerebral white matter or by the Virchow–Robin perivascular arachnoid spaces (Coons, 1999). Hence, fingerlike microprojections or detached foci of tumor cells from the main bulk of the tumor are found very frequently at the time of diagnosis. Failure to eradicate these satellite tumor cells is the key factor in the failure to cure glioblastoma by surgical treatment. Many genetic alterations have been documented during the transformation of glial cells and the subsequent tumor progression into the most malignant form, glioblastoma multiforme. Mutation or inactivation of the *p53* tumor suppressor gene is one of the key early genetic alterations that may confer a proliferative advantage to these cells and is associated with tumor progression (Fults et al., 1992; von Deimling et al., 1992; Sidransky et al., 1992). Because *p53* mutations are common in astrocytic gliomas, therapies aimed at restoring wild-type *p53* functions (Wieczorek et al., 1996) or specifically targeted at killing cells with mutant *p53* might be of benefit (Bischoff et al., 1996). However, even high-grade glioblastoma cells may have intact *p53* genes, and there may be molecular heterogeneity within the same tumor bed (Louis, 1993). In vitro studies showed gene transfer of wild-type *p53* into glioma cell lines expressing mutant *p53* leads to cell death by apoptosis (Gomez-Manzano et al., 1996; Li et al., 1997; van Meir et al., 1995), whereas in glioma cells with an intact *p53* gene, overexpression of *p53* has been associated with growth arrest (Gomez-Manzano et al., 1996; van Meir et al., 1995) or apoptosis (Li et al., 1997). Adenoviral vector system is one the major viral vectors used to date to deliver the therapeutic genes into glioblastoma cells. Adenoviral vector has the ability to infect both quiescent and dividing cells. It remains extrachromosomally at high-level transgene expression and can be produced in large scale with high titer. Previous in vitro experiments have shown that adenovirus-mediated gene transfer and overexpression of the wild-type *p53* tumor suppressor protein leads to cell death via apoptosis in the wild-type *p53* U87 MG human glioma cell line (Li et al., 1997). They reported the effects of adenovirus-mediated gene transfer of wild-type *p53* (AV*p53*) in an experimental model of human malignant glioma produced by intracerebral inoculation of human U87 MG cells into athymic *nu/nu* (nude) mice.

To monitor glioma cell growth in vivo, the U87 MG glioma cell line was genetically marked by stable transfection with the *Escherichia coli lacZ* gene that encodes β-galactosidase. The U87/*lacZ* cell line maintained strong β-galactosidase expression during at least 30 passages in vitro. Furthermore, U87/*lacZ* cells that were injected intracerebrally were capable of forming tumors that constitutively expressed β-galactosidase as revealed by histochemical staining of tumor tissue sections in the presence of the substrate X-gal (see Figs. 8.1A and 8.2). During subsequent experiments, the identification of single blue-stained glioma cells allowed a rapid and efficient evaluation of tumor growth and spread in brain tissue.

In view of the rapid apoptotic death of AV*p53*-transduced U87/*lacZ* cells in vitro, the hypothesis that directly intratumoral transduction with *p53* would cause tumor regression was tested. Tumors were established bilaterally by stereotactic injection into the caudate region of immunodeficient nude mice. Ten days after tumor cell injection, when the tumors were approximately $0.83 \pm 0.19 \text{mm}^3$ in volume, 6×10^8 particles of AV*p53* (or AV*GFP* that carries a green fluorescent protein, as a control) were injected into tumor beds using previously established coordinates. An examination of the brain coronal sections of mice euthanized 25 days after the injection showed that the tumor in the left hemisphere (injected with AV*p53*) had disappeared and had been replaced by areas of necrosis/gliosis (Fig. 8.1A). In contrast, the implanted tumor on the right side injected with the control adenoviral recombinant AV*GFP* had continued to grow (Fig. 8.1A).

To study in more detail the tumoricidal effect of AV*p53*, single tumors were established for 10 days, followed by injection of AV*p53* or AV*GFP*. Animals were euthanized at 2, 3, 4, 5, or 25 days after viral injection ($n = 4$ for each time point) to examine brains for the presence of tumor cells. As a result, all of the animals in the AV*GFP*-treated group had intact cerebral tumors (Figs. 8.2B, 8.2D, and 8.2F) that were characterized by blue-stained cytoplasm indicating the presence of β-galactosidase activity. Little necrosis was observed in these tumors, but there was a mild inflammatory response as well as some microhemorrhages. In the case of tumors treated with AV*p53*, focal necrosis and moderate inflammatory response were detectable as early as 2 days after virus injection (Fig. 8.2A); extensive necrosis/hemorrhages with fewer remaining tumor cells were apparent by 5 days (Fig. 8.2C). After 25 days, only a small number of residual cells surrounded the injection tract with a large area of necrosis/gliosis (Fig. 8.2E). Immunohistochemical analysis revealed that CD45[+] lymphocytes and Mac-1[+]

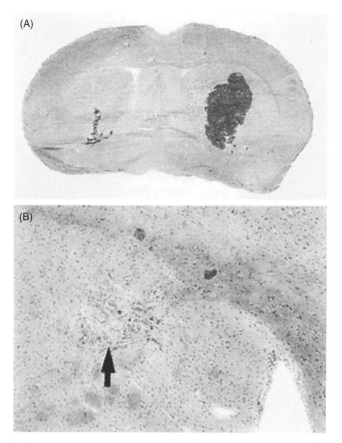

Figure 8.1. (A) Elimination of tumor cells after infection with AV*p53*.A, effect of infection with AV*p53* (left hemisphere) or AV*GFP* (right hemisphere) after bilateral implantation of U87//*lacZ* tumor cells. Tumor cells were allowed to grow for 10 days before recombinant virus injection. Animals were euthanized 25 days after treatment with recombinant viruses. Fluorescence microscopy showed that the tumor in the right hemisphere had robust, diffuse expression of GFP. Sections were stained for β-galactosidase activity (blue), followed by H&E staining. (B) Brain tissue section from an animal that died of unrelated causes 265 days after stereotactic injection of AV*p53* (10 days after the implantation of tumor cells). This gliotic area (arrow) did not contain any tumor cells. H&E staining. ×100 original magnification (Li et al., 1999). (Reproduced by permission of the American Association for Cancer Research Inc.) See insert for color representation of this figure.

macrophages were present within all of the tumor beds and in the immediately adjacent parenchyma, with the inflammatory reaction being most pronounced in the AV*p53*-treated animals. However, by 25 days after viral injection, the extent of cellular infiltration had declined significantly. At this time period, microscopic examination of semithin sections of Epon-embedded tissue showed that there was little evidence of damage to the adjacent neuropil from AV*p53* expression.

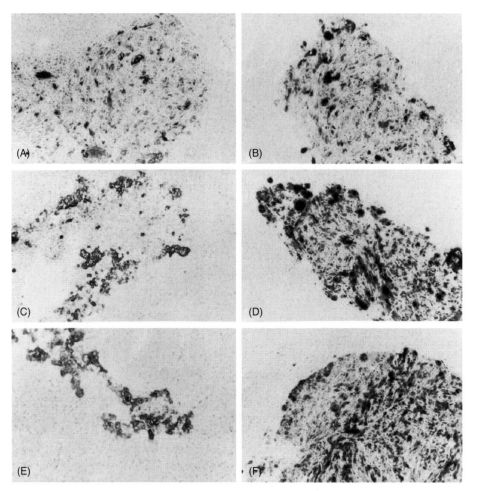

Figure 8.2. Rapid destruction of implanted U87/*lacZ* tumors after infection with AV*p53* (A, C, E) as compared to infection with AV*GFP* (B, D, F). Animals were euthanized at day 2 (A, B), 5 (C, D), and 25 (E, F) after treatment with AV. Sections were stained for β-galactosidase activity (blue), followed by H&E staining (Li et al., 1999). (Reproduced by permission of the American Association for Cancer Research Inc.) See insert for color representation of this figure.

Long-term experiments were then undertaken in nude mice implanted with U87/*lacZ* cells that were allowed to proliferate for either 10 days or 20 days to form tumors of different mass. The different groups of animals received either AV*p53*, AV*GFP*, or saline by stereotactic injection as outlined in Table 8.1. Mice injected with either saline or AV*GFP* were all dead by 65 days after glioma cell inoculation (Table 8.1). In contrast, mice injected on a single occasion with AV*p53* 10 days after tumor cell inoculation had a median survival time of 193 days

TABLE 8.1. Survival Times (in Days) of Different Experimental Groups

| Treatment | 10 Days[a] | 20 Days[a] | |
	Single Injection	Single Injection	Multiple Injections
Saline	$n = 7$	$n = 8$	
Range	47–60	45–65	
Median	52	58	
AV*GFP*	$n = 7$	$n = 10$	
Range	49–63	44–62	
Median	57	59	
AV*p53*	$n = 11$	$n = 12$	$n = 13$
Range[b]	81–	88–156	154–
Median	193[c]	124[c]	250[d]

[a]The number of days refers to the time after initial glioma cell inoculation.
[b]Incomplete range indicates animals did not die from tumor.
[c]Statistically significant ($P < 0.0001$) in relation to the saline and AV*GFP* groups by log-rank analysis of the Kaplan–Meier survival curve (Bonferroni correction).
[d]Statistically significant ($P < 0.0001$) in relation to the single injection group by log-rank analysis of the Kaplan–Meier survival curve (Bonferroni correction).

($P < 0.0001$). Nine months after inoculation, one of the three remaining survivors died of unrelated causes. Histological analysis of brain sections from this animal showed no tumor cells, but there was evidence of a small area of glial scar tissue in the original tumor bed (Fig. 8.1B) and along the needle tract. Two additional mice euthanized 1 year after intracerebral tumor implantation were also free of tumor cells.

The observed therapeutic effect of AV*p53* injection was dependent on the mass of the original tumor. Although animals in which tumor cells had proliferated for 20 days before a single adenoviral injection survived significantly longer than controls (median survival time of 124 days; $P < 0.0001$), they were all dead by 156 days (Table 8.1). However, in this experimental group, survival was improved significantly by performing multiple injections ($n = 4$) of AV*p53* at monthly intervals using the same initial coordinates of the implanted tumor. At 240 days, 61% of the mice were still alive; one mouse that died at 264 days of unrelated causes had only a glial scar remaining at the site of the original tumor, similar to what was observed in Figure 8.1B. After a 1-year period, 38% of the animals were free of tumor cells upon pathological examination at euthanasia (Table 8.1).

This study demonstrates that even a single injection of an adenoviral recombinant expressing wild-type *p53* leads to near complete eradication of an implanted intracerebral malignant glioma. However, it is evident in Figure 8.2E that a few tumor cells expressing β-galactosidase remain at 25 days after infection. Because these cells may form the nidus for recurrence of the tumor, multiple sequential injections with AV*p53* are likely to be required to eradicate the implanted tumors (Table 8.1).

The cell death within the implanted tumors was accompanied by a marked inflammatory response consisting mainly of macrophage infiltration, which abated with time. No edema developed, and the surrounding neuropil was largely unaffected, although there was evidence of generalized astrocytic and microglial activation. Because these experiments were carried out in immunodeficient animals, it is expected that the nature of the inflammatory response will be very different in immunocompetent animals in which the adenoviral particles themselves may elicit an immune reaction (Byrnes et al., 1995). This in itself may contribute to additional tumoricidal activity. Taken together, these experiments demonstrate that the adenovirus is very efficient in transducing these tumors and that adenovirus-mediated overexpression of *p53* may have therapeutic value in the treatment of astrocytic gliomas, irrespective of their molecular characteristics.

8.2.2. Gene Therapy in Drug Development

The efficacy of cancer chemotherapy approach is often hampered by an insufficient therapeutic index, lack of specificity, and the emergence of drug resistance. To date, the enzyme-activating prodrug gene therapy approach promises to enhance the selectivity and sensitivity of cancer chemotherapy for solid tumors (Moolten, 1986). The possibility of rendering cancer cells more sensitive to chemotherapeutics or toxins by introducing "suicide genes" was suggested in the late 1980s. The enzyme-activating prodrug therapy is based on the intracellular conversion of a systemically administered nontoxic prodrug into a highly cytotoxic molecule by an enzyme encoded by a gene introduced into the tumor cells by a viral vector (Manome et al., 1996). In the first step, the gene for a foreign enzyme is delivered and targeted in a variety of ways to the tumor where it is to be expressed. In the second step, a prodrug is administered that is selectively activated to the drug by the foreign enzyme expressed in the tumor. More importantly, a bystander effect was observed whereby the prodrug was cleaved to an active drug that kills not only the tumor cells in which it is formed but also neighboring tumor cells that do not express the foreign enzyme (Huber et al., 1994). The bystander effect would maximize the therapeutic efficacy as the expression of the foreign enzymes will not occur in all cells of a targeted tumor in vivo. There are two widely applied systems used for this approach: (1) *Escherichia coli* cytosine deaminase (CD) as the converting enzyme that converts the nontoxic prodrug 5-flurocytosine (5-FC) to the highly toxic 5-fluorouracil (5-FU). 5-FU is a well-known chemotherapeutic agent with high tumoricidal efficiency through inhibiting the enzyme thymidylate synthetase (Huber et al., 1994); and (2) herpes simplex virus thymidine kinase (HSV-tk) as the converting enzyme and gancyclovir (GCV) as the prodrug transformed into a cytotoxic agent, phosphogancyclovir (P-GCV), which leads to premature chain termination during DNA synthesis in tumor cells (Nagy et al., 2000).

The enzyme-activating prodrug systems proved to enhance the tumoricidal efficacy for lung cancer and peritoneal carcinomatosis when combined with cytokine gene therapy. Immunohistochemical analysis revealed that lymphoid CD4(+) and CD8(+) T cells as well as macrophages accumulated outside untreated tumor nodes while CD8(+) and CD25(+) activated T cells and macrophages heavily infiltrated the tumors after the treatments (Kwong, 1997; Lechanteur et al., 2000). In addition, based on the fact that a toxic metabolite of 5-FC, 5-fluorouracil, is a well-known radiation enhancer for the treatment of gastrointestinal and other tumors, 5-FC was found to enhance selectively the radiation cytotoxicity of human colorectal carcinoma cells expressing the CD gene. The addition of radiation would substantially improve the therapeutic potential of CD "suicide" gene therapy for the treatment of locally advanced colorectal carcinomas (Khil et al., 1996).

Direct in vivo tumor targeting with suicide viral vectors is limited by either inefficient gene transfer (i.e., retroviral vectors) or indiscriminate transfer of a conditionally toxic gene to surrounding nonmalignant tissue (i.e., adenoviral vectors). Retrovectors pseudo typed with the vesicular stomatitis virus G protein (VSVG) may serve as a remedy to this conundrum. Galipeau and colleagues (1999) developed a VSVG-typed retrovector (vTKiGFP) that proved to be able to efficiently express the tumor-specific herpes simplex virus thymidine kinase (TK) and green fluorescence protein (GFP) genes (Li et al., 1999). The in vivo antitumor activity of vTKiGFP retroparticles in a rat C6/*lacZ* glioma model of brain cancer was observed. Concentrated retrovector stock was injected stereotactically in preestablished intracerebral tumor. Subsequently, rats were treated with GCV for 10 days. Control rats (no GCV) had a mean survival of 38 days (range, 20 to 52 days). Sections performed on postmortem brain tissue revealed macroscopic intracerebral tumors with evidence of high-efficiency retrovector transfer and expression (as assessed by GFP fluorescence). Examination of fresh frozen brain sections by epifluorescence microscopy shows that in all animals, a predominant proportion of glioma cells fluoresce green (Fig. 8.3A), including distant micrometastasis. No green fluorescence was observed in untransduced brain tumors (Fig. 8.3C). In the experimental group (GCV treated), 8 of 12 GCV-treated rats remain alive and well >120 days after glioma implantation, two died within 10 days after drug treatment, presumably from direct GCV toxicity (both animals had brain tumors <1 mm in diameter on postmortem). Two rats developed tumor relapses at the initial injection site and died of progressive disease at day 82. Molecular pathology was used to examine brain tissue sections on these late relapses, revealed focal GFP expression in the tumors (Fig. 8.3E). GFP expression (Figs. 8.3A, 8.3C, and 8.3E) was compared with subsequent histochemical staining of C6/lacZ tumor cells with the substrate X-gal (Figs. 8.3B, 8.3D, and 8.3F). In conclusion, vTKiGFP is very efficient at transducing human glioma cell lines in vitro and leads to significant GCV sensitization.

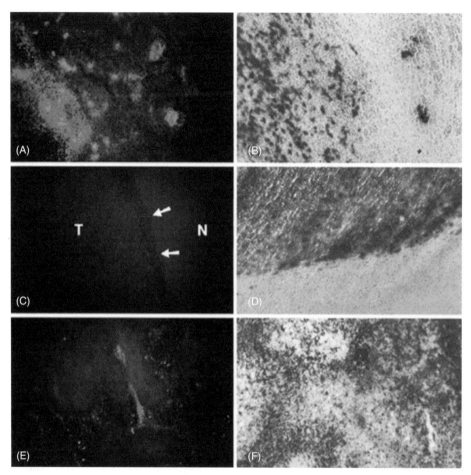

Figure 8.3. In vivo transduction of C6/*lacZ* tumors with vTKiGFP. Brain tumors were harvested postmortem as described previously. (A, B) Tumor from a control rat that received vTKiGFP without subsequent treatment with GCV (rat was sacrificed on day 30 after tumor implantation due to morbid state). (C, D) Tumor from a control rat that did not receive vTKiGFP but was treated with GCV (rat was sacrificed on day 43). (E, F) Tumor from a test rat that received vTKiGFP and subsequent treatment with GCV, which suffered symptomatic recurrent tumor (rat was sacrificed on day 82). GFP expression (A, C, E) was compared with subsequent histochemical staining of C6/*lacZ* tumor cells with the substrate X-gal (B, D, F). ×100. *T*, tumor; *N*, normal brain (Galipeau et al., 1999). (Reproduced by permission of the American Association for Cancer Research Inc.) See insert for color representation of this figure.

8.2.3. Immunogene Therapy

It has been observed that, in most instances, proliferating tumor cells escape the host antitumor immune responses. Essential to this process is the lack of responsiveness of the immune system toward antigens of neoplastic cells. Its mechanisms of genetic and pathological events involved in immune tolerance still remain largely unclear. Chemotherapy could direct cytotoxic actions on tumor cells but often result in immune suppression. Instead, gene therapy is less harmful to immune systems. Thus far, a number of different immunogene therapy strategies have been explored to stimulate host humoral and/or cellular reactions to tumor antigens and subsequently break immunological tolerance for tumors, which leads to tumor regression. Immunogene therapy may also serve as a neoadjuvant to surgical excision to control metastatic cancers. Immunomodulatory strategies include:

1. Vaccinating tumor cells with recombinant viral vectors encoding immune-augmenting cytokines such as interleukin (IL)-2, granulocyte-macrophage colony-stimulating factor (GM-CSF), interferon (IFN)-α, and IL-12
2. Vaccinating tumor cells engineered to express immunocostimulatory molecules, such as B7
3. Delivering antitumor vaccines by intratumoral injection of vectors
4. Engineering dendritic cells to express tumor antigens or tumor-derived RNA, naked DNA vaccines
5. Suppressing immunosuppressive gene expression

Cytokines play a crucial role in augmentation of host antitumor immunity. To date, viral vector-mediated gene delivery technology allows efficient transferring of cytokines into tumor cells. In vitro transduction of glioma cells by IL-2 has been shown to cause antitumor immune response as evidenced by expansion of the cytotoxic T lymphocyte (CD8$^+$) cell population and activation of CD3/CD16 epitope-bearing lymphocytes (Donson and Foreman, 1998).

Interleukin-2-mediated antitumor activity by modulating the host's immunological response to the neoplasm has been shown in advanced melanoma, non-Hodgkin's lymphoma, and other cancers (Sun et al., 1998; Takahashi et al., 2001). IL-2 stimulates the CD8$^+$ cells that are involved in antigen-specific cytotoxic activity to tumor cells. It also enhances the activity of natural killer/lymphokine-activated killer cells, which possess antitumor activity. Activation of both of these cell types most likely is required for the optimum opportunity for tumor rejection (Glick et al., 2000). Immunogenic-stimulating antitumor activity may be obtained by the introduction of genes into tumor cells that encode cytokines of IFN-α and IL-12 (Noguchi et al., 2001; Urosevic et al., 2007; Zhao et al., 2007; Kang et al., 2001; Sonabend et al., 2008) or GM-CSF (Janke et al., 2007; Hayashi et al., 1997) or MHC/co stimulatory factors such as B7-1 or B7-2 (Lakatosová-Andelová et al., 2008; Wu et al., 2001). Early promise in human phase I trials has been shown by immunizing patients with metastatic melanoma tumor vaccine using recombinant adenoviruses encoding MART-1 or gp100 melanoma antigens (Rosenberg et al., 1998) or using recombinant vaccinia virus and recombinant no replicating avipox virus to elicit anticarcinoembryonic antigen immune responses (Marshall et al., 2000). Tumor-derived immune suppression is a major impediment to successful immunogene cancer therapy. Attention has been given to the inhibition of immunosuppressive molecules such as transforming growth factor beta 1 or 2, which reinstalls the system immunity for antitumor rejection (Wu et al., 2001; Tzai et al., 1998). Recently, a novel strategy was reported to disrupt tumor-derived immune suppression by silencing a tolerogenic molecule of tumor origin, IDO, using small interfering ribonucleic acid (siRNA) (Zheng et al., 2006).

8.2.4. Oncolytic Viruses

Oncolytic viruses are replication-conditional viruses with capability to infect and lyse cancer cells, while leaving normal cells unharmed, making them potentially useful in cancer therapy. Current recombined DNA technologies allow the generation of tumor selectivity of oncolytic viruses. This can be achieved by either modifying the specificity of viral coat protein that increases entry into target cells while reducing entry to nontarget cells, or altering the genome of the virus so it can only replicate in cancer cells.

The most developed agent is a genetically engineered human herpes simplex virus (HSV) in which the *tk* gene is inactivated by deletion. This modified HSV remains replication competent only in cells that have endogenous *TK* activity, as in proliferating glioma cells, where the virus can exert cytolytic activity (Martuza et al., 1991). In neurons and glial cells the virus cannot replicate and does not show deleterious effects as evidenced by pathological findings (Ikeda et al., 1999). The multiattenuated herpes simplex virus-1 mutant (G207) was reported to exert selective cytotoxicity against epithelial ovarian cancer and colorectal cancer (Coukos et al., 2000; Kooby et al., 1999). Another promising oncolytic virus is the replication-competent adenovirus type 5 in which the cytotoxic E1A gene expression is driven by the prostate-specific antigen (PSA) gene (prostate-specific promoter/enhancer), thereby creating a prostate-specific enhancer containing virus. An in vitro study showed that this oncolytic virus expressed at high levels in human PSA-producing cells and led to remarkable regression of tumors in mouse xenograft models with a single intratumoral injection (Rodriguez et al., 1997). Synergistic antitumor efficacy without increasing toxicity was reported by applying the prostate cancer specific oncolytic adenovirus variant in combination with radiotherapy (Chen et al., 2001). Another class of oncolytic virus, which has shown clinical promise in many cancer types, consists of mutant adenoviruses that replicate only in tumor cells with mutant or deleted *p53*. A typical example is ONYX-015, an E1B gene deleted, *p53*-selective adenovirus mutant, which causes cytolysis selectively in tumors with mutant or deleted *p53* (Heise et al., 1997; Ries et al., 2000; Vollmer et al., 1999). Clinical promise has been seen in phase I and phase II studies of Onyx-015 in patients with advanced head and neck cancer (Ganly et al., 2000; Nemunaitis et al., 2000). Combined cancer therapy with adenovirus-mediated oncolysis and cytokine-mediated activation of host immune systems is considered one of the best current strategies for cancer molecular therapy (Tagawa et al., 2008). On one hand, the virus-mediated destruction of tumors, even a part of tumors, will induce the release of putative tumor antigens that, together with the introduction of cytokine(s), activate anti-tumor immune responses (Smyth et al., 2001). On the other hand, altering the host range or tissue specificity of any virus could have serious safety implications. Future studies need to focus on the better understanding of viral replication mechanisms and the host immune system (Chen et al., 2001).

8.2.5. Antiangiogenic Therapy

The current gene therapy strategies for cancer could be classified as either direct or indirect actions to tumor cells. The former includes previously discussed induction of apoptosis by restoration of tumor suppressor genes or inhibition of oncogenes and cytotoxicity mediated by suicide genes. The latter strategy is to regulate tumor growth through host responses, which include activation of immune systems and suppression of angiogenesis.

Angiogenesis is a process of new blood vessel formation, which is indispensable to the establishment of large solid tumors. Angiogenesis involves a complex series of events that likely include the coordinated action of several growth factors to produce new conduits of blood flow. Vasculogenesis, angiogenesis, and arteriogenesis are the three processes that may contribute to the growth of blood vessels (Laham et al., 2000). Therapeutic antiangiogenesis has emerged as a promising investigational strategy for the treatment of tumors. Gene therapy has been established as a potential method to induce suppression of angiogenesis and oxygen starvation in tumors. Numerous growth factors and transcription factors have been associated with physiologic and pathologic angiogenesis, which imply a pivotal role of these factors in the neovascularization to support the growth of a wide variety of solid tumors. The most studied growth factors include vascular endothelial growth factor (VEGF), angiopoietins, fibroblast growth factor (FGF), platelet-derived growth factor (PDGF), transforming growth factor-beta (TGF-beta), and metalloproteinases (MMPs) (Liu and Deisseroth, 2006). Transcription factors include integrins and interleukin-8 (IL-8) (Yuan et al., 2000). Angiopoietins and their receptors constitute another class of vascular growth regulators. Advancements in viral and nonviral vector technology including cell-based gene transfer have been applied to improve angiogenesis regulatory gene transmission and expression efficiency.

Vascular endothelial growth factor is a potent and selective vascular endothelial cell mitogen and angiogenic factor. VEGF is secreted by cells within necrotic/hypoxic areas, with a concomitant up-regulation of VEGF receptors on nearby endothelial cells (Plate et al., 1992). Very high levels of VEGF and its receptors have been recorded during growth of human glioblastoma (Plate et al., 1993). In this context, the inhibition of VEGF through an antisense (Im et al., 1999; Cheng et al., 1996) or antibody-based approach shows significant antitumor activity (Asano et al., 1995). Studies on the inactivation of VEGF-dependent angiogenesis by targeting VEGF receptor demonstrated the inhibition of growth and metastasis of human fibrosarcoma and glioblastoma (Goldman et al., 1998; Millauer et al., 1994). In these experiments, the truncated Flk-1 receptor produced by the transfected tumor cells interacted with the wild-type Flk-1 receptor expressed on neighboring endothelial cells, leading to formation of signaling incompetent heterodimers, thus preventing tumor vascularization. In addition, endothelial cell apoptosis induced by angiostatin, a proteolytic fragment of plasminogen, suppressed the growth of primary fiblosarcoma and human melanoma xenografts (Cao et al., 1998; Rodolfo et al., 2001; Feldman et al., 2001). Adenovirus-mediated gene transfer of endostatin in vivo resulted in the suppression of angiogenesis and significant reduction of the growth rates and the volumes of breast carcinoma and Lewis lung carcinoma. In addition, it also prevented the formation of pulmonary micrometastases in Lewis lung carcinoma. Immunohistochemical staining of the tumors demonstrated a decreased number of blood vessels in the treatment group versus the controls (Sauter et al., 2000).

In contrast, it is worthwhile to mention that therapeutic angiogenesis has provided a new avenue for cardiovascular gene therapy to increase blood flow to ischemic regions. The VEGF family and FGF family have been widely applied to ischemic disease clinical trials such as myocardial ischemia due to coronary artery disease and lower limb ischemia due to peripheral artery disorder. The platelet-derived growth factor (PDGF) has been reported to have potential treatment for foot ulcers caused by microvascular disease of diabetes.

8.2.6. Engineered RNA Gene Therapy

In the past decade, engineered RNAs that were used to silence undesired gene expression, now, they have become promising alternatives to traditional pharmacological antagonists. This new class of therapeutic RNAs includes antisense RNAs, ribozymes, and interfering RNAs (Drude et al., 2007).

Antisense RNA-mediated gene therapy aims to down-regulate the expression of a mutated gene. Antisense RNA is designed to be complementary to specific sites on a messenger RNA of mutated gene forming RNA:RNA hybrids. In contrast, antisense DNA strand can specifically bind to the sense strand of messenger RNA (mRNA) forming DNA:RNA hybrids. The binding of the antisense olignucleotides to the mutated mRNA therefore leads to the inhibition of the translation of a mutated protein. Antisense RNA is produced by using naked DNA-containing genes or using expression vectors that continuously synthesize antisense RNA inside the cell. An advantage of antisense RNA gene therapy over the more widely employed sense gene therapy is that the antisense RNA approach requires a knowledge and synthesis of only a small portion of the total gene sequence. Moreover, the promoter and other regulatory sequences on the gene need not be known (Weiss et al., 1999). Antisense oligonucleotides have been investigated to induce apoptosis in PC3 prostate cancer cells and in prostate cancer xenografts (Mercatante et al., 2002; Zellweger et al., 2001).

Ribozymes are RNA molecules that act as enzymes. Like antisense RNA, ribozymes are considered as another strategy to prevent the mutated gene from being translated into a protein by sequence-specific binding and cleavage of single-stranded mRNA encoded by the mutated gene. Cultured cell and animal model studies implied that ribozymes had promising therapeutic effects in the inhibition of HIV-1 (Sullenger and Gilboa, 2002), hepatitis B and C (HBV and HCV) infections (Morrissey et al., 2002; Lee et al., 2000), inactivating oncogenes such as BCR-ABL mRNA that is associated with chronic myelogenous leukemia (CML) (Tanabe et al., 2000) and inhibiting the growth of multitype solid tumors by targeting the human epidermal growth factor receptor type 2 (HER-2) mRNA (Lui et al., 2001; Thybusch-Bernhardt et al., 2001). Encouraging results were reported from early clinical trials of a ribozyme-made drug that was specially designed to degrade the mRNA of vascular endothelial growth factor receptor-1 (VEGFR-1) for patients with advanced solid tumors (Weng et al., 2005; Kobayashi et al., 2005). VEGFR-1 plays a pivotal role in tumor angiogenesis and metastasis.

The third strategy to inhibit target mRNA expression is mediated by RNA interference (RNAi). RNAi is a mechanism that blocks the expression of a chosen gene at the stage of translation or by hindering the transcription of gene by short double-stranded RNAs of 21 to 23 nucleotides in length. These small RNAs are classified as small interfering RNAs (siRNAs) and micro-RNAs (miRNAs). siRNAs are key to the RNAi process, and perfectly complementary bindings between the siRNA or miRNA sequences and the targeted mRNA strand result in breaking down of the mRNA strand that can no longer be translated into protein (Mallory et al., 2004; Lai, 2002). Mismatched reactions between the siRNA or miRNA sequences and the targeted mRNA strand lead to translational repression through incorporating into a multienzyme complex called RNA-induced silencing complex (RISC) (Castanotto et al., 2007). There is much ongoing work on how to deliver siRNAs and on chemical modifications to improve their stability and efficacy. The RNAi technique has moved remarkably rapidly toward applications. A number of preclinical investigations have shown promising results using siRNA or miRNA as a potential drug for the treatment of HIV, HBV/HCV infections (Novina et al., 2002; Chen et al., 2008), cancers, and metabolic disorders (Kao et al., 2004; Orlacchio et al., 2007).

8.3. MOLECULAR THERAPY CLINICAL TRIALS

The first human gene therapy trial on patients with advanced melanoma was conducted in 1989 (Rosenberg et al., 1990). There have been some serious adverse effects of human gene therapy. The first fatal systemic inflammatory response in an ornithine transcarbamylase-deficient patient following adenoviral gene transfer occurred in 1999 (Raper et al., 2003). Nevertheless, to date, over 1300 clinical trials using over 200 genes have been completed or are ongoing worldwide (Edelstein et al., 2007). According to the database from the *Journal of Gene Medicine Gene Therapy Clinical Trials* (http://www.wiley.co.uk/genmed/clinical), a vast majority of gene therapy clinical trials conducted up to 2007 were still phase I or I/II (80.9%), followed by 15.7% for phase II trials, and phase II/III and III trials occupied only 3.4%.

The large majority of gene therapy clinical trials have targeted cancer, cardiovascular disease, and inherited monogenic diseases. Nearly two-thirds of the clinical trial efforts thus far has been made on the treatment of such cancers as lung, skin, gastrointestinal, urological, neurological, and hematological tumors (Edelstein et al., 2007). Cardiovascular disease gene therapy counted approximately for 10% of all the trials aimed to increase blood flow to ischemic tissue via therapeutic angiogenesis, which proved to benefit myocardial protection, regeneration, and repair, as well as to prevent restenosis following angioplasty surgery and reblockage of coronary artery bypass grafts. Clinical efficacy has been demonstrated by transferring genes for vascular endothelial growth factor (VEGF)-1, VEGF-2, hypoxia-inducible factor (HIF), and fibroblast growth factor (FGF)-4 into ischemic myocardial muscle or ischemic lower limb (Gaffney et al., 2007; Lee et al., 2007). The third most popular gene therapy clinical trials have aimed to correct the inherited monogenic disorders. Inherited monogenic disorders are caused by a mutation in one single gene. Most monogenic disorders are severe and cureless. Gene therapy would provide hope for potential treatment. Clinical trials for some of the monogenic disorders, such as cystic fibrosis (CF) and the severe combined immunodeficiency (SCID) syndrome have been going on for many years and showing significant improvement of patient's health conditions (Moss et al., 2007; Rosenfeld, 2007; Cavazzana-Calvo and Fischer, 2007; Schmidt et al., 2005). A small number of trials have been conducted for infectious diseases such as HIV infection, neurological disorders such as multiple sclerosis, myasthenia gravis, Alzheimer's disease, and recently Parkinson's disease, as well as inflammatory bowel disease and rheumatoid arthritis (Edelstein et al., 2007).

Molecular therapy involves the introduction of therapeutic genes into target cells. Thereafter, the gene transfer vectors are becoming critical. The ideal gene transfer vector should transduce all the target cells, and, preferably, it should not infect normal adjacent cells. Nonviral approaches such as direct injection of naked DNA, cationic lipid/DNA complex, or ribozymes into certain type of tissues or cardiovascular system have been applied in nearly one-third of clinical trials (Kashani-Sabet, 2004; Shah and Losordo, 2005; Wolff et al., 2005). Viral vectors, however, are the most widely used vehicles to date in two-thirds of gene therapy clinical trials. Replication-defective adenovirus vectors can be produced at high titer, can efficiently infect dividing, as well as nondividing cells, and remain extrachromosomal. Therefore, adenoviruses are now the most commonly used vector in clinical trials. However, the first-generation adenoviral vectors also invoke intense local inflammation and stimulate potent cellular and humoral immune responses against both viral and transgene proteins (Vattemi and Claudio, 2006). Early human trials have demonstrated significant hepatic toxicity when large amounts of virus are delivered directly into the portal circulation (Raper et al., 2003). This problem may be alleviated with the newer generation of "gutless" adenoviral vector with all of the viral genes removed proved to reduce inflammatory and immunogenicity in preclinical studies (Alba et al., 2005).

Retroviral vectors were the first vectors applied in gene therapy. Retroviruses can integrate into host genome of target cells, and, if the initial infected cells survive, the daughter cells contain the therapeutic gene, which maximizes the therapeutic efficacy. The major disadvantages of retroviruses are that it can only infect dividing cells and some neoplastic cells in the nondividing period will not be infected and that the insertion of viral genes into host genome may cause carcinogenesis (Laufs et al., 2004). A new version of retrovirus, which is a vesicular stomatitis virus G protein pseudotyped retroviral vector, overcomes some of the disadvantages related to infectivity (Galipeau et al., 1999). Most recently, a type of retroviral vectors named lentiviral vectors are constructed based on HIV backbones. Unlike retroviruses, lentiviral vectors can infect both dividing and nondividing cells such as neuron and muscle cells. Lentiviruses appear to be noninflammatory and can mediate the expression of therapeutic gene in target cells for up to 6 months. A number of gene knock-down studies using lentiviral vector-mediated RNA interference (RNAi) have been reported (Sumimoto and Kawakami, 2007). Lentiviral vectors appear to be the next generation of viral vectors for human molecular therapy trials.

REFERENCES

Alba, R., Bosch, A., and Chillon, M. (2005). Gutless adenovirus: Last-generation adenovirus for gene therapy. *Gene Ther.* 12:S18–27.

Anai, S., Goodison, S., Shiverick, K., Iczkowski, K., Tanaka, M., and Rosser, C. J. (2006). Combination of PTEN gene therapy and radiation inhibits the growth of human prostate cancer xenografts. Hum. *Gene Ther.* 17:975–984.

Anderson, W. F. (1984). Prospects for human gene therapy. *Science* 226:401–409.

Anderson, W. F. (1992). Human gene therapy. *Science* 256:808–813.

Asano, M., Yukita, A., Matsumoto, T., Kondo, S., and Suzuki, H. (1995). Inhibition of tumor growth and metastasis by an immunoneutralizing monoclonal antibody to human vascular endothelial growth factor/vascular permeability factor 121. *Cancer Res.* 55: 5296–5301.

Bischoff, J. R., Kirn, D. H., Williams, A., Heise, C., Horn, S., Muna, M., Ng, L., Nye, J. A., Sampson-Johannes, A., Fattaey, A., and McCormick, F. (1996). An adenovirus mutant that replicates selectively in p53-deficient human tumor cells. *Science* (Washington DC) 274:373–376.

Bosco, E. E., Wang, Y., Xu, H., Zilfou, J. T., Knudsen, K. E., Aronow, B. J., Lowe, S. W., and Knudsen, E. S. (2007). The retinoblastoma tumor suppressor modifies the therapeutic response of breast cancer. *J. Clin. Invest.* 117(1):218–228.

Byrnes, A. P., Rusby, J. E., Wood, M. J. A., and Charlton, H. M. (1995). Adenovirus gene transfer causes inflammation in the brain. *Neuroscience* 66:1015–1024.

Cao, Y., O'Reilly, M. S., Marshall, B., Flynn, E., Ji, R. W., and Folkman, J. (1998). Expression of angiostatin cDNA in a murine fibrosarcoma suppresses primary tumor growth and produces long-term dormancy of metastases. *J. Clin. Invest.* 101: 1055–1063.

Castanotto, D., Sakurai, K., Lingeman, R., Li, H., Shively, L., Aagaard, L., Soifer, H., Gatignol, A., Riggs, A., and Rossi, J. J. (2007). Combinatorial delivery of small interfering RNAs reduces RNAi efficacy by selective incorporation into RISC. *Nucleic Acids Res.* 35:5154–5164.

Cavazzana-Calvo, M., and Fischer, A. (2007). Gene therapy for severe combined immunodeficiency: Are we there yet? *J. Clin. Invest.* 117:1456–1465.

Chatterjee, S. J., George, B., Goebell, P. J., Alavi-Tafreshi, M., Shi, S. R., Fung, Y. K., Jones, P. A., Cordon-Cardo, C., Datar, R. H., and Cote, R. J. (2004). Hyperphosphorylation of pRb: A mechanism for RB tumour suppressor pathway inactivation in bladder cancer. *J. Pathol.* 203:762–770.

Chen, Y., DeWeese, T., Dilley, J., Zhang, Y., Li, Y., Ramesh, N., Lee, J., Pennathur-Das, R., Radzyminski, J., Wypych, J., Brignetti, D., Scott, S., Stephens, J., Karpf, D. B., Henderson, D. R., and Yu, D. C. (2001). CV706, a prostate cancer-specific adenovirus variant, in combination with radiotherapy produces synergistic antitumor efficacy without increasing toxicity. *Cancer Res.* 15(61):5453–5460.

Chen, Y., Cheng, G., and Mahato, R. I. (2008). RNAi for treating hepatitis B viral infection. *Pharm. Res.* 25:72–86.

Cheng, S. Y., Huang, H. J., Nagane, M., Ji, X. D., Wang, D., Shih, C. C., Arap, W., Huang, C. M., and Cavenee, W. K. (1996). Suppression of glioblastoma angiogenicity and tumorigenicity by inhibition of endogenous expression of vascular endothelial growth factor. *Proc. Natl. Acad. Sci. U.S.A.* 93:8502–8507.

Clayman, G. L., El-Naggar, A. K., and Roth, J. A. (1995). In vivo molecular therapy with p53 adenovirus for microscopic residual head and neck squamous carcinoma. *Cancer Res.* 55:1–6.

Clayman, G. L., el-Naggar, A. K., Lippman, S. M., Henderson, Y. C., Frederick, M., Merritt, J. A., Zumstein, L. A., Timmons, T. M., Liu, T. J., Ginsberg, L., Roth, J. A., Hong, W. K., Bruso, P., and Goepfert, H. (1998). Adenovirus-mediated p53 gene transfer in patients with advanced recurrent head and neck squamous cell carcinoma. *J. Clin. Oncol.* 16:2221–2232.

Coons, S. W. (1999). Anatomy and growth patterns of diffuse gliomas. In *The Gliomas.* Berger, M. S., and Wilson, C. B. (Eds.). W. B. Saunders, Philadelphia, pp. 210–225.

Coukos, G., Makrigiannakis, A., Montas, S., Kaiser, L. R., Toyozumi, T., Benjamin, I., Albelda, S. M., Rubin, S. C., and Molnar-Kimber, K. L. (2000). Multi-attenuated herpes simplex virus-1 mutant G207 exerts cytotoxicity against epithelial ovarian cancer but not normal mesothelium and is suitable for intraperitoneal oncolytic therapy. *Cancer Gene Ther.* 7:275–283.

Densmore, C. L., Kleinerman, E. S., Gautam, A., Jia, S. F., Xu, B., Worth, L., Waldrep, J. C., Fung, Y. K., T'Ang, A., and Knight, V. (2001). Growth suppression of established human osteosarcoma lung metastases in mice by aerosol gene therapy with PEI-p53 complexes. *Cancer Gene Ther.* 8:619–627.

Donson, A. M., and Foreman, N. K. (1998). Adenovirus-mediated gene therapy in a glioblastoma vaccine model: Specific antitumor immunity and abrogation of immunosuppression. *J. Neuro-Oncol.* 40:205–214.

Drude, I., Dombos, V., Vauléon, S., and Müller, S. (2007). Drugs made of RNA: Development and application of engineered RNAs for gene therapy. *Mini. Rev. Med. Chem.* 7:912–931.

Eastham, J. A., Grafton, W., Martin, C. M., and Williams, B. J. (2000). Suppression of primary tumor growth and the progression to metastasis with p53 adenovirus in human prostate cancer. *J. Urol.* 164:814–819.

Edelstein, M. L., Abedi, M. R., and Wixon, J. (2007). Gene therapy clinical trials worldwide to 2007—an update. *J. Gene Med.* 9:833–842.

Feldman, A. L., Alexander, H. R., Hewitt, S. M., Lorang, D., Thiruvathukal, C. E., Turner, E. M., and Libutti, S. K. (2001). Effect of retroviral endostatin gene transfer on subcutaneous and intraperitoneal growth of murine tumors. *J. Natl. Cancer Inst.* 93:1014–1020.

Friedmann, T. (1989). Progress toward human gene therapy. *Science* 244:1275–1281.

Friedmann, T. (1992). A brief history of gene therapy. *Nature Genetics* 2:93–98.

Fueyo, J., Gomez-Manzano, C., Yung, W. K. A., Liu, T.-J., Alemany, R., Bruner, J. M., Chintala, S. K., Rao, J. S., Levin, V. A., and Kyritsis, A. P. (1998). Suppression of human glioma growth by adenovirus-mediated Rb gene transfer. *Neurology* 50:1307–1315.

Fults, D., Brockmeyer, D., Tullous, M. W., Pedone, C. A., and Cawthon, R. M. (1992). *p53* mutations and loss of heterozygosity on chromosomes 17 and 10 during human astrocytoma progression. *Cancer Res.* 52:674–679.

Gaffney, M. M., Hynes, S. O., Barry, F., and O'Brien, T. (2007). Cardiovascular gene therapy: Current status and therapeutic potential. *Br. J. Pharmacol.* 152:175–188.

Galipeau, J., Li, H., Paquin, A., Sicilia, F., Karpati, G., and Nalbantoglu, J. (1999). Vesicular stomatitis virus G pseudotyped retrovector mediates effective in vivo suicide gene delivery in experimental brain cancer. *Cancer Res.* 59:2384–2394.

Ganly, I., Kirn, D., Eckhardt, G., Rodriguez, G. I., Soutar, D. S., Otto, R., Robertson, A. G., Park, O., Gulley, M. L., Heise, C., Von Hoff, D. D., and Kaye, S. B. (2000). A phase I study of Onyx-015, an E1B attenuated adenovirus, administered intratumorally to patients with recurrent head and neck cancer. *Clin. Cancer Res.* 6:798–806.

Glick, R. P., Lichtor, T., and Cohen, P. E. (2000). Cytokine immunogene therapy. *Neurosurg. Focus* 9:1–9.

Goldman, C. K., Kendall, R. L., Cabrera, G., Soroceanu, L., Heike, Y., Gillespie, G. Y., Siegal, G. P., Mao, X., Bett, A. J., Huckle, W. R., Thomas, K. A., and Curiel, D. T. (1998). Paracrine expression of a native soluble vascular endothelial growth factor receptor inhibits tumor growth, metastasis, and mortality rate. *Proc. Natl. Acad. Sci. U.S.A.* 95:8795–8800.

Gomez-Manzano, C., Fueyo, J., Kyritsis, A. P., Steck, P. A., Roth, J. A., McDonnell, T. J., Steck, K. D., Levin, V. A., and Yung, W. K. (1996). Adenovirus-mediated transfer of the p53 gene produces rapid and generalized dealth of human glioma cells via apoptosis. *Cancer Res.* 56:694–699.

Hamada, K., Alemany, R., and Zhang, W.-W. (1996). Adenovirus-mediated transfer of a wild-type p53 gene and induction of apoptosis in cervical cancer. *Cancer Res.* 56:3047–3054.

Havlik, R., Jiao, L. R., Nicholls, J., Jensen, S. L., and Habib, N. A. (2002). Gene therapy for liver metastases. *Semin. Oncol.* 29:202–208.

Hayashi, S., Emi, N., Yokoyama, I., Namii, Y., Uchida, K., and Takagi, H. (1997). Inhibition of establishment of hepatic metastasis in mice by combination gene therapy using both herpes simplex virus–thymidine kinase and granulocyte macrophage-colony stimulating factor genes in murine colon cancer. *Cancer Gene Ther.* 4:339–344.

Heise, C., Sampson-Johannes, A., Williams, A., McCormick, F., Von Hoff, D. D., and Kirn, D. H. (1997). ONYX-015, an E1B gene-attenuated adenovirus, causes tumor-specific cytolysis and antitumoral efficacy that can be augmented by standard chemotherapeutic agents. *Nat. Med.* 3:639–645.

Huber, B. E., Austin, E. A., Richards, C. A., Davis, S. T., and Good, S. S. (1994). Metabolism of 5-fluorocytidine to 5-fluorouracil in human colorectal tumor cells transduced with the cytosine deaminase gene: Significant antitumor effects when only a small percentage of tumor cells express cytosine deaminase. *Proc. Natl. Acad. Sci. U.S.A.* 91:8302–8306.

Ikeda, I., Ishikawa, T., Wakimoto, H., Silver, J. S., Deisbock, T. S., Finkelstein, D., Harsh, G. R., Louis, D. N., Bartus, R. T., Hochberg, F. H., and Chiocca, E. A. (1999). Oncolytic virus therapy of multiple tumors in the brain requires suppression of innate and elicited antiviral responses. *Nature Med.* 5:881–887.

Im, S. A., Gomez-Manzano, C., Fueyo, J., Liu, T. J., Ke, L. D., Kim, J. S., Lee, H. Y., Steck, P. A., Kyritsis, A. P., and Yung, W. K. (1999). Antiangiogenesis treatment for gliomas: Transfer of antisense-vascular endothelial growth factor inhibits tumor growth in vivo. *Cancer Res.* 59:895–900.

Janke, M., Peeters, B., de Leeuw, O., Moorman, R., Arnold, A., Fournier, P., and Schirrmacher, V. (2007). Recombinant Newcastle disease virus (NDV) with inserted gene coding for GM-CSF as a new vector for cancer immunogene therapy. *Gene Ther.* 14:1639–1649.

Kang, W. K., Park, C., Yoon, H. L., Kim, W. S., Yoon, S. S., Lee, M. H., Park, K., Kim, K., Jeong, H. S., Kim, J. A., Nam, S. J., Yang, J. H., Son, Y. I., Baek, C. H., Han, J., Ree, H. J., Lee, E. S., Kim, S. H., Kim, D. W., Ahn, Y. C., Huh, S. J., Choe, Y. H., Lee, J. H., Park, M. H., Kong, G. S., Park, E. Y., Kang, Y. K., Bang, Y. J., Paik, N. S., Lee, S. N., Kim, S. H., Kim, S., Robbins, P. D., Tahara, H., Lotze, M. T., and Park, C. H. (2001). Interleukin 12 gene therapy of cancer by peritumoral injection of transduced autologous fibroblasts: Outcome of a phase I study. *Hum. Gene Ther.* 12:671–684.

Kao, S. C., Krichevsky, A. M., Kosik, K. S., and Tsai, L. H. (2004). BACE1 suppression by RNA interference in primary cortical neurons. *J. Biol. Chem.* 279:1942–1949.

Kashani-Sabet, M. (2004). Non-viral delivery of ribozymes for cancer gene therapy. *Expert Opin. Biol. Ther.* 4:1749–1755.

Khil, M. S., Kim, J. H., Mullen, C. A., Kim, S. H., and Freytag, S. O. (1996). Radiosensitization by 5-fluorocytosine of human colorectal carcinoma cells in culture transduced with cytosine deaminase gene. *Clin. Cancer Res.* 2:53–57.

Ko, L. J., and Prives, C. (1996). p53: Puzzle and paradigm. *Genes Dev.* 10:1054–1072.

Kobayashi, H., Eckhardt, S. G., Lockridge, J. A., Rothenberg, M. L., Sandler, A. B., O'Bryant, C. L., Cooper, W., Holden, S. N., Aitchison, R. D., Usman, N., Wolin, M., and Basche, M. L. (2005). Safety and pharmacokinetic study of RPI.4610 (ANGIOZYME), an anti-VEGFR-1 ribozyme, in combination with carboplatin and paclitaxel in patients with advanced solid tumors. *Cancer Chemother. Pharmacol.* 56:329–336.

Kooby, D. A., Carew, J. F., Halterman, M. W., Mack, J. E., Bertino, J. R., Blumgart, L. H., Federoff, H. J., and Fong, Y. (1999). Oncolytic viral therapy for human colorectal cancer and liver metastases using a multi-mutated herpes simplex virus type-1 (G207). *FASEB J.* 13:1325–1334.

Kwong, Y. L. (1997). Combination therapy with suicide and cytokine genes for hepatic metastases of lung cancer. *Chest* 112:1332–1337.

Laham, R., and Simons, M. (2000). Growth factor therapy in ischemic heart disease. In *Angiogenesis in Health and Disease*. Rubanyi, G. (Ed). Marcel Decker, New York, pp. 451–475.

Lai, E. C. (2002). Micro RNAs are complementary to 3′ UTR sequence motifs that mediate negative post-transcriptional regulation. *Nat. Genet* 30:363–364.

Lakatosová-Andelová, M., Jinoch, P., Dusková, M., Marinov, I., and Vonka, V. (2008). Live cell vaccines expressing B7.1, monocyte chemoattractant protein 1 and granulo-cyte-macrophage colony stimulation factor derived from mouse HPV16-transformed cells. *Int. J. Oncol.* 32:265–271.

Laufs, S., Nagy, K. Z., Giordano, F. A., Hotz-Wagenblatt, A., Zeller, W. J., and Fruehauf, S. (2004). Insertion of retroviral vectors in NOD/SCID repopulating human peripheral blood progenitor cells occurs preferentially in the vicinity of transcription start regions and in introns. *Mol. Ther.* 10:874–881.

Lechanteur, C., Delvenne, P., Princen, F., Lopez, M., Fillet, G., Gielen, J., Merville, M.-P., and Bours, V. (2000). Combined suicide and cytokine gene therapy for peritoneal carcinomatosis. *Gut* 47:343–348.

Lee, P. A., Blatt, L. M., Blanchard, K. S., Bouhana, K. S., Pavco, P. A., Bellon, L., and Sandberg, J. A. (2000). Pharmacokinetics and tissue distribution of a ribozyme directed against hepatitis C virus RNA following subcutaneous or intravenous administration in mice. *Hepatology* 32:640–646.

Lee, J. S., Kim, J. M., Kim, K. L., Jang, H. S., Shin, I. S., Jeon, E. S., Suh, W., Byun, J., and Kim, D. K. (2007). Combined administration of naked DNA vectors encoding VEGF and bFGF enhances tissue perfusion and arteriogenesis in ischemic hindlimb. *Biochem. Biophys. Res. Commun.* 360:752–758.

Li, H., Lochmuller, H., Yong, V. W., Karpati, G., and Nalbantoglu, J. (1997). Adenovirus-mediated wild-type p53 gene transfer and overexpression induces apoptosis of human glioma cells independent of endogenous p53 status. *J. Neuropathol. Exp. Neurol.* 56:872–878.

Li, H., Alonso-Vanegas, M., Colicos, M. A., Jung, S. S., Lochmuller, H., Sadikot, A. F., Snipes, G. J., Seth, P., Karpati, G., and Nalbantoglu, J. (1999). Intracerebral adenovi-rus-mediated p53 tumor suppressor gene therapy for experimental human glioma. *Clin. Cancer Res.* 5:637–642.

Louis, D. N. (1993). The p53 gene and protein in human brain tumors. *J. Neuropathol. Exp. Neurol.* 53:11–21.

Lu, W., Zhou, X., Hong, B., Liu, J., and Yue, Z. (2004). Suppression of invasion in human U87 glioma cells by adenovirus-mediated co-transfer of TIMP-2 and PTEN gene. *Cancer Lett.* 214:205–213.

Liu, Y., and Deisseroth, A. (2006). Tumor vascular targeting therapy with viral vectors. *Blood* 107:3027–3033.

Lui, V. W., He, Y., and Huang, L. (2001). Specific down-regulation of HER-2/neu medi-ated by a chimeric U6 hammerhead ribozyme results in growth inhibition of human ovarian carcinoma. *Mol. Ther.* 3:169–177.

Mallory, A. C., Reinhart, B. J., Jones-Rhoades, M. W., Tang, G., Zamore, P. D., Barton, M. K., and Bartel, D. P. (2004). MicroRNA control of PHABULOSA in leaf development: Importance of pairing to the microRNA 5' region. *EMBO J.* 23:3356–3364.

Manome, Y., Wen, P. Y., Dong, Y., Tanaka, T., Mitchell, B. S., Kufe, D. W., and Fine, H. A. (1996). Viral vector transduction of the human deoxycytidine kinase cDNA sensitizes glioma cells to the cytotoxic effects of cytosine arabinoside in vitro and in vivo. *Nat. Med.* 2:567–573.

Marshall, J. L., Hoyer, R. J., Toomey, M. A., Faraguna, K., Chang, P., Richmond, E., Pedicano, J. E., Gehan, E., Peck, R. A., Arlen, P., Tsang, K. Y., and Schlom, J. (2000). Phase I study in advanced cancer patients of a diversified prime-and-boost vaccination protocol using recombinant vaccinia virus and recombinant nonreplicating avipox virus to elicit anti-carcinoembryonic antigen immune responses. *J. Clin. Oncol.* 18:3964–3973.

Martuza, R. L., Malick, A., Markert, J. M., Ruffner, K. L., and Coen, D. M. (1991). Experimental therapy of human glioma by means of a genetically engineered virus mutant. *Science* 252:854–856.

Mercatante, D. R., Mohler, J. L., and Kole, R. (2002). Cellular response to an antisense-mediated shift of Bcl-x pre-mRNA splicing and antineoplastic agents. *J. Biol. Chem.* 277:49374–49382.

Millauer, B., Shawver, L. K., Plate, K. H., Risau, W., and Ullrich, A. (1994). Glioblastoma growth inhibited *in vivo* by a dominant-negative FlK-1 mutant. *Nature* 367:576–579.

Miller, A. D. (1992). Human gene therapy comes of age. *Nature* 357:455–460.

Miyashita, T., and Reed, J. C. (1995). Tumor suppressor p53 is a direct transcriptional activator of the human bax gene. *Cell* 80:293–299.

Miyashita, T., Krajewski, S., Krajewska, M., Wang, H. G., Lin, H. K., Liebermann, D. A., Hoffman, B., and Reed, J. C. (1994). Tumor suppressor p53 is a regulator of bcl-2 and bax gene expression in vitro and in vivo. *Oncogene* 9:1799–1805.

Moolten, F. L. (1986). Tumor chemosensitivity conferred by inserted herpes thymidine kinase genes: Paradigm for a prospective cancer control strategy. *Cancer Res.* 46: 5276–5281.

Morrissey, D. V., Lee, P. A., Johnson, D. A., Overly, S. L., McSwiggen, J. A., Beigelman, L., Mokler, V. R., Maloney, L., Vargeese, C., Bowman, K., O'Brien, J. T., Shaffer, C. S., Conrad, A., Schmid, P., Morrey, J. D., Macejak, D. G., Pavco, P. A., and Blatt, L. M. (2002). Characterization of nuclease-resistant ribozymes directed against hepatitis B virus RNA. *J. Viral Hepat.* 9:411–418.

Moss, R. B., Milla, C., Colombo, J., Accurso, F., Zeitlin, P. L., Clancy, J. P., Spencer, L. T., Pilewski, J., Waltz, D. A., Dorkin, H. L., Ferkol, T., Pian, M., Ramsey, B., Carter, B. J., Martin, D. B., and Heald, A. E. (2007). Repeated aerosolized AAV-CFTR for treatment of cystic fibrosis: A randomized placebo-controlled phase 2B trial. *Hum. Gene Ther.* 18:726–732.

Muller, M., Wilder, S., Bannasch, D., Israeli, D., Lehlbach, K., Li-Weber, M., Friedman, S. L., Galle, P. R., Stremmel, W., Oren, M., and Krammer, P. H. (1998). P53 activates the CD95 (APO-1/Fas) gene in response to DNA damage by anticancer drugs. *J. Exp. Med.* 188:2033–2045.

Nagy, H. J., Panis, Y., Fabre, M., Klatzmann, D., Houssin, D., and Soubrane, O. (2000). Suicide gene therapy of ovarian cancer: An experimental study in rats using retroviral-mediated transfer of herpes simplex virus thymidine kinase gene. *Anticancer Res.* 20:4633–4638.

Nemunaitis, J., Ganly, I., Khuri, F., Arseneau, J., Kuhn, J., McCarty, T., Landers, S., Maples, P., Romel, L., Randlev, B., Reid, T., Kaye, S., and Kirn, D. (2000). Selective replication and oncolysis in p53 mutant tumors with ONYX-015, an E1B-55kD gene-deleted adenovirus, in patients with advanced head and neck cancer: A phase II trial. *Cancer Res.* 60:6359–6366.

Noguchi, M., Imaizumi, K., Kawabe, T., Wakayama, H., Horio, Y., Sekido, Y., Hara, T., Hashimoto, N., Takahashi, M., Shimokata, K., and Hasegawa, Y. (2001). Induction of antitumor immunity by transduction of CD40 ligand gene and interferon-gamma gene into lung cancer. *Cancer Gene Ther.* 8:421–429.

Novina, C. D., Murray, M. F., Dykxhoorn, D. M., Beresford, P. J., Riess, J., Lee, S. K., Collman, R. G., Lieberman, J., Shankar, P., and Sharp, P. A. (2002). siRNA-directed inhibition of HIV-1 infection. *Nat. Med.* 8:681–686.

Orlacchio, A., Bernardi, G., Orlacchio, A., and Martino, S. (2007). RNA interference as a tool for Alzheimer's disease therapy. *Mini. Rev. Med. Chem.* 7:1166–1176.

Plate, K. H., Breier, G., Weich, H. A., and Risau, W. (1992). Vascular endothelial growth factor is a potential tumor angiogenesis. *Nature* 359:845–848.

Plate, K. H., Breier, G., Millbauer, B., Ullrich, A., and Risau, W. (1993). Up-regulation of vascular endothelial growth factor and its cognate receptors in a rate glioma model of tumor angiogenesis. *Cancer Res.* 53:5822–5827.

Pirollo, K. F., Hao, Z., and Rait, A. (1997). p53-mediated sensitization of squamous cell carcinoma of the head and neck to radiotherapy. *Oncogene* 14:1735–1746.

Raper, S. E., Chirmule, N., Lee, F. S., Wivel, N. A., Bagg, A., Gao, G. P., Wilson, J. M., and Batshaw, M. L. (2003). Fatal systemic inflammatory response syndrome in a ornithine transcarbamylase deficient patient following adenoviral gene transfer. *Mol. Genet. Metab.* 80:148–158.

Ray, S., Bullock, G., Nuñez, G., Tang, C., Ibrado, A. M., Huang, Y., and Bhalla, K. (1996). Adenoviral-mediated p53 tumor suppressor gene therapy of human ovarian carcinoma. *Oncogene* 12:1617–1623.

Ries, S. J., Brandts, C. H., Chung, A. S., Biederer, C. H., Hann, B. C., Lipner, E. M., McCormick, F., and Korn, W. M. (2000). Loss of p14ARF in tumor cells facilitates replication of the adenovirus mutant dl1520 (ONYX-015). *Nat. Med.* 6:1128–1133.

Rodolfo, M., Catò, E. M., Soldati, S., Ceruti, R., Asioli, M., Scanziani, E., Vezzoni, P., Parmiani, G., and Sacco, M. G. (2001). Growth of human melanoma xenografts is suppressed by systemic angiostatin gene therapy. *Cancer Gene Ther.* 8:491–496.

Rodriguez, R., Schuur, E. R., Lim, H. Y., Henderson, G. A., Simons, J. W., and Henderson, D. R. (1997). Prostate attenuated replication competent adenovirus (ARCA) CN706: A selective cytotoxic for prostate-specific antigen-positive prostate cancer cells. *Cancer Res.* 57:2559–2563.

Rosenberg, S. A., Aebersold, P., Cornetta, K., Kasid, A., Morgan, R. A., Moen, R., Karson, E. M., Lotze, M. T., Yang, J. C., and Topalian, S. L. (1990). Gene transfer into humans—immunotherapy of patients with advanced melanoma, using tumor-infiltrating lymphocytes modified by retroviral gene transduction. *N. Engl. J. Med.* 323:570–578.

Rosenberg, S. A., Zhai, Y., Yang, J. C., Schwartzentruber, D. J., Hwu, P., Marincola, F. M., Topalian, S. L., Restifo, N. P., Seipp, C. A., Einhorn, J. H., Roberts, B., and White, D. E. (1998). Immunizing patients with metastatic melanoma using recombinant adenoviruses encoding MART-1 or gp100 melanoma antigens. *J. Natl. Cancer Inst.* 90:1894–1900.

Rosenfeld, M. (2007). An overview of endpoints for cystic fibrosis clinical trials: One size does not fit all. *Proc. Am. Thorac. Soc.* 4:299–301.

Sauter, B. V., Martinet, O., Zhang, W. J., Mandeli, J., and Woo, S. L. (2000). Adenovirus-mediated gene transfer of endostatin in vivo results in high level of transgene expression and inhibition of tumor growth and metastases. *Proc. Natl. Acad. Sci. U.S.A.* 97:4802–4807.

Schmidt, M., Hacein-Bey-Abina, S., Wissler, M., Carlier, F., Lim, A., Prinz, C., Glimm, H., Andre-Schmutz, I., Hue, C., Garrigue, A., Le Deist, F., Lagresle, C., Fischer, A., Cavazzana-Calvo, M., and von Kalle, C. (2005). Clonal evidence for the transduction of CD34+ cells with lymphomyeloid differentiation potential and self-renewal capacity in the SCID-X1 gene therapy trial. *Blood* 105:2699–2706.

Shah, P. B., and Losordo, D. W. (2005). Non-viral vectors for gene therapy: Clinical trials in cardiovascular disease. *Adv. Genet.* 54:339–361.

Sidransky, D., Mikkelsen, T., Schwechheimer, K., Rosenblum, M. L., Cavenee, W. K., and Vogelstein, B. (1992). Clonal expansion of p53 mutant cells is associated with brain tumor progression. *Nature (Lond.)* 355:846–847.

Smyth, M. J., Godfrey, D. I., and Trapani, J. A. (2001). A fresh look at tumor immunosurveillance and immunotherapy. *Nat. Immunol.* 2:293–299.

Sonabend, A. M., Velicu, S., Ulasov, I. V., Han, Y., Tyler, B., Brem, H., Matar, M. M., Fewell, J. G., Anwer, K., and Lesniak, M. S. (2008). A safety and efficacy study of local delivery of interleukin-12 transgene by PPC polymer in a model of experimental glioma. *Anticancer Drugs* 19:133–142.

Spitz, F. R., Nguyen, D., and Skibber, J. M. (1996a). Adenoviral-mediated wild-type p53 gene expression sensitizes colorectal cancer cells to ionizing radiation. *Clin. Cancer Res.* 2:1665–1671.

Spitz, F. R., Nguyen, D., Skibber, J. M., Cusack, J., Roth, J. A., and Cristiano, R. J. (1996b). In vivo adenovirus-mediated p53 tumor suppressor gene therapy for colorectal cancer. *Anticancer Res.* 16:3415–3422.

Sullenger, B. A., and Gilboa, E. (2002). Emerging clinical applications of RNA. *Nature* 418:252–258.

Sumimoto, H., and Kawakami, Y. (2007). Lentiviral vector-mediated RNAi and its use for cancer research. *Future Oncol.* 3:655–664.

Sun, Y., Jurgovsky, K., Möller, P., Alijagic, S., Dorbic, T., Georgieva, J., Wittig, B., and Schadendorf, D. (1998). Vaccination with IL-12 gene-modified autologous melanoma cells: Preclinical results and a first clinical phase I study. *Gene Ther.* 5:481–490.

Swisher, S. G., Roth, J. A., Nemunaitis, J., Lawrence, D. D., Kemp, B. L., Carrasco, C. H., Connors, D. G., El-Naggar, A. K., Fossella, F., Glisson, B. S., Hong, W. K., Khuri, F. R., Kurie, J. M., Lee, J. J., Lee, J. S., Mack, M., Merritt, J. A., Nguyen, D. M., Nesbitt, J. C., Perez-Soler, R., Pisters, K. M., Putnam, J. B. Jr, Richli, W. R., Savin, M., Schrump, D. S., Shin, D. M., Shulkin, A., Walsh, G. L., Wait, J., Weill, D., and Waugh, M. K. (1999). Adenovirus-mediated p53 gene transfer in advanced non-small-cell lung cancer. *J. Natl. Cancer Inst.* 91:763–771.

Tagawa, M., Kawamura, K., Ueyama, T., Nakamura, M., Tada, Y., Ma, G., Li, Q., Suzuki, N., Shimada, H., and Ochiai, T. (2008). Cancer therapy with local oncolysis and topical cytokine secretion. *Front Biosci.* 13:2578–2587.

Takahashi, S., Yotnda, P., Rousseau, R. F., Mei, Z., Smith, S., Rill, D., Younes, A., and Brenner, M. K. (2001). Transgenic expression of CD40L and interleukin-2 induces an autologous antitumor immune response in patients with non-Hodgkin's lymphoma. *Cancer Gene Ther.* 8:378–387.

Tanabe, T., Kuwabara, T., Warashina, M., Tani, K., Taira, K., and Asano, S. (2000). Oncogene inactivation in a mouse model. *Nature* 406:473–474.

Thybusch-Bernhardt, A., Aigner, A., Beckmann, S., Czubayko, F., and Juhl, H. (2001). Ribozyme targeting of HER-2 inhibits pancreatic cancer cell growth in vivo. *Eur. J. Cancer* 37:1688–1694.

Tzai, T. S., Lin, C. I., Shiau, A. L., and Wu, C. L. (1998). Antisense oligonucleotide specific for transforming growth factor-beta 1 inhibit both in vitro and in vivo growth of MBT-2 murine bladder cancer. *Anticancer Res.* 18:1585–1589.

Urosevic, M., Fujii, K., Calmels, B., Laine, E., Kobert, N., Acres, B., and Dummer, R. (2007). Type I IFN innate immune response to adenovirus-mediated IFN-gamma gene transfer contributes to the regression of cutaneous lymphomas. *J. Clin. Invest.* 117:2834–2846.

van Meir, E. G., Roemer, K., Diserens, A. C., Kikuchi, T., Rempel, S. A., Haas, M., Huang, H. J., Friedmann, T. L., de Tribolet, N., and Cavenee, W. K. (1995). Single cell monitoring of growth arrest and morphological changes induced by transfer of wild-type p53 alleles to glioblastoma cells. *Proc. Natl. Acad. Sci. U.S.A.* 92:1008–1012.

Vattemi, E., and Claudio, P. P. (2006). Adenoviral gene therapy in head and neck cancer. *Drug News Perspect* 19:329–337.

Verma, I. M. (1990). Gene theory. *Sci. Am.* 263:68–72.

Vollmer, C. M., Ribas, A., Butterfield, L. H., Dissette, V. B., Andrews, K. J., Eilber, F. C., Montejo, L. D., Chen, A. Y., Hu, B., Glaspy, J. A., McBride, W. H., and Economou, J. S. (1999). p53 selective and nonselective replication of an E1B-deleted adenovirus in hepatocellular carcinoma. *Cancer Res.* 59:4369–4374.

von Deimling, A., Eibl, R. H., Ohgaki, H., Louis, D. N., von Ammon, K., Petersen, I., Kleihues, P., Chung, R. Y., and Wiestler, O. D. (1992). p53 mutations are associated with 17p allelic loss in grade II and grade III astrocytoma. *Cancer Res.* 52:2987–2990.

Weiss, B., Davidkova, G., and Zhou, L. W. (1999). Antisense RNA gene therapy for studying and modulating biological processes. *Cell Mol. Life Sci.* 55:334–358.

Weng, D. E., Masci, P. A., Radka, S. F., Jackson, T. E., Weiss, P. A., Ganapathi, R., Elson, P. J., Capra, W. B., Parker, V. P., Lockridge, J. A., Cowens, J. W., Usman, N., and Borden, E. C. (2005). A phase I clinical trial of a ribozyme-based angiogenesis inhibitor targeting vascular endothelial growth factor receptor-1 for patients with refractory solid tumors. *Mol. Cancer Ther.* 4:948–955.

Wieczorek, A. M., Waterman, J. L. F., Waterman, M. J. F., and Halazonetis, T. D. (1996). Structure-based rescue of common tumor-derived p53 mutants. *Nat. Med.* 2:1143–1146.

Wilson, J. (1999). Human gene therapy: Present and future. *Human Genome News* 10:1–2.

Wolff, J., Lewis, D. L., Herweijer, H., Hegge, J., and Hagstrom, J. (2005). Non-viral approaches for gene transfer. *Acta Myol.* 24:202–208.

Wu, G. S., Burns, T. F., McDonald, E. R. 3rd, Jiang, W., Meng, R., Krantz, I. D., Kao, G., Gan, D. D., Zhou, J. Y., Muschel, R., Hamilton, S. R., Spanner, N. B., Markowitz, S., Wu, S., el-Deiry, W. S. (1997). DR5 is a DNA damage-inducible p53-regulated death receptor gene. *Nature Genet.* 17:141–143.

Wu, R. S., Kobie, J. J., Besselsen, D. G., Fong, T. C., Mack, V. D., McEarchern, J. A., and Akporiaye, E. T. (2001). Comparative analysis of IFN-gamma B7.1 and antisense TGF-beta gene transfer on the tumorigenicity of a poorly immunogenic metastatic mammary carcinoma. *Cancer Immunol. Immunother.* 50:229–240.

Yuan, A., Yang, P. C., Yu, C. J., Chen, W. J., Lin, F. Y., Kuo, S. H., and Luh, K. T. (2000). Interleukin-8 messenger ribonucleic acid expression correlates with tumor progression, tumor angiogenesism patient survival, and timing of relapse in non-small-cell lung cancer. *Am. J. Respir. Crit. Care Med.* 162:1957–1963.

Zellweger, T., Miyake, H., Cooper, S., Chi, K., Conklin, B. S., Monia, B. P., and Gleave, M. E. (2001). Antitumor activity of antisense clusterin oligonucleotides is improved in vitro and in vivo by incorporation of 2′-O-(2-methoxy) ethyl chemistry. *J. Pharmacol. Exp. Ther.* 298:934–940.

Zhao, P., Zhu, Y. H., Wu, J. X., Liu, R. Y., Zhu, X. Y., Xiao, X., Li, H. L., Huang, B. J., Xie, F. J., Chen, J. M., Ke, M. L., and Huang, W. (2007). Adenovirus-mediated delivery of human IFNgamma gene inhibits prostate cancer growth. *Life Sci.* 81:695–701.

Zheng, X., Koropatnick, J., Li, M., Zhang, X., Ling, F., Ren, X., Hao, X., Sun, H., Vladau, C., Franek, J. A., Feng, B., Urquhart, B. L., Zhong, R., Freeman, D. J., Garcia, B., and Min, W. P. (2006). Reinstalling antitumor immunity by inhibiting tumor-derived immunosuppressive molecule IDO through RNA interference. *J. Immunol.* 177:5639–5646.

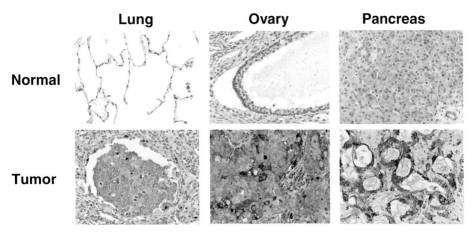

Figure 2.4. Immunohistochemical staining of a candidate cancer target. Differential expression of a protein associated with cancers shown by immunohistochemical staining of the target using specific antiserum on sections from tumor and normal tissue specimens derived from lung, ovarian, and pancreatic tissues. Intensity of staining (brown color) indicates the relative amount of the target protein in the tissue section. Sections are counterstained with hematoxylin and eosin to visualize cellular and tissue architecture. In the example shown, substantially more target protein is expressed in the tumor tissues for all three histotypes than is expressed in the corresponding normal tissues. An expression pattern like the one shown may indicate that tumors might be more dependent on the target activity than normal tissues. See page 31 for text discussion.

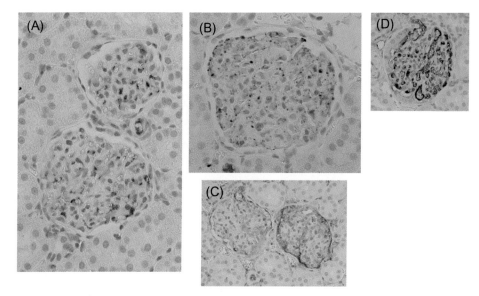

Figure 4.1. Kidney from a rat treated with VEGFR2 kinase inhibitor. Immunohistochemical label for albumin demonstrated globular (A) and punctate (B) deposits of positive material with glomerular mesangium, which correlated with increased mesangial eosinophilia. Additionally, positive labeling was present in the uriniferous space (C). Some glomeruli from vehicle-treated controls (D) demonstrated positive material lining endothelium of capillaries. See pages 89–90 for text discussion.

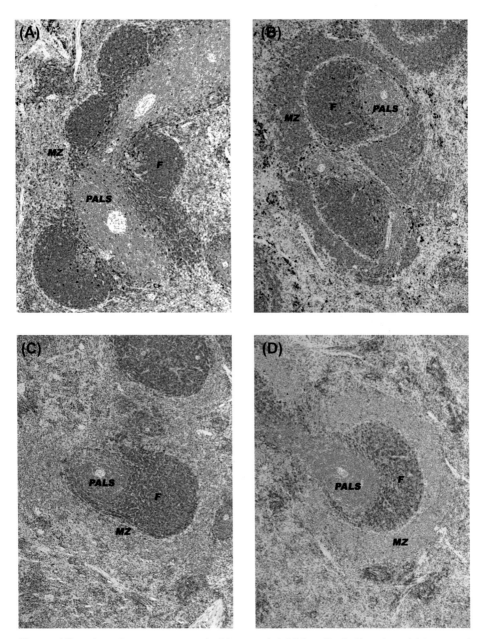

Figure 4.2. Spleen from a rat treated with a notch inhibitor (A, C, E) and a vehicle-treated control (B, D, F). Immunohistochemical stains for IgM (A, B), IgD (C, D), and CD8 (E, F). Target-related effects include decreased marginal zones, which in rats, is uniquely prominent and distinct from the PALS and follicles. (Legend: PALS = periarteriolar lymphoid sheath, MZ = marginal zone, F = lymphoid follicle.) See pages 91–92 for text discussion.

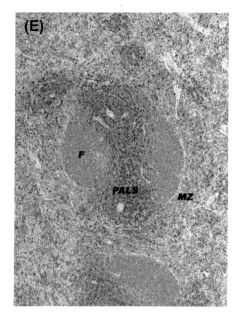

Figure 4.2. *Continued*

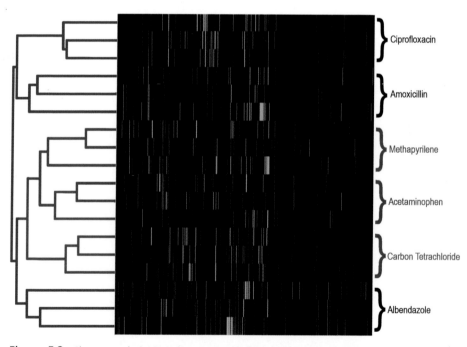

Figure 5.2. Cluster analysis. Rats in groups of three were treated with three hepatotoxins (methapyrilene 100 mg/kg, acetaminophen 972 mg/kg, carbon tetrachloride 400 mg/kg) and three nonhepatotoxic compounds (ciprofloxacin 72 mg/kg, amoxicillin 1100 mg/kg, albendazole 62 mg/kg) for 5 days except that carbon tetrachloride was a 7-day treatment. The figure shows a heat map of gene expression (red increased, green decreased expression) with the clustering hierarchy of compounds to the left. Gene expression for individual compounds clearly cluster together, and hepatotoxicants form a single cluster within the hierarchy (red). See pages 122–123 for text discussion.

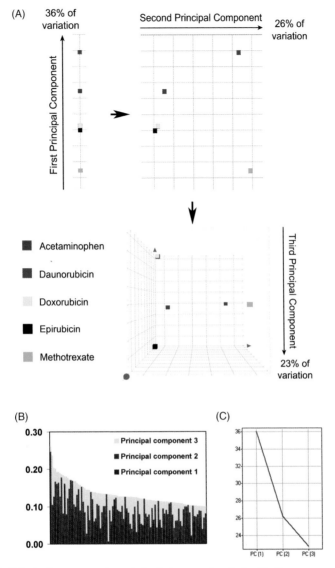

Figure 5.3. Principal component analysis. Rats were treated with five compounds at toxic doses for 5 days and microarray analysis on RNA isolated from liver was performed. (A) The first principal component (top left) represents 36% of all variation between the sample profiles and separates methotrexate and acetaminophen by the greatest difference. The second principal component (top right) represents 26% of all variation and distinguishes daunorubicin, doxorubicin, and epirubicin profiles from other gene profiles. The third principal component (bottom) represents 23% of all variation and separates the profiles of doxorubicin and epirubicin. (B) The relative weighting for each principal component for the top most weighted 100 genes out of a total of 2289. Note that individual genes may contribute to all three principal components. (C) Graph showing the relative contribution of each principal component to the total variation in the data set. The first three principal components describe 85% of the variation in the data set. See pages 122–124 for text discussion.

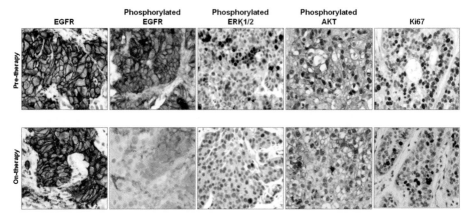

Figure 6.3. Pharmacodynamic effects on sequential tumor biopsies—baseline and after 28 days of therapy—from a patient treated with gefitinib at 250 mg/day. Baseline (upper panel) and on-therapy (lower panel) for EGFR, phosphorylated EGFR, phosphorylated ERK1/2, phosphorylated AKT, and Ki67 immunohistochemistry assays in a gastric carcinoma. On-therapy, inhibition of p-EGFR, p-ERK1/2 was detected, whereas only a reduction of p-AKT and proliferation was observed. No changes in total EGFR expression were present in tumor cells. See page 150 for text discussion.

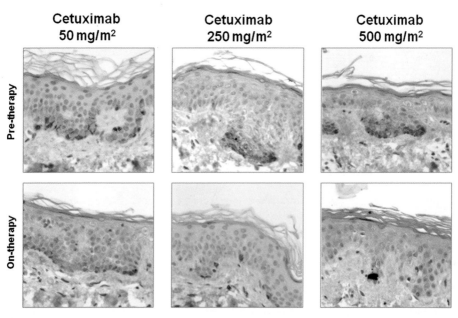

Figure 6.4. Dose-dependent pharmacodynamic inhibition of phosphorylated EGFR in sequential skin biopsies from patients treated with cetuximab at 50, 250, and 500 mg/m^2. Samples were obtained baseline and after 28 days of therapy. Baseline expression is mainly detected in basal keratinocytes by immunohistochemistry and reduced in a dose-dependent manner after treatment. See page 153 for text discussion.

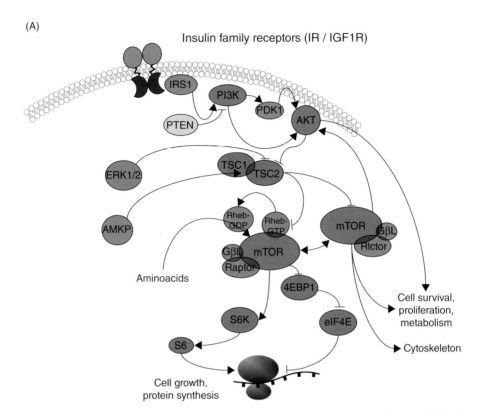

(A)

Insulin family receptors (IR / IGF1R)

Figure 6.5. (A) Regulation of mTOR activity by growth factors is mediated by the PI3K/AKT signaling pathway, leading to phophorylation and inhibition of tuberin (TSC2) by AKT and to the subsequent activation of Rheb, which activates mTOR. The mTOR also receives nutrient input signals. The Raptor/mTOR complex mediates the phosphorylation of eukaryotic initiation factor 4E (eIF-4E) binding protein (4E-BP1) and ribosomal protein S6 kinase (p70S6K1). 4EB-P1 and p70S6K1 are mTOR downstream effector molecules that function as regulators of ribosome biogenesis and protein translation. See page 157 for text discussion.

(B)

Phosphorylated
4E-BP1

Phosphorylated
S6

Pre-therapy

On-therapy

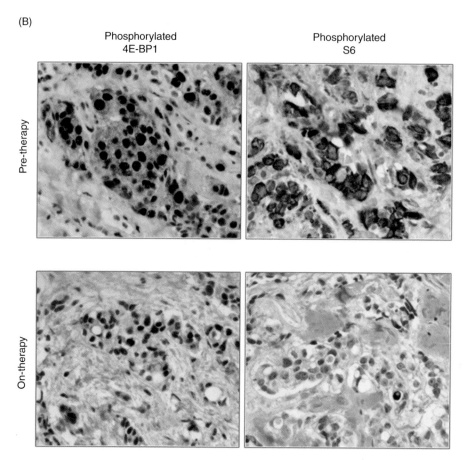

Figure 6.5. (*Continued*) (B) Pharmacodynamic effects on sequential tumor biopsies—baseline and after 28 days of therapy—from a patient treated with a rapamycin-analog mTOR inhibitor. Baseline (upper panel) and on-therapy (lower panel) for phosphorylated 4E-BP1 (p-4E-BP1) and phosphorylated S6 (p-S6) immunohistochemistry assays in a breast carcinoma. On-therapy, inhibition of p-4E-BP1 and p-S6 was detected in tumor cells. See page 157 for text discussion.

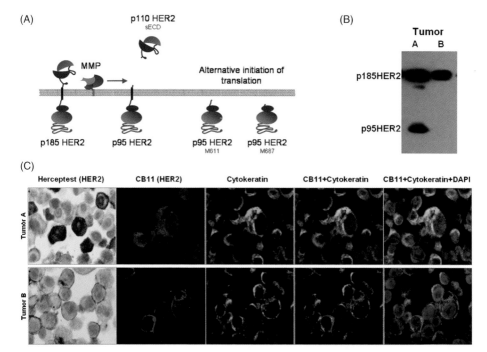

Figure 6.6. (A) HER2 receptor (p185HER2) undergoes a slow proteolytic shedding of its ectodomain that is detected in the serum of patients with advanced breast cancer. The shedding generates an NH2 terminally truncated fragment (p95HER2) that is membrane associated and has kinase activity. Membrane p95HER2 forms are largely synthesized by alternative initiation of translation from methionines 611 and 687, located before and after transmembrane region. The expression of truncated p95HER2 in breast cancer, detected by immunofluorescence assays, has been correlated with poor prognosis and resistance to trastuzumab. (B) Two infiltrating ductal breast carcinomas were subjected to Western blot analysis using an anti-HER2 antibody against intracellular domain of the receptor. Tumor A expresses both HER2 full-length receptor (p185) and truncated form receptor (p95). Tumor B expresses only the p185 HER2 receptor. (C) Two serial sections from tumors in (B) were assayed by immunofluorescence using an antibody to the extracellular domain of the receptor (ECD) and to the intracellular domain of HER2 (ICD), in red. Staining of cytoplasmic compartment was performed with an antibody anticytokeratin (green) and nuclei were stained with DAPI (blue). Tumor A shows membrane staining with the ECD but combined membrane and cytoplasmic staining with the ICD antibody, which co-localized with the anticytokeratin antibody (yellow). Tumor B shows only membrane staining with both antibodies. See pages 160–161 for text discussion.

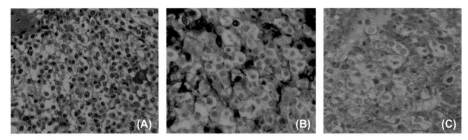

Figure 7.1. Oligodendroglioma. (A) Distinctive feature of oligodendrogliomas, perinuclear halos (a fixation artifact) highlight the uniform, perfectly round nuclei. (B) Occasional tumor cells with eosinophilic cytoplasm can be immunoreactive with GFAP. Most tumor cells are GFAP negative. (C) Low-grade oligodendrogliomas usually have very few MIB-1 immunopositive nuclei. See pages 174–175 for text discussion.

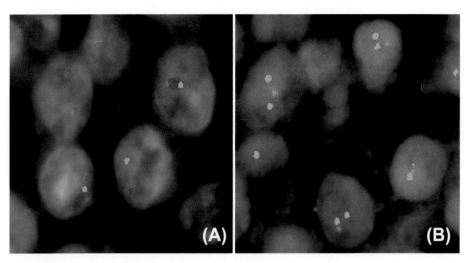

Figure 7.2. Representative FISH images. (A) and (B) are FISH images from an oligodendroglioma tumor. (A) 1p deletion is represented (the green signal is 1p32 and red is 1q42; mostly 1 green, 2 red signal pattern). (B) 19q deletion is represented (the green is 19p13 and red is 19q13.4 (mostly 2 green, 1 red pattern). (Courtesy of Dr. Arie Perry, St. Louis, Missouri.) See pages 174–175 for text discussion.

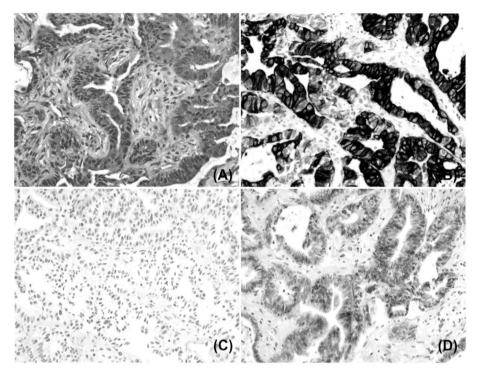

Figure 7.5. Colorectal adenocarcinoma. (A) Invasive moderately differentiated adenocarcinoma with a desmoplastic background. (B, C) Typical CD20+ (B)/CD7-(C) immunohistochemical profile. (D) Positive membranous/cytoplasmic EGFR staining. See page 179 for text discussion.

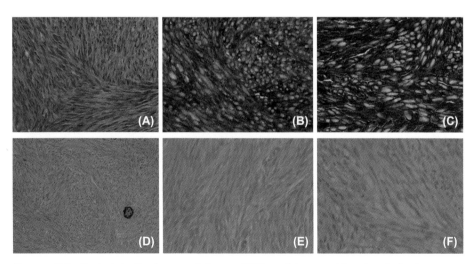

Figure 7.6. Gastrointestinal stromal tumor H&E and immunohistochemical phenotype. (A) Spindle cell neoplasm with moderate cellularity. (B) Strong membranous KIT positivity. (C) Extensive CD34 positivity. (D, E, F) Negative staining for SMA, desmin and S100, repectively. See pages 181–182 for text discussion.

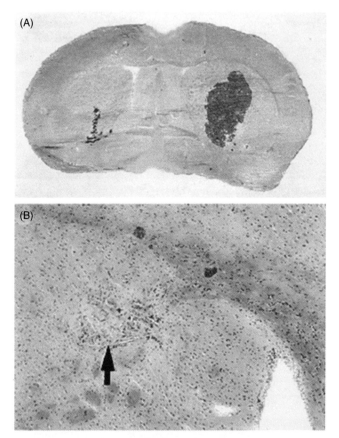

Figure 8.1. (A) Elimination of tumor cells after infection with AV*p53*.A, effect of infection with AV*p53* (left hemisphere) or AV*GFP* (right hemisphere) after bilateral implantation of U87/*lacZ* tumor cells. Tumor cells were allowed to grow for 10 days before recombinant virus injection. Animals were euthanized 25 days after treatment with recombinant viruses. Fluorescence microscopy showed that the tumor in the right hemisphere had robust, diffuse expression of GFP. Sections were stained for β-galactosidase activity (blue), followed by H&E staining. (B) Brain tissue section from an animal that died of unrelated causes 265 days after stereotactic injection of AV*p53* (10 days after the implantation of tumor cells). This gliotic area (arrow) did not contain any tumor cells. H&E staining. ×100 original magnification (Li et al., 1999). (Reproduced by permission of the American Association for Cancer Research Inc.) See pages 198–199 for text discussion.

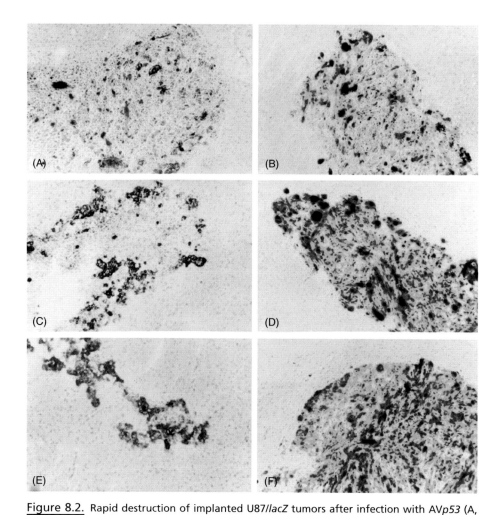

Figure 8.2. Rapid destruction of implanted U87/*lacZ* tumors after infection with AV*p53* (A, C, E) as compared to infection with AV*GFP* (B, D, F). Animals were euthanized at day 2 (A, B), 5 (C, D), and 25 (E, F) after treatment with AV. Sections were stained for β-galactosidase activity (blue), followed by H&E staining (Li et al., 1999). (Reproduced by permission of the American Association for Cancer Research Inc.) See pages 198–199 for text discussion.

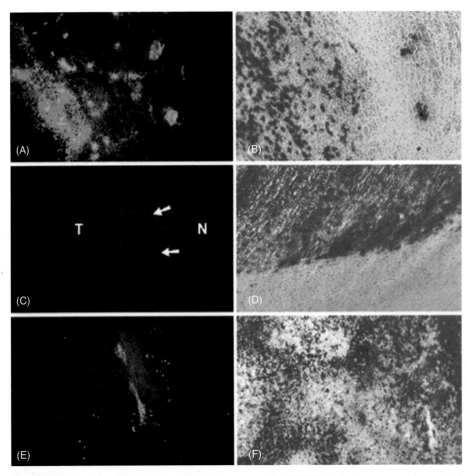

Figure 8.3. In vivo transduction of C6/*lacZ* tumors with vTKiGFP. Brain tumors were harvested postmortem as described previously. (A, B) Tumor from a control rat that received vTKiGFP without subsequent treatment with GCV (rat was sacrificed on day 30 after tumor implantation due to morbid state). (C, D) Tumor from a control rat that did not receive vTKiGFP but was treated with GCV (rat was sacrificed on day 43). (E, F) Tumor from a test rat that received vTKiGFP and subsequent treatment with GCV, which suffered symptomatic recurrent tumor (rat was sacrificed on day 82). GFP expression (A, C, E) was compared with subsequent histochemical staining of C6/*lacZ* tumor cells with the substrate X-gal (B, D, F). ×100. *T*, tumor; *N*, normal brain (Galipeau et al., 1999). (Reproduced by permission of the American Association for Cancer Research Inc.) See page 203 for text discussion.

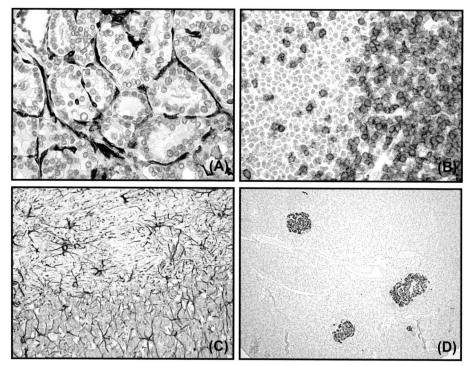

Figure 9.1. Identification of cell types using immunohistochemistry. (Top left) Angiogenesis. CD31 in thyroid carcinoma detects endothelial cells of blood vessels. (Top right) CD3 detects T cells in human tonsil. (Bottom left) Glial fibrillary acidic protein (GFAP) IHC staining of glial cells in rat cerebellum. (Bottom right) Insulin IHC in rat pancreas. Beta cells label in the islets of Langerhans label. Hematoxylin counterstain provides a blue nuclear stain (light) and DAB chromagen shows dark brown staining of the target protein (dark). See pages 222–223 for text discussion.

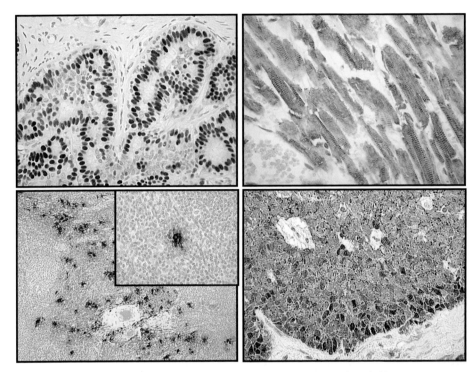

Figure 9.2. Examples of different subcellular localization patterns. (Top left) Estrogen receptor (ER) in a breast carcinoma. The nuclei of most tumor cells label. (Top right) Pan actin in
human heart showing striations in the cytoplasm of cardiomyocytes. (Bottom left) IHC stain
of tonsil using anti-mast-cell tryptase. Mast cells label with a cytoplasmic and extracellular
localization. Inset shows higher magnification image staining in tonsil. (Bottom right) dUTPase
in human colon carcinoma. Nuclear as well as cytoplasmic localization is detected. Hematoxylin
counterstain and DAB chromagen. See pages 222–224 for text discussion.

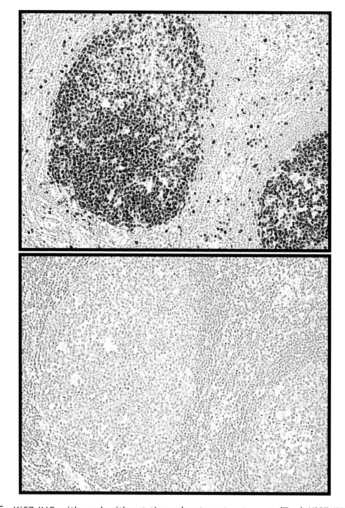

Figure 9.5. Ki67 IHC with and without tissue heat pretreatment. (Top) Ki67 IHC in section of human tonsil using steam heat pretreatment. Note strong nuclear staining of proliferating cells localized primarily to germinal centers. (Bottom) Ki67 IHC in a serial section of tonsil shown above. No steam heat pretreatment was performed. Only marginal nuclear staining is detected. Hematoxylin counterstain; DAB chromagen. See page 228 for text discussion.

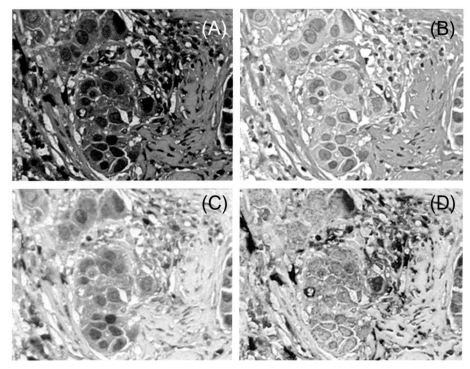

Figure 10.8. RGB image as seen in (A) the microscope field of view, and the color representation of the same field showing only the (B) hematoxylin, (C) DAB, or (D) Fast Red markers, after chromogen separation and electronic image synthesis. See page 276 for text discussion.

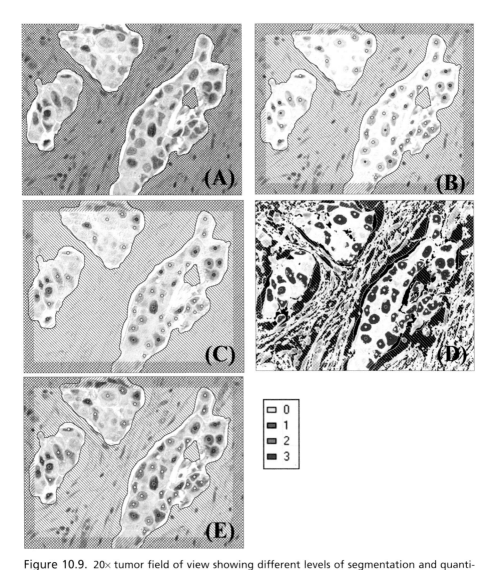

Figure 10.9. 20× tumor field of view showing different levels of segmentation and quantification based on the segmentation masks. (A) Field of view showing the tumor region automatically segmented based upon nucleus size, cell density, and marker content rules. (B, C) Same field of view showing the chromogen-separated images of the scene. (D) Nuclei masks segmented within the tumor regions. (E) Marker intensity labeling of cells based upon their marker intensity observed within the nucleus mask (0, negative; 1, weak; 2, mild; and 3, strong positive). See page 285 for text discussion.

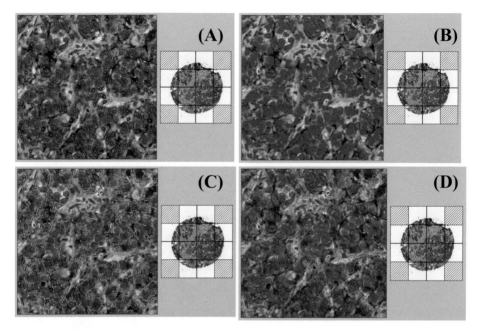

Figure 10.12. Cell segmentation of a given field of view extracted from the high-resolution image of a core within a TMA and processed using the chromogen separation engine: (A) image of the field of view and identification of each automatically found cell with their respective masks, (B) nucleus, and (C) positive HER2 membrane stain; (D) estimation of cytoplasmic boundaries based upon found membranes and iso-distance maps between nuclei of adjacent cells. See pages 287–289 for text discussion.

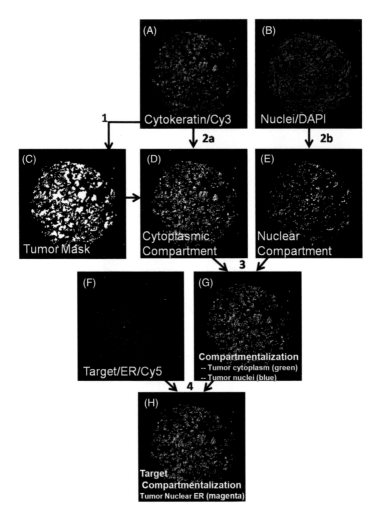

Figure 11.4. AQUA image analysis. Schematic representation of the AQUA analysis process for a typical experiment looking at biomarker expression in an epithelial cancer. (1) Tumor mask generation through pixel intensity thresholding (binary gating) and spatial image analysis procedures. (2a and 2b) Generation of cytoplasmic and nuclear-specific pixel mask through binary gating. (3) Combining cytoplasmic and nuclear-specific pixel masks in by 100% mutual exclusion. (4) Identification of coincidental target pixels with compartment pixels (for visualization only). See page 303 for text discussion.

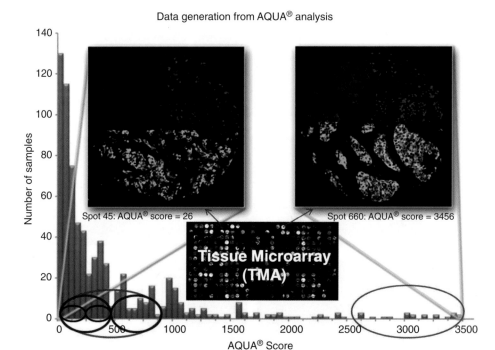

Figure 11.15. Typical AQUA analysis output. Frequency distribution from TMA analysis showing a low-resolution TMA image (inset) with example fluorescence images (inset). Different colored circles in frequency histogram delineated resolving capacity of AQUA scoring. See pages 314–317 for text discussion.

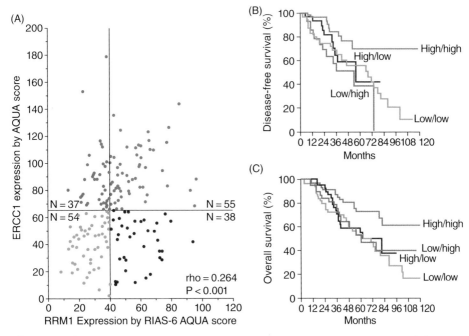

Figure 11.18. Ability of AQUA analysis to multiplex two independent biomarkers. (A) Scatter plot of AQUA scores for ERCC1 and RRM1 in stage I NSCLC with indicated cut points (groupings). KM analysis for (B) overall survival and (C) time to recurrence using groups established in (A) demonstrated increased overall survival and time to recurrence for patients with both high ERCC1 and high RRM1 expression as determined by AQUA analysis. (Adapted from Zheng et al., 2006.) See page 320 for text discussion.

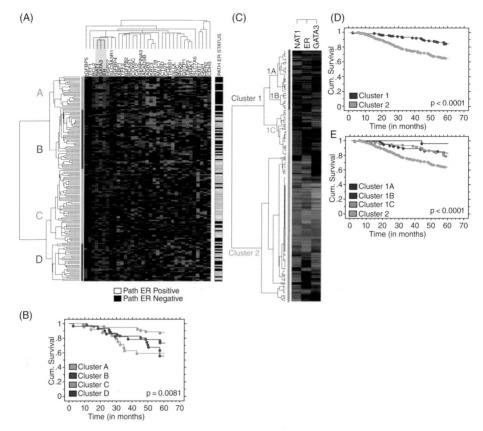

Figure 11.20. Hierarchical clustering analysis using AQUA analysis in breast cancer. (A) Unsupervised hierarchical clustering of 35 ER-related genes on 161 tumor samples with indicated cluster groupings. (B) KM survival analysis indicating a significant differentiation ($p = 0.0083$) of cluster groupings with respect to 5-year disease-specific survival. (C) Unsupervised hierarchical clustering analysis of ER and two most closely related genes from (A) and indicated cluster groupings (indicated: two main clusters, 1 and 2; and subsequent subcluster 1 groupings). (D, E) KM survival analysis of main clusters and cluster 1 subclusters indicate a significant association with 5-year disease-specific survival. (Adapted from Dolled-Filhart et al., 2006b.) See page 323 for text discussion.

9

MOLECULAR PATHOLOGY: IMMUNOHISTOCHEMISTRY ASSAYS IN DRUG DEVELOPMENT PERFORMED BY A CONTRACT RESEARCH LABORATORY

Frank Lynch and Steve Bernstein

Molecular pathology in drug development is not only performed within pharmaceutical and biotechnology companies but may also be outsourced to contract research organizations (CROs) that provide these important and highly valuable specialty services. This chapter focuses on the use of immunohistochemistry (IHC) assays and their applications to assist pharmaceutical and biotechnology companies in drug discovery and development from the perspective of a contract research organization.

Immunohistochemistry assays can be used in the spectrum of studies involved in drug discovery and development. These assays have applications ranging from basic research and preclinical studies through to clinical trial and diagnostic testing of patient samples. This chapter will provide a basic description of IHC assays and assay development in formalin-fixed, paraffin-embedded (FFPE) tissues and explain the interactions between a drug development company sponsor and a CRO specializing in IHC assays. The approach to these studies and the practical application of these assays will be discussed.

Molecular Pathology in Drug Discovery and Development, Edited by J. Suso Platero
Copyright © 2009 John Wiley & Sons, Inc.

9.1. IMMUNOHISTOCHEMISTRY IS THE TECHNIQUE OF MICROSCOPIC VISUALIZATION OF TARGET PROTEINS IN TISSUE SECTIONS USING SPECIFIC ANTIBODIES

Immunohistochemistry assays are performed on sections of tissue samples or cytology preparations that are placed onto glass microscope slides. Tissue samples may often be collected during various stages of drug discovery, ranging from evaluating animal treatment groups to testing tissue samples from patients enrolled in clinical studies. These tissues may be tested using a number of different assays including various "grind-and-find" assays in which analyses can typically only be inferred to the tissue level, as well as histologic and pathologic examination of sections of the intact tissue. With IHC techniques, various target proteins may be detected on the same specimen using different antibodies on serial sections of a tissue sample. IHC assays may be utilized to not only detect the expression of a target protein(s) but to determine the cell types that are expressing the target through binding of a primary antibody(s). Thus, the assay offers detection of a target protein with cell-specific and often subcellular resolution. The assay can often provide information on what cell type(s) is expressing the target; for example, in oncology studies: Is the target expressed in tumor cells or in other cell types such as stroma, infiltrating lymphocytes, or cells in adjacent normal tissue?

Several examples of IHC staining that identify cell types are provided in Figure 9.1. Examples include CD31, which is present on most blood vessels. This antibody can be used to assess angiogenesis or the vascularity of a tissue. Depending on the disease, drugs may be used to inhibit or promote angiogenesis, and this marker can be used to evaluate potential changes in tissue samples. T cells can be detected using an antibody to CD3, which is expressed on T cells. CD3 may be used in many applications to determine whether a cell is of T-cell lineage. For example, it can determine what cells are present at inflammatory sites in various diseases or whether a lymphoma is of T-cell origin. Glial fibrillary acidic protein (GFAP) is another example in the detection of β cells in islets of Langerhans in pancreas using antibodies to insulin, which is expressed in these cells (i.e., Fig. 9.1, bottom right, showing these cells in rat pancreas). The same antibody also recognizes insulin in human pancreas tissue sections.

In addition to assisting in the identification of cell types, IHC provides information regarding the specific cell compartment in which a protein is expressed. For example, is a protein localized to the nucleus, the cytoplasm or plasma membrane? Several images are provided in Figure 9.2 showing different types of subcellular localization patterns, including nuclear, cytoplasmic, and extracellular. Understanding subcellular localization is important in many applications, including basic science approaches when little is known about a particular target protein and where it is expressed. Subcellular localization may help provide some insight regarding the function of a protein and whether the localization changes under different experimental conditions. For example, when evaluating

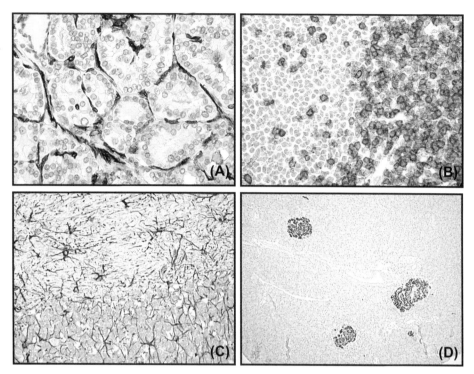

Figure 9.1. Identification of cell types using immunohistochemistry. (Top left) Angiogenesis. CD31 in thyroid carcinoma detects endothelial cells of blood vessels. (Top right) CD3 detects T cells in human tonsil. (Bottom left) Glial fibrillary acidic protein (GFAP) IHC staining of glial cells in rat cerebellum. (Bottom right) Insulin IHC in rat pancreas. Beta cells label in the islets of Langerhans label. Hematoxylin counterstain provides a blue nuclear stain (light) and DAB chromagen shows dark brown staining of the target protein (dark). See insert for color representation of this figure.

potential proteins for targeted drug therapies such as monoclonal antibody therapeutics, it is usually critical to demonstrate that the target is localized to the plasma membrane of the target cells. Other examples of localization patterns that are not shown include, but are not limited to, plasma membrane staining, Golgi-like or endoplasmic reticulum staining, perinuclear staining, vesicular staining as in lysosomes and peroxisomes, nucleolar staining, and chromatin staining. Each of these localization patterns can provide some information about the target protein being detected. Proper subcellular localization can assist in understanding whether the assay is indeed detecting the correct target.

Studying the expression pattern of the nucleotide metabolizing enzyme dUTPase, which cleaves dUTP to form dUMP, a substrate for thymidylate synthase, provides a good example of evaluating subcellular localization of a protein and linking it to the function of the protein. Prior to performing IHC, it was

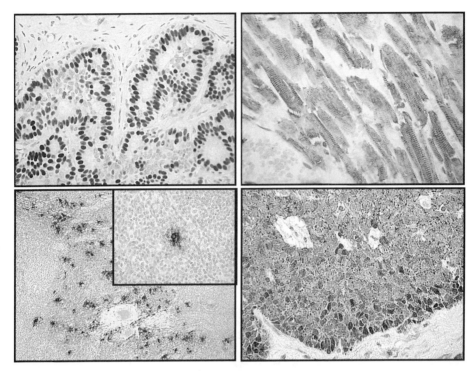

Figure 9.2. Examples of different subcellular localization patterns. (Top left) Estrogen receptor (ER) in a breast carcinoma. The nuclei of most tumor cells label. (Top right) Pan actin in human heart showing striations in the cytoplasm of cardiomyocytes. (Bottom left) IHC stain of tonsil using anti-mast-cell tryptase. Mast cells label with a cytoplasmic and extracellular localization. Inset shows higher magnification image staining in tonsil. (Bottom right) dUTPase in human colon carcinoma. Nuclear as well as cytoplasmic localization is detected. Hematoxylin counterstain and DAB chromagen. See insert for color representation of this figure.

assumed that the dUTPase protein was likely localized to the cell nucleus due to its function as a nucleotide metabolizing enzyme. IHC analysis revealed that staining was indeed present in some nuclei; however, cytoplasmic localization was also often observed. There was a great deal of speculation as to what this meant, and numerous tissue types and various tumor types were tested. The nuclear staining was generally found in proliferating cells, whereas the cytoplasmic stain was present in both proliferating and nonproliferating cells. Further biochemical and molecular biology analysis revealed that there were two isoforms to dUTPase, one that was targeted to the nucleus and another that was targeted to mitochondria (Ladner et al., 2000). This data supported what was observed by IHC, and a synthesis provided important information regarding the expression of dUTPase. Later, studies were performed in transfected cell lines with the specific isoforms, and distinct granular cytoplasmic staining was observed in cells transfected with the mitochondrial isoform and nuclear localization with the cells transfected with the nuclear isoform (Tinkelenberg et al., 2003).

The saying "a minute to learn and a lifetime to master" is quite fitting when describing IHC assays. Both the technical aspects of IHC staining as well as the interpretation of the stained tissue sections present many challenges. From the technical perspective, there are many considerations regarding the approach to assay development, from control tissues and the method of tissue pretreatment (antigen unmasking) to choosing the proper antibody and detection system. Once the assay is successfully performed, there are still more considerations when interpreting the staining results. There are nuances to the technique and analysis that are learned over time and through experience of testing many different antibodies and tissues. If the proper approach and controls are not used, it can be easy to get fooled when interpreting staining results. Thus, skilled, experienced professionals must be given the responsibility of the preparation and analysis of the assays.

9.2. BASICS OF THE IHC ASSAY

An IHC assay requires the specific binding and detection of a primary antibody to its target protein within a tissue section. This is achieved by a stepwise application of reagents on 4- to 6-μm-thick tissue sections in a series of incubation steps where the antibody is detected and visualized using an enzyme-linked chromagenic assay (see schematic in Fig. 9.3 and the flowchart in Figure 9.4). Figure 9.3 outlines the main steps of a routine IHC protocol using a simple ABC technique as an example (Hsu et al., 1981). Each of the steps is described in more detail below.

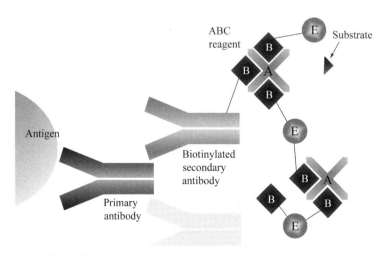

Figure 9.3. Schematic showing basic ABC detection method.

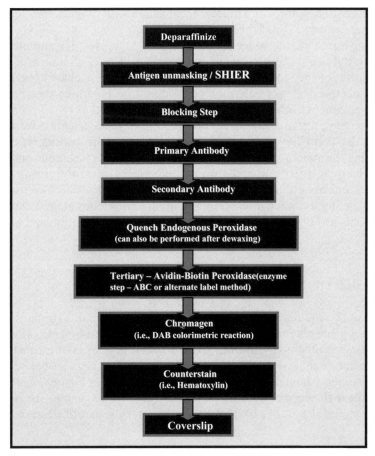

Figure 9.4. Basic steps of IHC protocol (ABC) method.

9.2.1. Formalin Fixation and Paraffin Embedding of Tissues

Immunohistochemistry assays can be performed on tissues in various forms, including FFPE tissues, frozen tissues, and cytological preparations or smears. The purpose behind freezing the tissues or embedding in paraffin is to make them harder so that 4- to 6-µm-thick sections may be prepared. Sections are prepared with a cryostat for frozen sections or a microtome for paraffin sections. Sections that are 4 to 6 µm in thickness allow light to readily pass through the tissue when mounted on a glass microscope slide. In most cases, FFPE tissues are used because they provide optimal morphology and are easy to handle and store. Tissues are fixed in 10% neutral buffered formalin for about 24 hours and then dehydrated through a series of alcohol and xylenes and then infiltrated in melted paraffin wax. These tissues are then oriented in blocks of paraffin, and these blocks are placed on a microtome for sectioning. When using FFPE tissues for

IHC assays, the paraffin must first be removed to return the tissue to an aqueous state and allow proper binding of the primary antibody detection reagents. Deparaffinization is achieved by incubating slides with tissue sections in xylenes. Xylene is an organic reagent that acts as a solvent to remove the paraffin from the tissue section. The tissue sections are then hydrated through a descending alcohol series to water.

9.2.2. Tissue Pretreatment/Antigen Unmasking

One of the potential drawbacks of using FFPE tissues in IHC assays is that the formalin fixation and paraffin embedding may adversely affect the antigenicity of the tissue by altering or changing a target epitope for an antibody (Battifora, 1991). Antigen-unmasking methods were developed to help reverse the negative effects of formalin fixation and paraffin embedding (Shi et al., 1991). This tissue pretreatment procedure is performed after tissue sections are dewaxed. The method heats the tissue sections in the presence of various buffers using various sources of heat, such as microwave, steamer, pressure cooker, and water bath. This process has revolutionized IHC in FFPE tissues. allowing for better detection of most target antigens (Gown et al., 1993; Shi et al., 2001). This process has also been termed HIER for heat-induced epitope retrieval (Riera et al., 1997). An example of IHC staining with and without Antigen Unmasking (HIER) is shown in Figure 9.5. Prior to these methods, various enzyme digestion procedures and alternate fixatives were used to allow for better IHC staining (Battifora and Kopinski, 1986).

Many different tissue pretreatments should be tested to determine which pretreatment provides the best access of the antibody to the epitope. Several pretreatment solutions are available commercially. Some of the pretreatment solutions include sodium citrate, ethylenediaminetetraacetic acid (EDTA), Tris, urea, sucrose, and other proprietary commercial solutions such as Target Retrieval Solution (DAKO, Carpinteria, CA), as well as others. These buffers may also include a range of different pH levels. The length of time for the heat pretreatment varies, but 20 minutes is a good estimate. After tissue sections are heated, they should be allowed to cool before performing subsequent steps. After cooling, slides are placed in phosphate-buffered saline (PBS) or Tris buffer, which will be used in the IHC protocol.

9.2.3. Blocking Step

A blocking reagent is incubated on the tissue section so that the primary and secondary antibodies do not bind nonspecifically. The blocking reagent includes nonspecific proteins and more specifically serum protein from the species in which the secondary antibody is made. For example, if the secondary antibody in a protocol is made in goat, then a normal goat serum should be included in the blocking step so that the secondary antibody, which usually contains a label, does not bind nonspecifically to the tissue section. The blocking step usually includes an incubation of about 5 to 30 minutes.

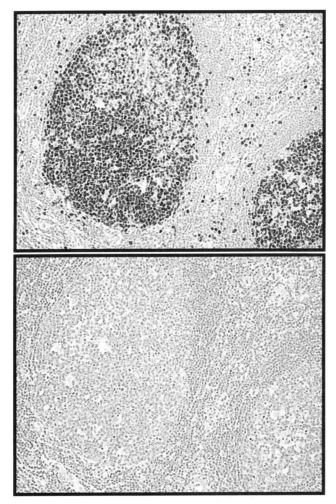

Figure 9.5. Ki67 IHC with and without tissue heat pretreatment. (Top) Ki67 IHC in section of human tonsil using steam heat pretreatment. Note strong nuclear staining of proliferating cells localized primarily to germinal centers. (Bottom) Ki67 IHC in a serial section of tonsil shown above. No steam heat pretreatment was performed. Only marginal nuclear staining is detected. Hematoxylin counterstain; DAB chromagen. See insert for color representation of this figure.

9.2.4. Primary Antibody

The primary antibody is an immunological reagent that is used in IHC assays to bind to a specific target antigen or epitope in the tissue section. Primary antibodies can be monoclonal or polyclonal and made in various species. The most commonly used primary antibodies are from mouse, rabbit, and goat. Polyclonal antibodies must be immunoaffinity purified against the recombinant protein or peptide from which it was generated. Nonspecific clones in an unpurified antibody will yield background staining and these must be removed.

Primary antibody incubations vary in time and temperature. For single-day IHC protocols the antibody incubation time may range from 10 minutes to 1 hour. These incubations can be performed at room temperature or at 37 °C to accelerate binding. Some antibodies provide better detection when incubated overnight in order to extend the time the antibody incubates on the tissue section. Overnight incubations can be performed at room temperature or at 4 °C. The concentration of the primary antibody in IHC assays usually ranges from about 0.5 to 5.0 μg/ml. High concentrations, that is, over 10 μg/ml often yield nonspecific staining. After primary incubation is completed, the antibody is removed and the tissue section is rinsed in buffer to make sure that any unbound antibody is removed.

9.2.5. Secondary Antibody

The secondary antibody in most detection systems includes a label and is directed against the primary antibody. If the primary antibody is made in mouse, the secondary should bind to the mouse antibody. In many detection systems, a labeled goat IgG antibody is used. For example, if the primary is mouse, the secondary would be goat–anti–mouse IgG. Goat serum would also be used in the blocking step. If the primary antibody is made in goat, then the secondary needs to be made in another species such as rabbit (rabbit–anti–goat IgG). The label on the secondary is often biotin, but other labels such as fluorescein isothiocyanate (FITC) may be used, especially to circumvent problems of endogenous biotin background. The secondary may also be labeled with an enzyme used in the colorimetric reaction, such as horseradish peroxidase; or the secondary may include a polymer that increases the sensitivity of the detection system. In the ABC technique described in the flowchart in Figure 9.4, the secondary is biotinylated. Secondary antibody incubation steps are usually about 10 to 30 minutes in duration and can be performed at room temperature or at 37 °C. Buffer rinses are performed after incubation is complete.

9.2.6. Hydrogen Peroxide Block

When a peroxidase detection method is being used, endogenous peroxidase activity needs to be blocked so that it does not react with the chromogen. Normally, incubation for about 5 minutes in 3.0% hydrogen peroxide will quench endogenous peroxidase activity. This blocking can be performed at other times during the protocol but must be performed prior to the peroxidase enzyme incubation. Buffer rinses are performed after incubation is complete.

9.2.7. Avidin–Biotin Complex Peroxidase

This step includes a labeling reagent, such as ABC peroxidase. The avidin of the ABC binds to biotin on the secondary antibody. A biotinylated peroxidase enzyme is also part of the ABC complex and can bind to avidin of other complexes forming a larger complex. Thus, at this juncture of the protocol the detection enzyme is now bound to the secondary, which is bound to the primary, which is bound to its target antigen. In other detection methods, the peroxidase enzyme may be linked to molecules other than an ABC complex, such as streptavidin, or may be linked to a polymer. The ABC reagent forms a complex that allows many peroxidase enzymes to be bound to the secondary. The peroxidase enzyme may also be substituted with other enzymes. Alkaline phosphatase detection systems have also been commonly used. The length of this step may range from about 10 to 30 minutes at room temperature or 37 °C. Buffer rinses are performed after incubation is complete.

9.2.8. Chromagen

DAB (3′, 3′-diaminobenzidine) is often used as chromagen in IHC assays. This molecule is converted to a dark brown insoluble precipitate when it reacts with the peroxidase enzyme in the presence of hydrogen peroxide. DAB chromagen usually yields a discreet localization pattern that provides high-quality resolution, which is important when trying to discern the subcellular localization of a target. The length of time in DAB is usually about 5 minutes. Longer or shorter incubation times will provide stronger or weaker detection, respectively. Other chromagens are also commercially available. Buffer rinses are performed after incubation is complete.

9.2.9. Counterstain

At this point in the protocol, the target antigen has been detected. The tissue section now needs to be counterstained so that the morphology of the cells and tissues can be observed. Hematoxylin is the most commonly used counterstain in IHC assays. This molecule binds the acidic components in the nucleus resulting in a purplish-blue nuclear stain. The length of the hematoxylin counterstain step will vary depending on the hematoxylin used, but the step is brief, usually about one minute. Buffer or water rinses are performed after incubation is complete.

9.2.10. Coverslip

After the completion of the IHC protocol, the stained slides are sealed with a cover glass and mounting media. For DAB chromagen, the slides can be permanently coverslipped in a number of different commercially available mounting medias. Slides are dehydrated through a series of increasing alcohols and then rinsed in xylenes and coverslipped and can be scanned under a light microscope and stored indefinitely.

There are many different commercially available detection kits from many different vendors that can be used for IHC assays. These include biotin and nonbiotin-based kits as well as kits that provide various levels of sensitivity. Each kit should be used according to the manufacturer's directions and should be adjusted to suit the needs and staining platform of the investigator.

In most situations the tissues used in these studies are FFPE tissues. These tissues have many benefits over frozen tissues, particularly due to the superior morphology they provide. In addition, formalin fixation offers sample stability, preserving the integrity of the sample. Paraffin-embedded tissues are easily stored for extended periods at ambient temperatures. These advantages are particularly important when samples are collected at many sites for clinical studies. Less sample handling and greater sample stability are preferable to obtain samples that are useful. When more difficult procedures or delicate handling of samples is required, there is a greater risk of damage and potential loss of sample integrity. However, FFPE tissues have some drawbacks in that some antibodies do not react well and protein and ribonucleic acid (RNA) extraction may be adversely affected compared to fresh frozen material.

9.3. IMMUNOHISTOCHEMISTRY ASSAY DEVELOPMENT

Immunohistochemistry assay development is an important and sometimes time-consuming process that requires a great deal of experience. This step is absolutely critical because, once developed, this assay will ultimately be tested on experimental or clinical samples from drug development studies. If the assay is not properly developed, the study may not generate quality data and may not adequately answer the questions of the study. To ensure that a high-quality IHC assay is developed, there are a number of parameters to test. These include the antibodies to be tested, dilutions and incubation times for these antibodies, tissue pretreatments or antigen-unmasking techniques, IHC detection systems, target tissue types to be tested, and testing of appropriate positive and negative controls. Positive controls may include positive and negative cell lines as well as FFPE tissues. Each testing component is important and can affect the outcome of the assay. The CRO needs to take a stepwise approach to testing these parameters in order to develop an optimal assay.

More than one antibody should be tested to detect a specific marker for two basic reasons. The first is that not all antibodies, particularly monoclonal antibodies, will react well in IHC assays in FFPE tissues. Thus, testing multiple antibodies increases the chances of finding an antibody that reacts well. The second and perhaps most important reason to test multiple antibodies is to demonstrate similar IHC reactivity in tissues from at least two different antibodies generated against the same target. For example, if two antibodies demonstrate plasma membrane staining of a similar subset of cells in various tissues, this provides a very high level of confidence that the assay is indeed detecting the target protein. Antibodies to the same target often yield different results due to their affinities, the microenvironment of their epitopes, and the position of the epitope on the target protein.

Tissue pretreatments or antigen-unmasking techniques can make the difference between quality IHC staining and no staining at all. The purpose of this step is to promote the ability of the antibody to find and bind to its target epitope within the tissue section. Numerous methods are available, which include heating the tissue sections in the presence of various buffers and enzyme digestion of the tissue section. These various approaches should be tested on tissues known to express the target antigen and the approach that provides the best result should be chosen, that is, the staining pattern most consistent with the expected expression of the target.

The optimal IHC assay should then be tested on a panel of tissue samples to provide an understanding of the staining pattern. The tissues tested should include the target tissues of a particular study. For example, if a clinical study is testing a therapeutic in breast cancer, the assay should be tested in a panel of breast tumors prior to testing the clinical study samples. Testing this panel beforehand provides an idea of the staining expected in the study and also how this assay will be scored.

In some cases, the sponsor has a working IHC protocol that it would like to transfer to the CRO. The CRO needs to work closely with the sponsor to make sure that the existing assay is acceptable and, if so, properly transferred. In many cases, different automated IHC platforms may be used at the two sites, and the assay will likely need to be modified for each. The same tissue sections should be stained and the results compared to ensure near identical staining.

When is an IHC assay fully developed or validated? This is an important question and a topic of discussion in the field. The degree of testing may vary depending on the application of the assay. The time and cost of developing a fully validated assay may not be justified in early studies but may be critical in late-stage clinical studies where the IHC assay may serve as a companion diagnostic to a therapeutic. The CRO needs to understand the sponsor's needs and the level of assay development needs to be agreed upon during the proposal stage. A specific and reproducible assay should be adequate for most studies. However, further validation of an assay may be required, and these guidelines should be addressed in the proposal and contract. IHC assay validation requires a greater investment of time and resources and test material. Once an IHC assay is developed by the CRO, it should be shared with the sponsor prior to testing clinical samples. Normally, this is achieved via a report describing the assay development process. This is further described in Section 9.6.8.

9.4. SENDING A STUDY TO A CONTRACT LABORATORY VS. RUNNING IN-HOUSE

Drug development can be a rather long and costly process, and pharmaceutical and biotechnology companies work diligently to collapse time frames and accelerate the studies wherever possible in this competitive field. Speeding up studies may not only save money but may also provide a competitive financial and marketing edge if other groups are developing competing therapeutics. The term "outsourcing" is often used to refer to contracted work that is performed by another individual or company outside the company sponsoring the work. Some companies that perform this outsourced work are referred to as contract research organizations, or CROs. The amount of work that is performed by these CROs for biotechnology and pharmaceutical companies is growing, and this trend is expected to continue for years to come (Anscomb A., 2008). Outsourcing certain studies such as molecular pathology assays, particularly IHC assays, to CROs may allow facets of a study to be completed more quickly and effectively, thus saving time and money, while generating quality data.

The reasons why a pharmaceutical or biotechnology company would send out a study are quite variable and depend on the sponsor's size, capability, competitive situation, financial status, and business philosophy as well as the specific type of work or study being performed. Table 9.1 presents a list of potential reasons to outsource IHC studies along with explanations and considerations for each. Additional detail covering each point is discussed further in the text below.

9.4.1. Turn-around Time

Perhaps one of the most common reasons to outsource a study is turn-around time, or the time in which it takes to initiate and complete a study and deliver results. It is obvious that the sponsoring company would like results as quickly as possible, as decisions and actions regarding the development of a drug can be made faster. The sponsor needs to consider whether timing is critical and, if so, can an outside laboratory or CRO provide results more quickly than what can be done in-house. For molecular pathology assays, the CRO may already have a number of assays in place. Thus, the somewhat lengthy process of assay development may already be complete or may only require minimal refining. For example, if a particular drug development program needs to assess proliferation and apoptotic pathways by IHC, the CRO may have these in place already and can quickly provide these services. If assay development or assay transfer from the sponsor to the CRO is required, additional time will be necessary and will effect turn-around time. The sponsor needs to carefully evaluate the study and communicate it to the CRO in a detailed fashion. The CRO needs to consider all aspects involved in completing the study and provide honest timelines for completing all components of the study. The sponsor must then determine the best option to save time. Although turn-around time is a critical consideration, the decision to outsource a study may be related to a mixture of many other factors or business pressures. Some other reasons are provided below.

9.4.2. In-house Expertise

Quality IHC assay development, staining, and analysis require an experienced staff. The biotechnology or pharmaceutical sponsor needs to assess projects and determine the level of expertise required to properly fulfill its needs. In some cases, the sponsor may not fully understand the intricacies involved in these

TABLE 9.1. Outsourcing IHC Studies: Reasons and Considerations

Reason to Outsource	Explanation	Considerations
Turn-around time	The time it takes to complete a study from start to finish. One goal in outsourcing is to complete a study faster than it would take if the study were performed in-house.	Carefully review the study and make honest decisions on time and manpower to complete. The sponsor must consider the time it will take to get the CRO up to speed (develop or transfer assay) and to ask the CRO for expected timelines.
In-house expertise	The sponsor needs to identify the skill set required for a study and determine if in-house personnel meet these needs.	Experience and appropriate application of skills must be considered in light of the scope of a study, which may be outside the comfort zone or in-house skill set. Some in-house expertise is preferred to allow proper communication with CRO.
Limited in-house throughput capacity and range of services	The sponsor needs to understand the amount of work and types of projects the in-house group can perform. The in-house group may also be limited in the types of IHC services they can support.	Large studies and multiple priorities may overwhelm the in-house group. Outsourcing studies may help meet intermittent needs and deadlines and bridge staffing issues. The CRO may offer a specific type of service not performed in-house.
Laboratory infrastructure	The basic laboratory space, instrumentation, and personnel required to provide these services	What are the basic resources required and how will they change in the future and will outsourcing be an option to consider?
Lab certifications/ qualifications	Current good laboratory practices (cGLP), clinical laboratory improvement amendments (CLIA), College of American Pathology (CAP), etc.	What are study requirements and how does the in-house lab meet these needs. cGLP is required when data is generated that will accompany or support many FDA filings. CLIA and CAP may be needed if HIPAA (45CFR160, 2003) compliance for patient privacy is required.
Third-party testing	Activities performed by organizations independent of the drug development company.	Third-party testing provides a nonbiased view and thus a better confidence in the test results.
Costs	The total amount of money required to perform IHC assays to support drug development needs	The sponsor must evaluate current and future needs and associated costs, including proper staffing, instrumentation, and cost of entry.
Future work or partnering	Build a relationship with a CRO or IHC service company to prepare for future business options. There is the potential for a long-term relationship that can grow over time.	The sponsor gets to know a company now so that they can easily expand relationship in the future, e.g., performing phase I and then subsequent phase II and III studies and perhaps developing companion diagnostics or other commercial products.

studies and may underestimate the level of expertise required. IHC assays have many applications, and it is important to not only run these assays and evaluate the results properly, but it is also critical to be able to properly integrate results. Just because the in-house staff can run some IHC assays does not necessarily translate in their ability to develop and apply appropriate assays, design experiments to address specific study needs, or manage a study effectively. There are many technical nuances to these studies as well as challenges in developing and scoring IHC assays. For example, the sponsor may have planned a research or clinical study that requires the development of multiple novel assays on many different tissue types, and these assays may require specialized or unique methods of analysis. This project may require a different approach that may be outside the comfort zone of the in-house staff, and results could be compromised due to inexperience or a lack of understanding of the study. In summary, the sponsor must carefully consider the level of expertise required to support IHC assays and determine whether the in-house group can meet its needs or whether it should outsource. It is also important to note that not all CROs that offer IHC services have the appropriate expertise. Choosing a proper laboratory will be addressed in Section 9.5.

Immunohistochemistry assays are not necessarily contracted out simply because the sponsoring company is lacking the expertise to run the studies. In many cases, companies that possess skilled scientists with IHC expertise may be more likely to outsource this work. Companies that understand the value these assays bring to their drug discovery efforts may be more likely to use these assays and thus there may be a greater in-house demand. In-house expertise at the sponsoring laboratory allows sponsors to choose the right laboratory. In-house expertise is important for a successful relationship with a CRO, particularly when many studies need to be outsourced. Having in-house expertise allows for a better transition of information as well as allowing the sponsor to better understand what the CRO is proposing and making sure that study objectives are clear on both sides.

9.4.3. Throughput Capacity and Range of Services

As mentioned above, the IHC services required by a drug development company may increase over time and overwhelm the in-house resources. There may be times when several studies need to be performed at the same time or when in-house staff is limited due to vacation or other personnel reasons. The reasons may vary, but the outcome is the same, that is, the study results will not be delivered in a time frame consistent with the desired timeline of the drug development team. For example, one very large study requiring assay development and the testing of thousands of slides can be beyond the capacity of the in-house IHC group, or that a single study may require all in-house resources and all other studies would need to be placed on hold or delayed. In-house IHC groups generally support drug development activity for many different drug programs and areas of drug development and preclinical and clinical teams. Thus, the potential for conflicting use of in-house resources is a likely possibility, and the in-house laboratory may have a difficult time determining what study to give priority. Outsourcing these studies to a CRO can help meet the increasing demands and intermittent needs for IHC services and thus help decrease conflict and meet deadlines.

The range of services that the in-house group provides may be limited to specific types of studies. For example, an in-house group may be staffed to provide IHC assay support related to toxicology and research and development primarily in animal tissues, but may not support clinical study services. Performing clinical studies requires specific staffing, such as clinical pathologists, and potentially different procedures and work flow. In some cases clinical studies may require rapid turn-around when evaluating patient samples for entry into a trial. The in-house group may not be set up to provide these services. The in-house group would need to decide whether to add clinical study services to the range of services they provide or elect to outsource these types of studies. In addition, the in-house group may require specific tissues and not want to build a tissue bank. The services offered by a CRO may include testing of various tissues that they can provide, thus obviating the need for building an in-house tissue bank.

9.4.4. Laboratory Infrastructure

The pharmaceutical or biotechnology company sponsor must evaluate its current and future infrastructure levels that can be assigned to molecular pathology assays. The sponsor must first determine what resources are necessary to meet the demands for these assays and then decide what is currently available and what will be available in the future. Infrastructure considerations include laboratory space, appropriate staffing of skilled personnel, instrumentation, and any specialized materials such as the potential need for a tissue bank.

Space and personnel requirements usually require good planning, as these cannot be readily changed on short notice. If a large increase in these assays is expected in one year but there is uncertainty in the next, outsourcing may be a good option to bridge the demands. Proper staffing must take critical mass into consideration and must determine what level of personnel support is required to handle all projects when there are changing priorities, increases in workload, and proper coverage for vacations and personal leave. The proper relationship with a quality CRO may assist in building this critical mass without carrying excess number of full-time employees (FTEs) or consultants. Drug discovery and development is a changing and dynamic process, and the use of CROs may assist in keeping in-house liabilities low from a personnel perspective.

Another item to consider is infrastructure for the correct laboratory instrumentation. Laboratory instrumentation may change depending on the type and number of assays that the in-house group is expected to support. The potential for increasing instrumentation should also be considered when evaluating space requirements. IHC assays often require the testing of a variety of different tissue samples. The number and type of tissues will vary depending on the studies being performed. If a tissue bank needs to be built, it may also require additional personnel, space, and storage facilities. If clinical sample testing is to be performed in-house, proper storage such as heat-resistant safes and/or $-80\,°C$ freezers may be necessary. Both of these items can take up large amounts of space.

9.4.5. Costs

Costs are a primary concern in any business decision. The sponsor needs to consider all costs involved with performing IHC molecular pathology assay studies in-house versus outsourcing. Defining the total cost of these studies can be difficult, as there are many considerations to take into account. Many of the costs involved in running these assays in-house may be straightforward such as fixed costs and the operating cost of instrumentation, supplies, and reagents. Other costs may be less apparent, such as forecasting the changing needs and level of staffing required to perform IHC assays effectively. Lastly, there is another type of cost to consider that may be less tangible but is critical, that is, the opportunity cost. This section details costs to evaluate when considering outsourcing a study.

Fixed Costs. These are costs such as the cost for space and utilities. These costs are likely well understood in a company in terms of the cost per square foot of space. These costs can be determined based on the square footage allotted and what it costs the company to maintain. Management at the company must consider how much space can be allocated for this particular area of work now and in the future. Increasing demands in other areas of the biotechnology or pharmaceutical company may limit space availability. Outsourcing the increasing molecular pathology needs gives the sponsor more flexibility to allocate resources and accommodate in-house changes.

Variable Operating Costs. Besides fixed costs the sponsor must also consider variable operating costs related to performing IHC assays. These costs include the number of FTEs (discussed further below) dedicated to this area, and the cost of instrumentation and supplies and reagents. The costs of performing IHC assays will vary depending on the amount and complexity of work on hand. The number and different types of instrumentation may change. These instruments not only carry their initial price tag, but most require service contracts that must also be added annually to these costs. In addition to FTEs the in-house laboratory may still require additional staffing resources such as pathologists who may be needed as part-time or as project-dependent consultants.

Start-up Costs. There are a number of initial costs if a company is starting an in-house group from scratch to support IHC assays. This is a significant investment, and the company must forecast a long term need in this area of work to make it economically feasible. Starting a molecular pathology group not only requires finding skilled specialists but also includes outfitting a laboratory.

Instrumentation requirements may include histology equipment to process and embed and perform microtomy on tissue samples, automated IHC platforms, microscopes and digital cameras, and imaging systems. In addition, a tissue bank may need to be built or purchased. Lastly, quality systems need to be designed and implemented. This requires a large investment of time and energy and is discussed later in Section 9.6.9. In summary, starting a laboratory is a considerable investment that requires a good amount of time before it is operational. For smaller companies or companies that are not yet well funded, this cost of entry may serve as a significant barrier. In this case, outsourcing to a specialty CRO will be a more cost-effective option and may also serve the immediate needs in this area of drug development. Larger or well-funded companies may be more apt to invest in building an in-house group and only consider outsourcing to provide additional support.

Opportunity Cost. The other "cost" a drug development company in need of IHC assay support should consider is the opportunity cost related to performing these studies in-house. The time and resources devoted to building in-house groups and developing these processes could be used for other areas of the drug development that could collapse time frames and possibly accelerate drug development, which may provide a competitive marketing edge. In addition, the sooner a decision is made to stop pursuing a drug the more resources are saved and can be used to focus on other options in the drug pipeline that may provide better business opportunities.

9.4.6. Lab Certifications

Lab certifications may be required when dealing with studies in which the data will be submitted and reviewed by agencies for acceptance or approval. The Food and Drug Administration (FDA) has in place regulations titled "current Good Laboratory Practices" commonly known as cGLPs. The cGLPS are in the Code of Federal Regulations (CFRs). For a more detailed discussion see the Code of Federal Regulations: 21CFR58—Good Laboratory Practices for Nonclinical Laboratory Studies (21CFR58, 2008). In short, 21CFR58 outlines required GLP practices for studies that support or are intended to support applications for research or marketing permits for products regulated by the FDA. If a study will be used for these purposes the laboratory, whether in-house or CRO, should follow cGLP guidelines. The cGLP guidelines do not require any outside agency certification but do require what is tantamount as a "self-certification" that the laboratory is following cGLP guidelines. It should be incumbent on any company to ensure that the laboratory providing a service that will be used in an FDA submission is following cGLPs and has a dedicated quality assurance group. It is good practice for the sponsoring company to audit a contracting laboratory prior to initiating any service in which the data generated is to be used in support of submissions. The intended use of the laboratory work product should be clearly understood by both the sponsor and CRO prior to the commencement of the study.

In addition to cGLPs there are CLIA and CAP certifications. CLIA certifications ensure that the clinical laboratory follows the Clinical Laboratory Improvement Amendments (CLIA, 1988). The College of American Pathology (CAP) certification ensures that the laboratory has procedures in place that allows for greater consistency between testing laboratories. While these certifications are necessary for the clinical diagnostic laboratories, they are not necessary certifications for laboratories' data submissions to the FDA. It is up to the sponsoring company to decide whether these certifications are necessary for the study to be outsourced.

9.4.7. Third-Party Testing

The term third-party testing encompasses the function of a CRO. However, beyond the CRO being an extra "pair of hands" to complete work on time and on budget, it is also an organization that is independent from the sponsor or any affiliates, suppliers, and the like. The independence of the CRO makes it unique in that the testing and/or analysis can be accomplished with an unbiased view as to the result. The independent laboratory's result can be viewed by both the sponsor and agencies with the knowledge that the data submitted is "unencumbered" by a relationship. Oftentimes the data that is generated can be used not only to advance a study but also to cancel a study or move the study into another unexpected direction. An independent laboratory generates the result and is not swayed by anticipated results.

9.4.8. Future Considerations for Partnering

Another reason to outsource some studies is to prepare for the future. Building a relationship with a CRO can take time. Working with a CRO allows a drug development company to get acquainted with a CRO and determine whether they can work well together. Having an established relationship on a smaller scale will make it easier to expand on the relationship in the future without taking as much time and reducing risk. Most drug development companies are trying to identify biomarkers to help them better understand their drug mechanisms and the patient response during clinical studies. The sponsor may eventually need to partner with a CRO or other company if a particular biomarker assay has the potential to serve as a companion diagnostic and needs to be developed to support a drug therapy. For example, an IHC companion diagnostic test may determine which patients should be placed on therapy. In most cases pharmaceutical and biotechnology companies do not have this expertise. A reliable company may need to be selected as a partner and if the sponsor has worked with the company during earlier stages of clinical development this process may proceed more smoothly.

The working relationship between the sponsor and CRO has the potential to continue and grow for years. The company may start by outsourcing a single study and if the relationship proves to be a good fit, other studies are likely to follow. Testing around a single drug can lead to many studies from small phase I studies through to large phase III studies and possibly the development of companion diagnostics depending on the success of the drug and the types of assays necessary. This potentially lengthy relationship underlines the importance of picking the right laboratory from the start. If the relationship is not a good fit, the sponsor will have to pursue other companies, and this will cost time and money while the CRO gets up to speed on the projects. In summary, the reasons why a drug development company would decide to send out a study to a CRO vary depending on the situation and on the in-house resources available to complete studies.

9.5. CHOOSING AND WORKING WITH AN OUTSIDE LABORATORY—KEYS FOR A SUCCESSFUL RELATIONSHIP— WHAT TO DO BEFORE A SLIDE IS STAINED

Once the sponsoring laboratory decides to use a CRO to perform an IHC study, the next step is to find and choose a laboratory that is capable of satisfactorily completing the study. The sponsor should not only choose a laboratory that has the appropriate expertise to meet the needs of the study in a timely fashion but also should consider other aspects of working with an outside laboratory. Once a CRO or outside laboratory is chosen, the next step is to build a successful relationship.

9.5.1. Finding the Right Laboratory, Asking the Right Questions

Where does the sponsor look to find an IHC specialty company? The sponsor can find CROs that provide IHC services in Internet searches and exhibiting at scientific trade shows. Like any business, word of mouth can be a good channel to find a company that has been successful elsewhere. However, what may have been adequate for one company may not suit the needs of another. Choosing the right laboratory is not a simple task and can be time consuming, but it is worth the investment. The sponsor should develop a list of questions based on its current and future needs and start the process by interviewing the CRO. A list of some potential questions often asked is provided in Table 9.2. Questions should be designed to learn as much about a company as possible. After the interview process the sponsor may want to consider a pilot study with a small number of companies. Since IHC is such a specialty requiring a large amount of expertise, the pilot study will demonstrate whether a laboratory is equipped to develop these assays. Even after selecting a laboratory, it may be a good idea to start with smaller projects to ensure that work is of the highest quality, completed on time, and that the interactions with the CRO are positive. If it is possible to do this, there will be no surprises with larger studies. Most of all, the sponsor should clearly understand the level of service it can expect and the CRO must understand the level of service that is to be supplied. A great deal of energy goes

TABLE 9.2. Potential Questions for Evaluating IHC Laboratories

- How long has the company been in business?
- How long has the staff been there? Comment on turnover. Comment on expertise and experience at levels of technicians, scientists, pathologists, data management, and quality assurance.
- Is providing IHC services the core business?
- What is the business model? How are services charged?
- What is the range of services provided, e.g., preclinical and clinical?
- Does the company follow GLP and have SOPs in place for all laboratory operations?
- What type laboratory certifications do you possess, i.e., GLP, CLIA, CAP?
- Has a sponsor ever audited the quality systems?
- What is your throughput capacity and size of the lab? How many staff are dedicated to IHC assays? What is the breakdown by job description?
- Describe a typical project and provide estimated turn-around time.
- Can the laboratory take on studies that last up to several years?
- How much experience in developing assays? Discuss the company's assay development approach.
- Can a list of assays be provided that have been developed by the company?
- Does the laboratory specialize in a particular area, i.e., preclinical or clinical studies or oncology vs. neuroscience?
- What type of reports and other deliverables, including digital images are provided?
- What are the laboratories imaging capabilities?
- What are the qualifications of management, i.e., study directors, project managers, and pathologists?
- Does the company have a tissue bank? If so, what is the composition and is it available for testing?
- Provide some examples of studies with proven success stories.
- How does management see the growth of the company?
- Can a list of references be provided?

into this choice because the results of the study can help guide the course of therapy and can be the difference in determining whether a drug is effective or not. Thus it is energy well spent.

9.5.2. What to Look for When Choosing/Evaluating a Laboratory to Outsource IHC Studies

Choosing the appropriate outside laboratory is critical when outsourcing an IHC study, particularly studies that test clinical samples collected from clinical studies. Choosing the correct laboratory can be the difference of getting the study completed on time with quality results versus missing a deadline or getting poor quality data. Picking the right laboratory can make the process uneventful versus stressful. Essentially, the right laboratory has the technical and practical experience as well as the right personnel to allow for a good relationship with smooth interaction and minimal headaches. Many of the points to consider when choosing a laboratory are similar to the points made in Section 9.4 regarding the reasons to consider outsourcing. For example, turn-around time, expertise, throughput capacity, and range of services provided. These and others are discussed below.

Expertise and Experience. A team of experienced individuals is required to fully support the broad range of IHC applications in drug development. From a technical perspective the laboratory needs a staff of experienced technicians that can effectively perform and troubleshoot IHC assays using automated platforms. The technicians should also have a basic understanding of histology to initially evaluate control and test tissues. In addition, the technicians should be versed on how to develop IHC assays. Not so surprisingly this takes a great deal of experience to obtain a good working knowledge. From a professional perspective, the laboratory should have staff skilled in evaluating antibody reactivity, developing scoring schemes, performing pathology analysis, and interpreting results and reporting them to the sponsor. Of great importance is a functional quality assurance unit that understands the processes and integrates easily with the scientific team. Since IHC is such a specialty, it can be surmised that not all CROs that offer IHC services have the appropriate expertise. Well-qualified individuals who understand the broad applications of IHC assays are rare, as there are no formal training programs. The ideal technical and professional staff will possess a synthesis of research and clinical experience. Even if a laboratory may be able to stain an IHC slide and have a pathologist interpret it, it does not mean the laboratory has the expertise to develop the appropriate, assays, develop scoring methods, score the samples appropriately, and manage a clinical study. For example, a reference laboratory that runs IHC slides for diagnostic purposes may not be able to deliver results in a "project-based" approach required for most clinical studies especially when novel antibodies are employed. In addition to the staff described above, other experienced individuals are also necessary to be able to properly provide support IHC services. The CRO specializing in IHC requires skilled histotechnicians that can process, embed, and cut tissue sections, a sample and data management group to oversee samples and transfer data, and quality assurance personnel that ensure that the studies remain in control. The various roles of the personnel involved are discussed in Section 9.5.3.

Capacity and Range of Services. The sponsor needs to evaluate the range of services and capacity of the IHC lab. Some laboratories may specialize in specific areas of IHC expertise, for example, basic research, preclinical and toxicology, or clinical studies. Other IHC companies may be primarily set up as clinical reference laboratories and may not be equipped to manage large studies in a project manner. The size of a company or the number of employees can be deceiving as the company may offer many types of services beyond IHC support. It is important to determine the number of individuals that are dedicated to supporting this niche IHC business. There are different skill sets involved in each and experience is necessary in the area of work that is being considered for outsourcing. For example, a university laboratory may provide IHC services but may not have the depth of staff or proper certifications to properly manage a study.

The sponsor should carefully evaluate immediate and future needs and determine whether the outside laboratory can fulfill these needs. If many studies or large studies are planned, the lab should have the appropriate staff and infrastructure to complete these studies and be able to grow with the sponsor's needs. For example, the sponsor may start off outsourcing a small phase I clinical study, but this could lead to much larger phase II and III studies and possibly the need for developing commercial products.

Potential Pitfalls. Sponsors should be cautious of the "sales pitch." Some CRO laboratories may have sales representatives that do not fully understand the processes required for a successful IHC study since they are typically not experts. They may sell many types of products and services and not have the proper technical grasp of a project. Care should be taken to ask the right questions to make sure that the CRO can handle a study in the manner expected by the sponsor (see Table 9.2). This is another reason why having some in-house expertise at the sponsor is key. The quotation and contract should be very specific as to how the work will be performed, under what timelines, and with what type of deliverables.

Payment for Services. The sponsor outsourcing the study needs to understand the manner in which the CRO, or outside laboratory, conducts its business and how it expects to be compensated for its services. Most laboratories will offer a "fee-for-service" approach whereby the sponsor pays the contracted laboratory a specific amount for a study and the sponsor has no other obligation to the contracted laboratory. Some companies may be willing to provide services at no charge or at a reduced rate in exchange for other rights related to the study, future studies, or potential commercial products. The business relationship should be discussed upfront and then clearly defined in the contractual agreement between the sponsor and the outside lab. The sponsor and outside contracted laboratory should discuss the manner in which payments are made in a fee-for-service agreement and make sure they are in agreement. Discussion topics should include percentages of upfront payments and payment milestones.

9.5.3. Relationship between Sponsor and Contract Laboratory

Building and Maintaining the Relationship. Building and maintaining a strong relationship between the sponsor and the contracted IHC laboratory is critical for continued success. A great deal of time and energy from both parties goes into starting the relationship and additional input is required to make sure the relationship thrives and delivers the best possible results. The IHC assays established during the early portions of a study can greatly impact the future of a drug target or whether a drug is successful in clinical trials; and, as mentioned previously, some studies have the potential to go on for years. Thus, it is a worthwhile investment for both parties to build a synergistic relationship that will produce dependable quality results based on open communications.

Expectations. From the beginning of the relationship, the sponsor and contract laboratory should clearly understand what is expected of each other. Both parties need to be aware of their respective responsibilities so that there are no surprises as the relationship progresses. There are many details that need to be identified, such as the when and how samples should be stained and if specific deadlines exist. These responsibilities should be defined in proposals and contracts prior to study initiation.

Communication. Proper communication is paramount in the success of the relationship. There should be clearly defined open lines of communication so that both parties understand the status of the study. These lines of communications can occur at numerous levels depending on the stage of the relationship and the stage of a specific study. Once a study is started, a point person should be assigned at the sponsor and the contract laboratory. A contact at the sponsor with IHC expertise is extremely valuable so that from a scientific perspective the two parties can speak the same language and better communicate results. Also, if a scientific question needs to be asked by the sponsor, he or she should be able to speak directly to a scientist at the contract laboratory who is knowledgeable about the study rather than speaking to an administrator. During a study the method of communication may require a mix of in-person meetings, teleconferences, and e-mail exchanges.

As with any research-oriented endeavor, changes or problems may arise before or during a study that were not anticipated. It is the responsibility of both the sponsor and the contract laboratory to communicate any changes as quickly as possible so that a new course of action can be planned. A lack of communication or miscommunication can be the source of many problems and could be the source of potential conflict and/or a lack of confidence. It is important not to jump to conclusions before the situation is completely understood. A good working relationship between the sponsor and contract laboratory should allow for better communication and a greater confidence and trust in each other, and, likewise, good communication promotes a good working relationship.

9.5.4. Roles for a Successful Relationship

There are a number of people who fill the many roles involved in properly outsourcing IHC assays in drug discovery. In particular, when conducting the testing of samples from patients enrolled in clinical studies, there are a number of different areas of expertise required at both the sponsor and the CRO. In addition, personnel at other institutions may also be involved. Some of these roles are listed in Table 9.3, and a brief description of each is provided. In some cases, an individual can fill more than one role. This list of the many potential roles underlines the need for a critical mass of experienced personnel and the type of

TABLE 9.3. Roles for Successful Relationship When Outsourcing Clinical Studies

Sponsor	IHC CRO	Other
Clinical director	Study director	Central laboratory
In-house scientist with IHC expertise	Project manager	Contacts at clinical sites
Scientific lead for a study	Lab technicians/histologists	Contacts at vendors
Clinical research associates	Pathologist	Consultants
Data management	Data management	Third parties
Quality assurance	Quality assurance	
Contact in biomarker group	Sample handling/receiving	
Contract personnel and legal	Business development contact/salesperson	

organization required to manage these studies. Many of these roles may also apply to preclinical or research studies as well.

Roles at Sponsor

- The clinical director is responsible for overseeing the study and interfacing with numerous in-house and external groups.
- In-house scientist with IHC expertise: This role is to be able to serve as a liaison with the IHC CRO to make sure the information is of high quality and that it is transferred properly. This person can provide insight to the in-house team.
- Clinical research associates (CRAs): Interfaces with the sponsor and clinical sites to make sure the sites are well informed and conducting the protocols as directed.
- Data management: Sets up databases according to study requirements and integrates data from the CRO.
- Quality assurance: Makes sure that study protocols are being followed; audits studies; maintains standard operations procedures (SOPs).
- Contact in biomarker group: Works on identifying specific markers for clinical studies with in-house groups and what information these markers may provide when tested in clinical studies. May interface with CRO on how these markers may be tested in IHC assays.
- Contract personnel and legal: Interfaces with the CRO and in-house scientific personnel and legal group to request and finalize proposals and contracts for conduct of studies.

Roles at CRO

- The study director is assigned to a study and is responsible for the overall conduct of the study at the CRO. He makes sure that the study is being performed properly according to designated protocols, the study is properly documented and is available to interface with the sponsor.

- Project manager: The CRO assigns a project manager to each study that works with the study director and oversees the day-to-day technical and administrative details of the study.
- Laboratory IHC technicians: Perform IHC slide staining, generally using automated platforms. Under the direction of study director or project manager, performs assay development experiments and stains IHC slides.
- Histologists: Perform various aspects of sample handling, processing, and embedding of submitted samples and microtomy of tissue sections onto glass slides.
- Pathologist: Reviews stained tissue sections for pathology evaluation and IHC reactivity. Other scientists skilled in the art of evaluating histological sections and IHC reactivity also can review and score stained slides.
- Data management: Maintains databases and interfaces with the study director, project manager, and quality assurance to transfer data generated at the CRO into appropriate formats required by the sponsor.
- Quality assurance: Oversees the quality aspect of the study. Ensures that studies are performed according to standard operating procedures with scheduled audits of the study protocols, deviations, data, and reports.
- Sample handling/receiving: Receives clinical samples from the sponsor and clinical sites according to appropriate SOPs, enters sample data into databases and submits samples for processing and storage.
- Business development contact/salesperson: Interfaces with various personnel at the CRO to build relationships and design proposals and contracts that reflect costs associated with the services requested by the sponsor.

Other Roles outside the Sponsor and CRO

- Central Laboratory: A laboratory that the sponsor contracts to provide a broad array of services to support clinical studies. This may include various types of testing as well as providing collection kits and labels to clinical sites to manage patient samples.
- Contacts at clinical sites: Various individuals at sites who are participating in a clinical trial. Roles may vary from medical to administrative and center around enrolling and treating patients on a protocol.
- Contacts at vendors: Individuals at companies providing reagents or services related to the clinical studies.
- Consultants: Specialists providing services or guidance to the sponsor or CRO.
- Third parties: Other companies involved in the sponsor and CRO relationship, for example, instrumentation or diagnostic companies, or partners of the sponsor.

9.6. RUNNING AND MANAGING OUTSOURCED CLINICAL STUDIES

Once the sponsor has decided that IHC services are required to support a study and that the work will be outsourced, what are the practical steps involved? The flowchart in Figure 9.6 highlights these steps. This section will focus on the process of performing clinical studies at a CRO and each step is briefly discussed.

9.6.1. Confidentiality Agreement

Prior to sending the request for proposal (RFP), the sponsor and CRO should execute a two-way confidentiality agreement, which protects the intellectual property of both parties and allows the groups to discuss the specifics of a study so that a more thorough proposal can be submitted. It is important to provide the CRO with adequate information about the study so that the best approach can be taken.

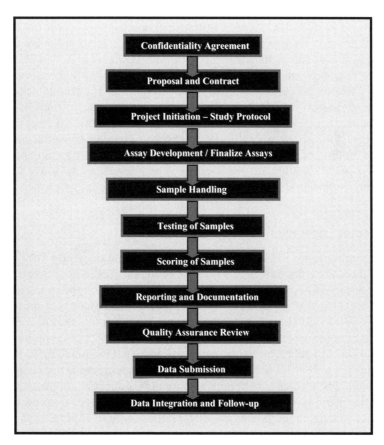

Figure 9.6. Basic steps in running an outsourced clinical study.

9.6.2. Proposals and Contracts

The sponsor may elect to obtain several bids from various CROs that have the capacity to complete the study. The sponsoring company may often draft an RFP, which outlines the study objectives and the specific services that are required of the CRO. Participating labs submit proposals that include costs and timelines to address the details of the RFP. If applicable, the CRO may make suggestions regarding the particular assays to be run or the manner in which the study will be conducted. The sponsor reviews the proposals and chooses the best proposal, which may not always be the least expensive, but perhaps the one that demonstrates a better approach to the study or demonstrates expertise in the area of interest. In some cases a CRO is selected without going to bid if the lab has previously worked on the same assays in another trial such that limited assay development is required or if the sponsor and laboratory already have built a successful relationship.

Once a proposal is accepted and a CRO is selected, the next step is to prepare a contract. The purpose of the contract is to clearly describe the work that will be performed and specific timelines as well as the compensation for the services. It also should protect the interests of both parties. In many cases the final proposal is included as an appendix or exhibit that is referred to in the contract. The compensation schedule is usually built around milestones in a study and is part of the contract. For example, one milestone may cover assay development and another milestone may include collection of samples or the testing of submitted samples and delivery of a report. Once both parties agree to the terms of the contract, it is dually executed and the study is ready to start. In most cases, the legal group of the sponsor drafts the contract. If changes arise during a study, these may be reflected in an amendment or change order to the contract. For example, if more samples are received or if additional or fewer assays or biomarkers are required, these are reflected in the amendment or change order.

9.6.3. Project Initiation and Study Protocol

Once the contracts are in place, the next step is to begin the study. The CRO that is awarded the contract now needs to activate the project in-house. This involves assigning appropriate personnel, including study director, project manager, and technicians. The goals of the study need to be captured in a study protocol that allows the CRO staff to understand the flow and design of the study. This document may be solely used in-house at the CRO or may be shared and signed-off by the sponsor, depending on the type of study and what is agreed upon. This document should describe the testing to be performed, including assays that need to be developed and the types of samples that will be collected and tested, and any reagents that need to be supplied by the sponsor or procured commercially.

Project management begins at study initiation and continues throughout the study. The conduct of the study needs to be constantly monitored so that studies are performed properly and according to designated timelines and quality guidelines. The project manager or study director at the CRO should provide periodic sponsor updates so that the sponsor understands the status of the study and can make in-house plans accordingly.

9.6.4. IHC Assay Development/Finalize Assays for Study

The IHC biomarker assays are typically determined by the sponsor; however, the CRO may suggest additional assays based on previous experience. The IHC assays may already be in place at the CRO, which can save time. If the assays are not in place or have not been tested in appropriate tissue types, the CRO will develop the assays. The basic approach to assay development has been described in Section 9.3. Before the assays are tested on any of the clinical study samples, the CRO should make sure the sponsor is in agreement with the assay.

9.6.5. Sample Handling

Sample handling and management is critical when performing clinical studies. The test samples received from patients on clinical studies are priceless and great care needs to be taken with all aspects of their handling. Samples are normally collected at numerous clinical sites and sent to the CRO or sponsor who will properly document their receipt. If samples are delivered directly to the CRO from the clinical sites and the sponsoring drug development company is bypassed, it is important for the CRO to properly communicate sample receipt to the sponsor and also alert it to any potential issues surrounding the samples. Samples should be securely stored and protected until ready for analysis. Details of sample handling and management have been described elsewhere (Lynch et al., 2008).

9.6.6. Testing of Study Samples

Once a set number of samples have been received, they are tested with the assays generated in assay development. In some cases the samples are all tested together at the end of the study or the sponsor may request one or more interim analyses, particularly when studies enroll over long periods of time or for dose escalation studies when data is needed for a specific cohort of patient samples before moving to the next. Prior to testing the samples, a quality control run should be performed on control tissues. These same control tissues as well as appropriate serum negative controls are tested with the specific IHC assays. After staining, all controls and test slides are evaluated for proper staining, and it should be determined whether any samples need to be repeated to obtain a higher quality stain.

9.6.7. Scoring of Study Samples

When scoring IHC assays, a one-size fits all approach does not work. The staining pattern observed needs to be carefully evaluated and as much information as possible should be captured. This is not always an easy or straightforward task as various patterns may be observed in different cell and tissue types. Testing a multitude of tissues in the assay development stage of the study generally allows for a good understanding of the range of staining patterns expected with the assay. This information should be incorporated into a scoring scheme and shared with the sponsor before the scoring is performed. The sponsor needs to agree with the method of analysis and also needs to understand the specifics in order to build appropriate databases for data transfer and statistical analysis.

The facets of staining to be captured by the scoring scheme may include the cell types staining, the subcellular localization of the stain, relative intensity of the stain, and the percentage of cells staining. For example, in oncology studies, the percentage of positive tumor cells may be scored as a range from 0 to 100. Other methods such as the standard pathology scoring system of 0 to 3 may be used as well. It is important to score the samples with a method that provides the best data resolution possible without overlooking or masking any critical patterns. In some cases image analysis may be required. Lastly, scoring is generally performed under blinded conditions, that is, the individual scoring the sample should have no information regarding the specifics of patient treatment.

9.6.8. Reporting and Documentation of Outsourced IHC Studies

All studies that are a part of the drug development process need to be performed and reported in a controlled manner so that the resulting data is reliable and properly integrated with other data. The need for controlled documentation and reporting is crucial in outsourced studies since the sponsor is not involved in the day-to-day operation of the study and needs to feel confident that the proper work is being performed. If the resulting data is to be used as part of a submission to the FDA, this documentation is required to be compliant with regulations. This section will focus on the reporting process, project management, sample handling, data interpretation, data management, and overall documentation of outsourced molecular pathology IHC studies.

Reports. The method and description of data reporting should be determined in the proposal and contract stage of the outsourcing process. The type, content, format, frequency, and timelines of reports should be clearly set forth by the sponsor and outlined in the proposal and contract so that both parties understand report requirements and expectations. The reports generated in IHC studies performed in the drug development process can usually be broken down into two types: an assay development/validation report that details the assay for IHC biomarkers to be tested and a report of the results of the application of the IHC biomarker assays on experimental tissues or clinical samples from patients enrolled in a study.

ASSAY DEVELOPMENT/ASSAY VALIDATION REPORTS. As discussed previously, the approach and extent of assay development and validation for IHC studies can vary depending on the needs of the study and should be determined before the study starts. Thus, the resulting assay development report should meet the needs of the study and sponsor. The ultimate goal of the assay development report is to relay the specifics of an IHC assay for the detection of a specific biomarker and to determine if the assay can be used to test experimental tissues or samples from a clinical study. The report should indicate the protocol and reagents used in the study, including incubation times, sources, lot numbers, and the like. The report should also include representative images of stained tissues, particularly those of the target tissue for a study. For example, if an IHC biomarker assay is being developed for a drug to treat colon cancer and colon cancer samples will be collected or tested in the study, then colon cancer samples should be evaluated in the assay development process. The report should also include appropriate control tissues and potentially recommend control tissues to be used in the clinical study. Lastly, the assay development report should consider the method of scoring that will be performed on the experimental or clinical samples.

Besides the optimized or validated assay, what else should be reported? It is important to relay the results of all testing performed. For example, several antibodies may be tested in an effort to find the best candidate antibody and IHC assay for a specific target biomarker. Some of these antibodies may not react well in the IHC assay, and others may provide supporting data for specificity of reactivity. Positive results as well as negative or less than adequate results should be reported. All antibodies to a target that were tested should be reported, so that the sponsor is aware of the results and can make better decisions in the future. Proper and complete reporting allows studies to be reviewed by the sponsor at a later date and still provide an understanding of the testing that was performed along with the results, long after the study has been completed and even after inevitable staff changes.

CLINICAL STUDY REPORTS. The resulting IHC biomarker assays from the assay development/validation stage are subsequently used to test experimental or clinical samples. These qualified assays and appropriate positive and negative controls are used to measure levels or changes in IHC biomarkers. The reporting necessary for these studies depends on the type of study and the questions being asked in the study. There are many types of IHC biomarkers—some are tested on baseline or diagnostic samples and others are tested in pre- and posttreatment samples or on samples from various time points. The sponsor defines what needs to be reported prior to commencement of the study; however, there may be additional data the CRO can provide after evaluating the study samples. Reports may be provided at the end of the study as a final report or with interim reports. The format depends on how a study is structured. For GLP studies, the report format should include all elements as defined by regulatory agency guidelines.

9.6.9. Quality Assurance Review of GLP Studies

Quality assurance (QA) personnel at the IHC CRO should review all data and reports prior to submitting to the sponsor. The data is checked to make sure the raw data is in agreement with data transferred to the report and to other formats being submitted to the sponsor. The QA staff audits the overall study to ensure that the study protocol was followed, that study deviations were prepared as needed, and that all documentation is complete and signed by the appropriate staff. The ensuing final report is also audited to ensure that all elements defined by regulatory agency guidelines are included and are in agreement with all study documentation. Quality assurance should prepare a signed statement as proof of the study audit. After quality assurance audit is complete the study director signs the report, which is then ready for submission to the sponsor.

9.6.10. Data Submission

After the quality assurance staff approves data, it can be sent to the sponsor. The sponsor normally assigns a data manager from the sponsor to interface with the CRO. Before any data is generated, representatives from the sponsor and CRO usually meet to discuss the type of information that will be transferred and the manner in which it will be transferred. For example, several IHC biomarkers may be tested with different scoring criteria. The data for each assay needs to be determined along with the format of the data. The CRO should take into account the data needs of the sponsor when implementing its in-house data management approach. Any data that is generated by the CRO needs to be properly documented, and relevant information needs to be transferred to the sponsor. The type of data to be generated in a study is usually understood at the beginning of the study, but additional data needs may arise as a study progresses.

The format for the data transfer is generally the responsibility of the sponsor. Once the format is finalized, the CRO normally sends a test file to the sponsor to make sure the data loads properly into the sponsor's databases. When successful, this same format will be used to generate computer files that reflect the data from the IHC staining. Results in spreadsheet format are often transferred as comma, tab, or space delimited files, but other formats such as the CDISC standard may also be used. Security of data is of the utmost importance. The method of transfer may be via password-protected or encrypted files sent electronically (via e-mail, secure email, or to a Web-based secure site) or via courier on password-protected and/or encrypted CD-ROM.

9.6.11. Data Integration and Follow-up

The study director and/or project manager at the CRO interface with the sponsor to make sure that data was transferred properly and to also make sure that the results are clearly understood. Some discussion may be necessary with other members of the clinical and research teams at the sponsor so that all parties are in agreement with the interpretation of study results.

9.7. APPLICATIONS OF IHC IN DRUG DISCOVERY AND DEVELOPMENT PROCESS

The applications of IHC assays in the drug discovery process are broad and can be applied in many areas of research and clinical studies. These include basic science, preclinical and toxicology studies, and phase I to III clinical studies, as well as commercialization of an IHC assay in association with a therapeutic. The remainder of this chapter will focus on some of the applications of IHC in clinical studies and provide some examples.

9.7.1. Target Validation

Immunohistochemistry assays may be used in helping determine whether a protein is a good target for drug development. In this application, IHC is used to localize a target protein to better understand its cellular expression in normal and disease tissue as well as its subcellular localization pattern. In these early studies in the drug discovery process the sponsor would be interested in having the CRO develop an IHC assay for a particular target and test a series of normal and disease tissues. For oncology drug discovery an ideal candidate target would be one that is expressed in tumor cells, but not in normal tissue. Figure 9.7 shows a marker found when looking for targets in prostate cancer. Many of the targets evaluated labeled normal tissue as well as tumor tissue. IHC provides the cell-specific resolution to be able to determine that the marker is localized on tumor cells (Xu et al., 2000). For a monoclonal antibody therapeutic it may be critical that the target protein is expressed on the plasma membrane of target cells, thus allowing access of the therapeutic antibody to bind the target positive cells. Figure 9.7 also provides an example of a monoclonal antibody target protein that is expressed on the plasma membrane of tumor cells. This testing is usually performed on sections from banked tissues rather than experimental tissues. The IHC data may help the drug development company decide whether to proceed with developing a targeted therapy or to discontinue work on the target. Outsourcing this work to an independent CRO laboratory provides a third-party unbiased review of the cell and tissue-specific expression of the target.

9.7.2. Preclinical Testing

Immunohistochemistry testing is commonly used in evaluating the expression of target proteins or biomarkers in sections of drug-treated and untreated tissue samples. Early in the drug development program testing is generally performed in experimental animal models, which may include xenografts in oncology programs. The purpose of these studies is to use IHC to evaluate any changes in expression of a target biomarker upon treatment with a therapeutic agent. These studies may provide baseline information as to whether the target therapeutic is

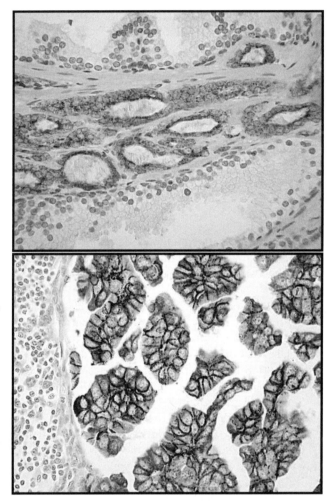

Figure 9.7. IHC–target validation. (Top) AMACR IHC in prostate carcinoma. This antibody labels tumor cells but not the normal epithelium. (Bottom) Detection of a target antigen localized to the plasma membrane of tumor cells in an ovarian carcinoma. Lymphocytes are negative. Hematoxylin counterstain; DAB chromagen.

having an effect on the tumor cells. Xenograft models provide a good opportunity to evaluate whether certain target proteins may be used as biomarkers in clinical studies. The treated and untreated samples are sent to the CRO, and the CRO develops assays in these tissue types and determines whether any changes are observed in the markers. For example, a therapeutic that affects an apoptosis pathway may be tested for an increase in apoptosis or necrosis in treated samples compared to untreated samples. The CRO may often be blinded to treatment in order for the sponsor to obtain an unbiased view of study results.

9.7.3. Phase I through Phase III Clinical Studies

In phase I to III clinical studies tissues from patients on the novel therapy are often tested using IHC methodology. These samples may be tested using IHC staining for a number of different purposes, depending on the design of the study and the types of biomarkers the sponsor is interested in testing. For example, IHC biomarker analysis may be used to help determine optimal dosing of a drug therapy in dose escalation studies. Pharmacodynamic biomarkers may be tested in pre- and posttreatment tissue samples collected from patients enrolled in the study. These markers are used to evaluate the mechanism of action of the drug, and IHC may be used to determine if the expected changes in biomarker expression are being observed. For example, if one of the expected outcomes of a drug therapy is to inhibit cellular proliferation, then Ki67 (a proliferation marker) IHC may be performed on pre- and posttreatment samples to determine if proliferation is decreased. For these type studies surrogate tissues such as skin may be valuable since the epidermis of skin possess proliferating cells and obtaining skin sample biopsies is less invasive than excising tumor samples (Albanell et al., 2002). Figure 9.8 shows an example of a decrease in proliferation in the posttreatment skin biopsy.

Predictive biomarkers are another type of biomarker that is often tested using IHC. These markers may be very powerful if they can be used to help determine which patients may be likely to respond to a specific therapy. Drug development companies may use these markers to help enroll patients that will likely respond to a therapy or stratify patient populations on the study. Predictive biomarkers are also important in targeted therapy whereby only patients expressing the target of the drug are enrolled in the study. Her2/neu falls into this category and has been shown to be an important IHC biomarker test (Dowsett et al., 2003; Garcia-Caballero et al., 2006). In some cases these predictive markers may be tested from sections of the patient diagnostic blocks or baseline samples, and posttreatment samples may not need to be obtained during the study. A number of targeted therapies are currently being developed in which associated IHC tests are used to test patient samples. For example, several companies are developing monoclonal antibody therapeutics to Insulin Growth Factor 1 Receptor (IGF-1R).

Typically, when IHC is used for either dose escalation or as an enrollment criterion a fast turn around of results is necessary. These studies may be best performed by a CRO laboratory staffed to handle these tight timelines. For dose escalation, results may be required several times over the course of the study. IHC biomarkers that are used to determine enrollment (acceptance or stratification) need to be turned around in a matter of days.

9.7.4. Companion Diagnostics

The FDA has recommended that drug development companies incorporate biomarker testing into clinical studies to help better treat patients (CDER, 2001). If the therapeutic and associated tests are successful in clinical trials, the test may

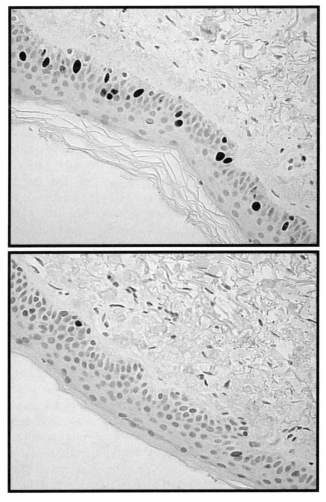

Figure 9.8. Pharmacodynamic markers—Ki67 in treated and untreated skin samples. (Top) Ki67 in pretreatment sample. Proliferating cells located in the basal region of the epidermis label with a nuclear localization. (Bottom) Ki67 in posttreatment sample. There are fewer positive cells in this sample. Hematoxylin counterstain; DAB chromagen.

need to be made commercially available. Tests such as the HercepTest for Herceptin therapy have been called companion diagnostics. Due to the number of targeted therapies in development, these tests are expected to become more and more common (FDA, 2005).

Immunohistochemistry testing may be an ideal platform for developing companion diagnostics. This is due to the fact that many targets are localized to the plasma membrane of cells and thus are not generally secreted and not candidates for serum testing. Other reasons that support IHC testing include:

- IHC provides cell-specific resolution; avoids questions about source of expression and tissue heterogeneity.
- IHC detects the target protein, not RNA.
- IHC can detect posttranslation modifications, for example, phospho-specific antibodies.
- IHC is a standard working test in clinical laboratories and hospitals.

The importance of IHC tests in clinical studies and as potential companion diagnostics underlines the need to choose the right laboratory when outsourcing the development and analysis of these tests.

9.8. CONCLUSION

Molecular pathology assays such as IHC are an important testing platform with wide application in the drug development process. Performing IHC assays requires a team of skilled technicians and scientists with varied expertise. Outsourcing IHC assays to specialty CROs is a viable option that provides flexibility and time and cost savings to drug development companies. Choosing the right laboratory to outsource IHC assays is critical, and the results generated can have a significant impact on the future of a therapeutic candidate.

REFERENCES

21CFR58, (2008), Good Laboratory Practices for Nonclinical Laboratory Studies, Code of Federal Regulations, Title 21, Part 58, 2008.

45CFR160, (2003), General Overview of Standards for Privacy of Individually Identifiable Health Information, Code of Federal Regulations, Title 45, Part 160.

Albanell, J., Rojo, F., Averbuch, S., Feyereislova, A., Mascaro, J. M., Herbst, R., LoRusso, P., Rischin, D., Sauleda, S., Gee, J., Nicholson, R. I., and Baselga, J. (2002). Pharmacodynamic studies of the epidermal growth factor receptor inhibitor ZD1839 in skin from cancer patients: Histopathologic and molecular consequences of receptor inhibition. *J. Clin. Oncal.* 20:110–124.

Anscomb, A. (2008). *Outsourcing in Drug Discovery*, 3rd ed., May, 2008, Kalorama Information, Rockville MD.

Battifora, H. (1991). Assessment of antigen damage in immunohistochemistry. The vimentin internal control. *Am. J. Clin. Pathol.* 96:669–671.

Battifora, H., and Kopinski, M. (1986). The influence of protease digestion and duration of fixation on the immunostaining of keratins. A comparison of formalin and ethanol fixation. *J. Histochem. Cytochem.* 34:1095–1100.

CDER (2001). CDER Guidance for Industry—Bioanalytical Method Validation, May (2001). Guidance document prepared by the Biopharmaceutics Coordinating Committee in the Center for Drug Evaluation and Research (CDER) in cooperation with the Center for Veterinary Medicine (CVM) at the Food and Drug Administration.

CLIA (1988). Clinical Laboratory Improvement Amendments of 1988, Pub. L. No. 100–578, 102 Stat. 2903; 42 U.S.C. § 263a.

Dowsett, M., Bartlett, J., Ellis, I. O., Salter, J., Hills, M., Mallon, E., Watters, A. D., Cooke, T., Paish, C., Wencyk, P. M., Pinder, S. E. (2003). Correlation between immunohisto-chemistry (HercepTest) and fluorescence in situ hybridization (FISH) for HER-2 in 426 breast carcinomas from 37 centres. *J. Pathol.* 199:418–423.

FDA, (2005). Draft Drug-Diagnostic Co-Development Concept Paper, Department of Health and Human Services (HHS)F & Food and Drug Administration (FDA), April 2005.

Garcia-Caballero, T., Menendez, M. D., Vazquez-Boquete, A., Gallego, R., Forteza, J., and Fraga, M. (2006). HER-2 status determination in breast carcinomas. A practical approach. *Histol. Histopathol.* 21:227–236.

Gown, A. M., de Wever, N., and Battifora, H. (1993). Microwave-based antigenic unmasking. A revolutionary new technique for routine immunohistochemistry. *Appl. Immunohistochem.* 1:256–266.

Hsu, S. M., Raine, L., and Fanger, H. (1981). Use of avidin-biotin-peroxidase complex (ABC) in immunoperoxidase techniques: A comparison between ABC and unlabeled antibody (PAP) procedures. *J. Histochem. Cytochem.* 29:577–580.

Ladner, R. D., Lynch, F. J., Groshen, S., Xiong, Y. P., Sherrod, A., Caradonna, S. J., Stoehlmacher, J., and Lenz, H. J. (2000). dUTP nucleotidohydrolase isoform expression in normal and neoplastic tissues: Association with survival and response to 5-fluoruracil in colorectal cancer. *Cancer Res.* 60:3493–3503.

Lynch, F., Bernstein, S., and Battifora, H. (2008). IHC testing and analysis of clinical specimens using validated assays 49–72. In *Validation of Cell-Based Assays in the GLP Setting*, Prabhahar, U., and Kelley, M. (Eds.). John Wiley & Sons Ltd. West Sussex, England.

Riera, J. R., Astengo-Osuna, C., Longmate, J. A., and Battifora, H. (1997). The immuno-histochemical diagnostic panel for epithelial mesothelioma: A reevaluation after heat-induced epitope retrieval. *Am. J. Surg. Pathol.* 12:1395–1398.

Shi, S.-R., Key, M. E., and Kalra, K. L. (1991). Antigen retrieval in formalin-fixed, paraffin-embedded tissues: An enhancement method for immunohistochemical stain-ing based on microwave oven heating of tissue sections. *J. Histochem. Cytochem.* 39:741–748.

Shi, S.-R., Cote, R. J., and Taylor, C. R. (2001). Antigen retrieval techniques: Current perspectives. *J. Histochem. Cytochem.* 49:931–937.

Tinkelenberg, B. A., Lynch, F. J., and Ladner, R. D. (2003). Identification of sequence determinants of human nuclear dUTPase isoform localization. *Exp. Cell Res.* 287:39–46.

Xu, J., Stolk, J. A., Zhang, X., Silva, S. J., Houghton, R. L., Matsumura, M., Vedvick, T. S., Leslie, K. B., Badaro, R., and Reed, S. G. (2000). Identification of differentially expressed genes in human prostate cancer using subtraction and microarray. *Cancer Res.* 60:1677–1682.

10

QUANTIFICATION OF MOLECULAR PATHOLOGY: COLORIMETRIC IMMUNOHISTOCHEMISTRY

Raphael Marcelpoil

The practice of anatomic and clinical pathology traditionally requires understanding of general concepts and technologies that are common to specific applications in each area of the clinical laboratory. Increasing knowledge of the molecular basis of disease, advances in technology for analyzing nucleic acids and gene products, the explosion of information regarding inherited susceptibility to disease are changing pathology practice. Pathology is being transformed by new knowledge in molecular pathology and human genetics and by advances in the application of molecular biotechnology. As this trend accelerates, the importance of integrating robust and comprehensive data gained via nucleic-acid-based technology with other laboratory and clinical information available in the care of patients is emphasized (Williams et al., 1999).

Recognizing these needs, large interdisciplinary programs such as the Biomedical Informatics (BMI) program of the European Research Consortium for Informatics and Mathematics (ERCIM) have been developed to provide a framework for developing, integrating, and sharing biomedical knowledge related to human health from very different research disciplines such as genomics, proteomics, clinical research, and epidemiology. The ultimate objectives of BMI are to support molecular medicine and personalized health care. The advances in information and communication technologies (ICT), coupled with the increased

Molecular Pathology in Drug Discovery and Development, Edited by J. Suso Platero
Copyright © 2009 John Wiley & Sons, Inc.

knowledge about the human genome, have opened new perspectives for the study of complex diseases. There is a growing need to integrate and translate the knowledge about human genome into concrete benefits for all citizens such as more effective disease prevention mechanisms, individualized medicines and treatments, and many other aspects of future citizen-centered health-care systems (Zobel, 2005). Among the most promising research areas is biomedical imaging, a multidisciplinary field aiming at effective analysis and processing of biological/ genetic data. Biomedical imaging can also be considered as one of the emerging areas in biomedical informatics, emanating from synergies among algorithmic research, medical informatics, medical imaging, and molecular biology. Built on previous engineering knowledge, modern technology and complex algorithmic solutions, the aim of this field is to develop robust analysis frameworks for maximizing the information content of biological data.

Our focus in this chapter will emphasize the methodological aspect of colorimetric immunohistochemistry quantification, benefits, and constraints of the recent developments of these techniques.

10.1. INTRODUCTION

Pathology is a discipline crucially dependant on the interpretation of images for diagnosis and prognostication of diseases. When historical interpretation techniques relied heavily on the subjective analysis of specimens, with variable intra- as well as interobserver agreement, modern interpretation makes use of both molecular input and machine objective quantification. Figure 10.1 illustrates the difficulty for the human eye/brain system to analyze objectively an object within a scene, regardless of its contextual information (e.g., the perception of a given object may be very different according to its context), emphasizing the need of computer-aided microscopy when pathology is turned into molecular pathology.

The assessment and analysis of tissues is the classical domain of pathology. Although methodological and technological developments have turned digital image analysis into one of the most efficient tools to assist pathologists in their eagerness to interpret images more and more accurately, a large gap separates classical pathology from computer-assisted molecular pathology (Brugal, 1984). Histological interpretation techniques based on image analysis were initially confined to technologies developed for the analysis of a single marker (e.g., DNA-like analyses using Feulgen stain). For this purpose, if possible, the tissue samples were enzymatically disaggregated (Hedley et al., 1983), and the task of analyzing tissue was reduced to the evaluation of a cytological slide, or the three-dimensional character of the histological section was roughly taken into account through the introduction of a stereological correction factor (Mairinger and Gschwendtner, 1996).

With the evolution and easy availability of high-performance computers, advances in information and communication technologies, database and storage

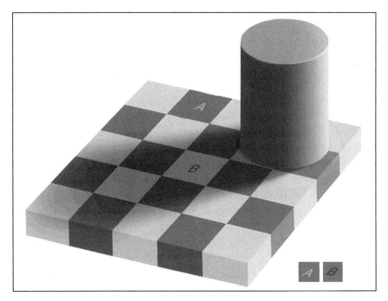

Figure 10.1. The squares marked A and B are the same shade of gray, yet they appear different. (Image rendered by Edward H. Adelson.)

technology, and affordable high-resolution digital cameras, the situation has now changed. More sophisticated algorithms, which for lack of CPU power could never before be applied to tissue sections in a routine environment, can now be used to assess and quantify tissue-specific features related to the molecular quantification of mixed markers in colorimetric studies. At the same time a far more comprehensive support for a reproducible and more standardized assessment of tissue sections has become available based on the initial step in image analysis, the creation and management of digital images. This is especially true in the fields of quality control, quality assurance, and standardization. Digital images of difficult cases can be exchanged with reference pathologists via telepathology or Internet to get a second opinion (Krupinski et al., 1993). They can be effectively used for proficiency testing. Digital images are the basis of powerful image reference databases, which can be accessed via network (intra- and Internet), and they play an increasingly important role in the documentation of cases and evaluation of results, especially in comprehensive electronic or printed reports.

Effective analysis of microscopic images is essential particularly for detection and quantification of molecular material, such as genetic material [genes, messenger ribonucleic acid (mRNA)] or the expression of this genetic information in the form of proteins, for example, gene amplification, gene deletion, gene mutation, number of mRNA molecules, or protein expression analyses. Gene amplification is the presence of too many copies of the same gene in one cell, wherein a cell usually contains two copies, otherwise known as alleles, of the same gene. Gene deletion indicates that less than two copies of a gene can be found in a cell. Gene mutation indicates the presence of incomplete, nonfunctional, or hyperactive genes. Messenger RNAs are molecules of genetic information, synthesized from DNA (deoxyribonucleic acid) reading, that serve as templates for protein synthesis. Protein expression is the production of a given protein by a cell. If the gene coding for this protein is up-regulated or too many copies of the gene or mRNA are present, the protein may be overexpressed. If the gene is down-regulated or deleted, the protein expression level may be low or absent.

Normal cellular behaviors are precisely controlled by molecular mechanisms involving a large number of proteins, mRNAs, and genes. Gene amplification, gene deletion, and gene mutation are known to have a prominent role in abnormal cellular behaviors through abnormal protein expression. The range of cellular behaviors of concern includes behaviors as diverse as, for example, proliferation or differentiation regulation. Therefore, effective detection and quantification in gene amplification, deletion, and mutation, mRNAs levels, or protein expression analyses is necessary in order to facilitate useful research and diagnostic and prognostic tools.

There are numerous laboratory techniques dedicated to detection and quantification in gene amplification, deletion and mutation, mRNA levels, or protein expression analyses. For example, such techniques include Western, Northern and Southern blots, polymerase chain reaction (PCR), enzyme-linked immunoseparation assay (ELISA), and comparative genomic hybridization (CGH) techniques. However, microscopy is routinely utilized because it is an informative technique, allowing rapid investigations at the cellular and subcellular levels, which may be implemented at a relatively low cost.

When microscopy is the chosen laboratory technique, the biological samples usually first undergo specific detection and revelation preparations. Once the samples are prepared, a human expert analyzes the samples with a microscope alone or with a microscope coupled to a camera and a computer, allowing both a more standardized and quantitative study. The microscope may be configured for fully automatic analysis, wherein the microscope is automated with a slide loader, motorized stage and focus, motorized objective changers, automatic light intensity controls, and the like. The preparation of the samples for detection may involve different types of preparation techniques that are suited to microscopic imaging analysis, such as, for example, hybridization-based and immunolabeling-based preparation techniques. Such detection techniques are coupled with appropriate revelation techniques, for example, fluorescence-based or color-reaction-based techniques within the visible spectrum range.

In situ hybridization (ISH), colorimetric or silver-based (CISH and SISH, respectively), and fluorescent in situ hybridization (FISH) are detection and revelation techniques used, for example, for detection and quantification of genetic information amplification and mutation analyses. The similarities to immunohistochemistry (IHC) are obvious. Because of the familiarity of the format, IHC is the molecular technique that has the greatest attraction for diagnostic histopathology laboratories. Both ISH and FISH can be applied to histological or cytological samples. These techniques use specific complementary probes for recognizing corresponding precise sequences. Depending on the technique used, the specific probe may include a colorimetric or silver-based (ISH) marker, or a fluorescent (FISH) marker, wherein the samples are then analyzed using a transmission microscope or a fluorescence microscope, respectively. The use of ISH or FISH depends on the goal of the user, each type of marker having corresponding advantages over the other techniques.

In case of protein expression analyses, IHC and immunocytochemistry (ICC) techniques are widely used to help in the diagnosis and prognosis of cancer. IHC is the application of immunochemistry to tissue sections, whereas ICC is the application of immunochemistry to cultured cells or tissue imprints after they have undergone specific cytological preparations, for example, liquid-based preparations. ICC or IHC refer, respectively, to the process of localizing proteins in isolated cells and cells of a tissue section exploiting the principle of antibodies binding specifically to antigens in biological tissues (Russ, 2006). ICC and IHC take their names from the roots *immuno*, in reference to antibodies used in the procedure, and *cyto*, meaning cell, or *histo*, meaning tissue. Specific molecular markers are characteristic of particular cancer types. IHC is also widely used in basic research to understand the distribution and localization of biomarkers in different parts of a tissue.

Immunochemistry is a family of techniques based on the use of a specific antibody, wherein antibodies are used to specifically target molecules inside or on the surface of cells. There are two strategies used for the immunohistochemical detection of antigens in tissue, the direct method and the indirect method. The direct method is a one-step staining method and involves a labeled antibody reacting directly with the antigen in tissue sections. This technique utilizes only one antibody and the procedure is therefore simple and rapid. However, it can suffer problems with sensitivity due to little signal amplification and is in less common use than indirect methods. The indirect method of immunohistochemical staining uses one antibody against the antigen being probed for, and a second, labeled, antibody against the first. The indirect method involves an unlabeled primary antibody (first layer) that reacts with tissue antigen, and a labeled secondary antibody (second layer) that reacts with the primary antibody. (The secondary antibody must be against the IgG of the animal species in which the primary antibody has been raised.) This method is more sensitive due to signal amplification through several secondary antibody reactions with different antigenic sites on the primary antibody. The second layer antibody can be labeled with a fluorescent dye or an enzyme. In a common procedure, a biotinylated secondary antibody is coupled with streptavidin–horseradish peroxidase. This is reacted with 3,3′-diaminobenzidine (DAB) to produce a brown staining wherever primary and secondary antibodies are attached in a process known as DAB staining. Using nickel can enhance the reaction, producing a deep purple/gray staining.

Immunohistochemistry is an excellent detection technique and has the tremendous advantage of being able to show exactly where a given protein is located within the tissue examined. This has made it a widely used technique in the biosciences, enabling researchers to examine protein expression within specific tissues. Its major disadvantage is that, unlike immunoblotting techniques where staining is checked against a molecular weight ladder, it is impossible to show in IHC that the staining corresponds with the protein of interest. For this reason, primary antibodies must be well validated in a Western blot or similar procedure. The technique is even more widely used in diagnostic surgical pathology for typing tumors (e.g., carcinoma vs. melanoma).

In both hybridization and immunolabeling studies, chromogens of different colors are used to distinguish the different markers. However, the maximum number of markers that may be used in a study is restricted by several factors. For example, the spectral overlapping of the colors used to reveal the respective markers may be a limiting factor because dyes may absorb throughout a large portion of the visible spectrum. Accordingly, the higher the number of dyes involved in a study, the higher the risk of spectral overlapping. Further, the spectral resolution of the acquisition device may be a limiting factor, and the minimal color shift that the device is able to detect must be considered.

In addition the quantification accuracy of these techniques may be dependent upon several factors. For instance, the type of reaction used may play a role in the accuracy of the technique since the linearity of the relationship between ligand concentration and the intensity of the immunochemical staining reaction may strongly depend on the reaction type. The cellular localization of the markers may also affect accuracy where, for example, if membrane and nuclear markers spatially overlap, the resulting color is a mixture of the respective colors. Accordingly, since the corresponding quantification is subjective, the accuracy of the determination may be affected. In addition, a calibration standard (cells with known features, gels with given concentrations of the marker, or the like) may be required where a developed analysis model is applied to a new and different case. Staining kits are generally available that incorporate calibration standards. However, the calibration standard is usually only applicable to a particular specimen, such as a specific cell category or a structure of a specific type, that is known to exhibit constant features with respect to the standard and may be of limited utility when applied to a sample of a different nature. Another major source of variation in the observed and measured intensity of the marker is linked to the reproducibility and robustness of the staining protocol itself, involving both aspects of specimen storage and preparation techniques, as well as staining instrument efficiency and laboratory "good practice" standards.

Overall, the described "colorimetric" studies present sample analysis information in color and facilitate processing and quantification of the information to thereby help to provide a diagnosis or to form a prognosis for the particular case. For illustration, the detection and quantification of the HER2 protein expression and/or gene amplification may be assessed by different approaches used in quantitative microscopy. HER2 is a membrane protein that has been shown to have a diagnostic and prognostic significance in metastatic breast cancer. Because HER2-positive patients were shown to be more sensitive to treatments including Herceptin (a target treatment developed by Genentech), the definition of the

HER2 status of metastatic breast cancers has been proven to be of first importance in the choice of the appropriate treatment protocol. This definition of the
HER2 status was based on a study of samples treated with either hybridization
(FISH, ISH) or immunolabeling (IHC) techniques. In such studies, using FISH
with, for example, a Food and Drug Administration (FDA)-approved kit such as
PathVysion produced by Vysis, requires an image analysis protocol for counting
the number of copies of the *HER2* gene present in every cell. In a normal case,
two copies of the gene are found in each cell, whereas more than four copies of
the gene in a cell indicate that the gene is amplified. Alternatively, using IHC
with, for example, an FDA-approved kit such as Herceptest produced by DAKO,
requires an image analysis protocol that classifies the cases into four categories
depending on the intensity and localization of the HER2-specific membrane
staining. Current studies tend to show that these two investigation techniques
(hybridization and immunolabeling) may be complementary and may help
pathologists in tumor subtype diagnosis when combined.

10.2. IMAGING DEVICES AND SYSTEMS

Computer-aided microscopy systems have been designed and developed to help
pathologists understand diseased cells. As the image of a particular region of
interest (ROI) is captured, the system simultaneously captures its x-y coordinates
and processes the field of view (FOV) to measure the marker content of the
cells located in the region of interest. Equipped with this information and a
motorized stage, the microscope can repeatedly return to any previous ROI the
pathologist has selected. Such a system is based on a semiautomated microscope
equipped with a digital camera, encoded turret, and motorized stage. The VIAS
(see Fig. 10.2) represents such a system. It includes a personal computer (PC)
with a frame-grabber board running BD-TriPath's proprietary image-analysis
software.

The digital microscope integrated into the VIAS is a custom version of the
Axio Imager.M1 from Carl Zeiss Micro Imaging, equipped with a motorized
stage from Märzhäuser Wetzlar. It uses a 100-W halogen bulb for illumination
and contains five objective lenses on its turret, providing 2.5×, 5×, 10×, 20×, or
40× magnifications. The turret is encoded to ensure that all ROI images in a
particular sequence of images are captured with the same objective. The system
can provide quantitative results for images captured at either 10×, 20×, or 40×
(SISH) magnifications.

Colorimetric studies require extensive sample preparation and procedure
control. When disposing of an adapted staining protocol, it is critical to be able
to verify that the staining for each sample matches the particular model used
in the image acquisition and processing device such that accurate and useful
results are obtained from the gathered information. In a typical microscopy
device based on image acquisition and processing (see Fig. 10.2), the magnified
image of the sample must first be captured and digitized with a camera. Generally,

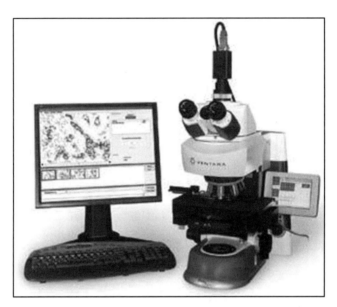

Figure 10.2. Typical imaging workstation: The Ventana Image Analysis System (VIAS) is a semiautomated microscopy system that helps pathologists understand diseased cells. This interactive histology imaging system, launched in 2005, offers anatomic pathology laboratories a solution utilizing on-demand digital imaging, direct visualization of IHC stained slides, and real-time quantitative analysis of tissue samples.

charge-coupled device (CCD) digital cameras are used in either bright-field or fluorescence quantitative microscopy. Excluding spectrophotometers, two different techniques are generally used to perform such colorimetric microscopic studies. In one technique, a black-and-white (BW) CCD camera may be used. In such systems, a gray-level image of the sample is obtained, corresponding to a monochromatic light having a wavelength specific to the staining of the sample to be analyzed. The specific wavelength of light is obtained either by filtering a white source light via a specific narrow bandwidth filter or by directly controlling the wavelength of the light source, using either manual or electronic controls. Accordingly, using this technique, the analysis time increases as the number of colors increases because a light source or a filter must be selected for every different sample staining or every different wavelength. Therefore, many different images of the sample, showing the spectral response of the sample at different wavelengths, must be individually captured in a sequential order to facilitate the analysis. When multiple scenes or fields of view must be analyzed, the typical protocol is to automate the sequence in a batch mode to conserve processing time.

According to a second technique, a color CCD digital camera is used (3CCD), wherein three gray-level images of the sample are simultaneously captured and

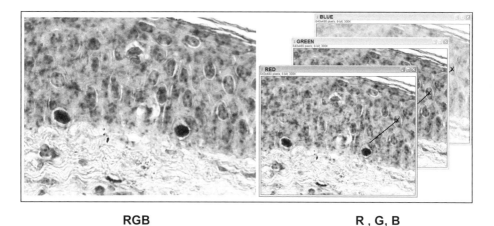

RGB   **R , G, B**

Figure 10.3. RGB field of view and its pseudocolor decomposition in R, G, and B channels.

obtained. Each gray-level image corresponds to the respective red, green, and blue channel (RGB) of the color CCD camera (see Fig. 10.3). The images are then analyzed directly in the RGB color space by restricting the analysis to the pixels located in a specific region of the RGB cube (where pixels from a training database were also located) or, after mathematical transform of the RGB color space, in one of the many color spaces defined by the CIE (*Commission Internationale de l'Eclairage*) such as, for example, an HLS (hue, luminance, and saturation) space. Alternatively, some camera manufacturers produce specific CCD cameras wherein narrow bandwidth filters targeting specific wavelengths may replace the usual broad red, green, and blue filters. In such an instance, the camera allows a fast image capture of the three spectral components of a scene in a parallel manner. However, cameras modified in this manner may be restricted to specific spectral analysis parameters because the filters cannot be exchanged and therefore cannot be adapted to address a unique dye combination used for the sample. Thus, the second technique generally relies upon either the detection of contrast between the species of interest and the remainder of the sample or the analysis of the sample over a narrow bandwidth.

Techniques used in colorimetric analyses of prepared samples are of limited use in the detection and quantification of species of interest due to several factors such as, for example, spectral overlapping, mixing of colors due to spatial overlap of membrane, cytoplasmic and nuclear markers, chromatic aberrations of the optical path, limited spectral resolution of the acquisition device, subjectivity of the detection and quantification process, and inconsistencies between human operators.

The image-processing step of colorimetric analysis techniques has histori-cally been directed to the subjective detection of contrast within the prepared sample or to a complex and voluminous analysis of the sample at different specific wavelengths using a combination of light sources and filters. Therefore faster, simpler, and more effective colorimetric analysis techniques had to be developed to overcome detection and quantification limitations when compared to former techniques, providing superior information about the sample, reducing subjectivity and inconsistency in the sample analysis.

Colorimetric immunohistochemistry (C-IHC) detection methods and subcellular imaging algorithms based upon multispectral analysis are now available to optimize and standardize the reading of colorimetric markers. Such markers may be used to detect and/or quantify gene amplification, gene deletion, gene mutations, and abnormal protein expression that may be visible upon analyzing a tissue section slide treated with an appropriate marker chosen to highlight the abnormal cellular activity that may aid in the diagnosis and/or determination of prognosis for a disease such as cancer. These methods are useful for obtaining a valuable quantitative measurement of a target molecular species within a given tissue sample. Additional molecular species can be highlighted within the same tissue sample or on consecutive tissue sections by additional biomarkers. Such assays or "multiplexed assays" are designed in order to more systematically analyze a tissue sample so as to allow a clinician to provide a more accurate diagnostic/prognosis for patients suffering from a complex disease such as cancer or to evaluate the impact of a new drug on key cellular functions in the targeted cellular population and its side effects in other organic tissues.

10.3. QUANTIFICATION: INTRODUCTION TO COLORIMETRIC IMAGE ANALYSIS

Color perception is mainly constrained by the number of spectral measurements, the spectral resolution. Due to the limited space available on the retina, evolution was forced to trade-off between the number of different spectral receptors and their spatial distribution. For humans, spectral vision is limited to three color samples and a tremendous amount of spatial samples. Daylight has driven evolution to set the central wavelength of color vision at about 520 nm and a spectral range of about 330 nm. For any colorimetric system, measurement is constrained by these parameters (Geusebroek, 2000).

Microscope image processing and analysis is a broad term that covers the use of digital image processing techniques to capture, process, analyze, and present images and report comprehensive data obtained from a microscopic image. Image processing techniques are now widely used in a number of fields as diverse as medicine, biological research, cancer research, pharmacology, drug testing, and the like. Image processing for microscopic applications begins with fundamental techniques intended to most accurately reproduce the information contained in the microscopic sample. This includes adjusting the optical path of the microscope and camera according to Koehler illumination standards, adjusting the dynamic range of the camera and light brightness, maximizing signal-to-noise ratio, correcting the image for chromatic aberrations, correcting for illumination nonuniformities, and validating the linearity of the camera.

10.3.1. Image Acquisition

Today, acquisition is usually done using a CCD camera mounted in the optical path of the microscope. The camera may be full color (3CCD) or monochrome. Very often, high-resolution cameras are employed to gain as much direct information as possible. Cryogenic cooling is also possible among other techniques to minimize noise. Often digital cameras used for these applications provide pixel intensity data to a resolution of 12 to 16 bits, among which the most appropriate 8 or 10 bits dynamic range is selected. In order to best suit the expected image processing to be performed, the camera/objective couple must be well selected. Below we will develop some aspects of the difficult match between image sensor and microscope objective to best suit the application.

10.3.2. Resolution and Magnification

The field resolution, or Abbe diffraction limit of the microscope, depends on the objective numerical aperture (NA):

$$\text{Field resolution} \quad r_{\text{field}} = \frac{1.22\lambda}{\text{NA}_{\text{obj}} + \text{NA}_{\text{cond}}} \tag{10.1}$$

with λ the wavelength (typically 550 nm, green), NA_{obj} and NA_{cond} the numerical aperture of the objective and condenser, respectively. Recent developments in fluorescent microscopy (Westphal and Hell, 2005) have shown that this limit can theoretically be bypassed; however, bright-field microscopic resolution remains dependent upon this limit.

The selection of the camera sensor must be done according to the sampling theory (Nyquist sampling criterion). The sampling frequency must be twice the highest frequency present in the signal. If the sampling frequency is too low, the digital conversion will loose details. If it is too high, it will create unnatural/false information ("aliasing") and the image processor will process more pixel than necessary. It means that the camera pixel size must be selected so that it is as close as possible to half the image resolution (twice the highest possible frequency). The image resolution takes the magnification into account and the pixel size of the camera sensor while the field resolution takes into account only the numerical aperture of the objective. Image Resolution:

$$r_{\text{image}} = \frac{\text{pixel size}}{\text{magnification}} \tag{10.2}$$

Table 10.1 shows the resolution for the most popular 10× Zeiss objectives and their theoretical optimum camera pixel size according to the sampling theory.

TABLE 10.1. 10× Zeiss Objective and Optimal Camera Matching Pixel Size

Objective Type	Mag.	NA	Object Res. (μm)	Image Res. (μm)	Optimum Camera Pixel Size (μm)
Achroplan	10×	0.25	1.34	13.4	6.7
Plan Neofluar	10×	0.3	1.12	11.2	5.6
Plan Apochromat	10×	0.45	0.75	7.5	3.75

TABLE 10.2. Field Size as Function of Objective Magnification and Sensor Dimension

Objective	⅓″ Camera	½″ Camera	⅔″ Camera
5×	960 × 720 μm	1280 × 960 μm	1760 × 1320 μm
10×	480 × 360 μm	640 × 480 μm	880 × 660 μm
20×	240 × 180 μm	320 × 240 μm	440 × 330 μm

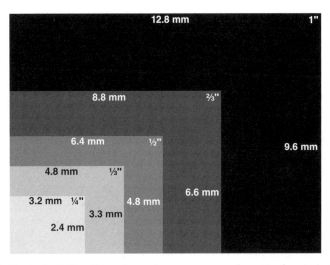

Figure 10.4. Physical relative dimensions of camera sensors from ¼ of an inch to 1 full inch.

10.3.3. Sensor Size

The image resolution depends on the magnification and the physical pixel size on the sensor. For historical reasons (photography standard), camera sensor sizes are somehow standardized (⅓″, ½″, ⅔″, ... , see Fig. 10.4).

It is straightforward (see Table 10.2) to get the field size in the object plane (sensor size/magnification). In order to capture a given region of interest of the sample, the number of fields to be scanned and captured is directly linked to the field size. Intuitively, the bigger the field size, the lower the number of field to scan. Provided the image resolution is kept, it is possible to replace, for example, a ⅓″ (640 × 480 pixels) camera by a ⅔″ (1280 × 960 pixels). As the number of pixels increases on the camera, we have to pay attention to the digital standard in use (i.e., FireWire, USB 2.0, LVDS, CameraLink) as the bandwidth to transfer data becomes a key factor in application speed.

10.3.4. Two Major Camera Technologies Available for Color Image Acquisition

3CCD Progressive Scan Camera. The 3CCD camera is the golden standard for color image acquisition since the three channels (red, green, and blue) have the exact same characteristics in terms of resolution. The biggest problem with 3CCD cameras is the limiting size of the sensor and size/cost issue. Most of the cameras are available in ⅓″ in XVGA standard (1024 × 780).

Bayer Progressive Scan Camera. Another way to produce color images is to use one-chip CDD [or complementary metal–oxide semiconductor (CMOS)] equipped with a special filter (Bayer pattern; see Fig. 10.5). A color interpolation algorithm is implemented to retrieve red, green, and blue information from each pixel. This process averages out the color values of appropriate neighboring pixels to guess. As long as the colors in the image change slowly in the spatial dimension relative to the filter pattern, color interpolation works extremely well. However, for edges of objects, or fine details, color may be interpolated incorrectly and artifacts can result. For example, a small white dot in a scene might illuminate only a single blue pixel. The white dot might come out blue if it is surrounded by black or some other color, depending on what comes out of the interpolation.

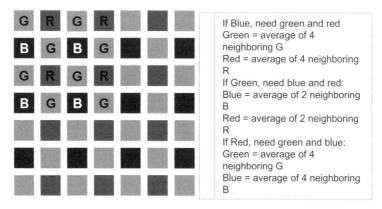

Figure 10.5. CMOS Bayer pattern architecture and color interpolation algorithm for RGB image reconstruction.

Most monochip cameras support the RAW data mode. A RAW image file contains minimally processed data from the image sensor. The RAW image format's purpose is to record exactly what the sensor "saw" or "sensed" (the data), and the conditions surrounding the recording of the image (the metadata). This mode makes it possible to optimize the frame rate by asking the frame grabber to recompose the RGB color information from the raw data produced by the camera. The raw data represent three times less data than the final image.

10.4. MEASURING COLORIMETRIC INFORMATION

10.4.1. Lambert–Beer Law

As mentioned above, the acquisition system must be appropriately designed for image quantization and images corrected in accordance with the key law of image processing, the Lambert–Beer law, an empirical relationship that relates the absorption of light to the properties of the material through which the light is traveling. The Lambert–Beer law is typically expressed as:

$$OD = \varepsilon l C \tag{10.3}$$

where OD is the optical density of the solution, ε is the proportionality constant called molar extinction or absorption coefficient, l is the thickness of the sample, and C is the concentration of the molecular specie. The absorption coefficient ε is specific to the molecular specie and is typically expressed in units of liters/male/centimeter (L/mol/cm).

In optics, the Lambert–Beer law generally describes a proportionality that can be observed between the concentration of molecules in a solution (the concentration of the "molecular specie" or the "sample") and the light intensity measured through the solution at a given wavelength. This proportionality relationship defined by the Lambert–Beer law has been verified under several conditions including, for example, monochromatic light illuminating the sample, low molecular concentration within the sample, generally no fluorescence or light response heterogeneity (negligible fluorescence and diffusion) of the sample, and lack of chemical photosensitivity of the sample. Furthermore, an additional requirement includes, for instance, correct Koehler illumination of the sample under the microscope.

10.4.2. Koehler Illumination

Koehler illumination is offered on almost all modern microscopes. It provides the most even illumination in the image plane and allows for effective contrast control. Koehler illumination is critical for densitometry analysis. Correct Koehler illumination is typically provided by, for example, a two-stage illuminating system for the microscope in which the source is imaged in the aperture of the substage condenser by an auxiliary condenser. The substage condenser, in turn, forms an image of the auxiliary condenser on the object. An iris diaphragm may also be placed at each condenser, wherein the first iris controls the area of the object to be illuminated, and the second iris varies the numerical aperture of the illuminating beam.

The procedure for Koehlering the microscope optical path is detailed next. Correct adjustment of the condenser aperture diaphragm is one of the most critical aspects for obtaining superior image quality because it controls the numerical aperture, resolving power, depth of field, and the overall image character.

A typical Koehler setting protocol includes the following steps:

1. Swing in the front lens of the condenser.
2. Move the condenser to its highest position.
3. Swing in the 20× objective (objective typically used for image processing).
4. Focus the objective on some cellular material on the slide.
5. Close the condenser diaphragm until it becomes visible through the oculars.
6. Use both centering screws to center the condenser diaphragm in the live image window.
7. Lower the condenser until the edge of the condenser diaphragm appears in focus.
8. If necessary, repeat steps 6 and 7 to improve the centering and the focus of the condenser diaphragm in the live image window.
9. Open the condenser diaphragm until its edge just disappears from the FOV.
10. Set the condenser diaphragm aperture:
    a. Remove one eyepiece from its tube.
    b. Look into the tube with your naked eye.
    c. Use the condenser's sliding knob to set the aperture diaphragm to approximately ⅔ to ⅘ of the objective exit pupils in diameter (covering 44 to 64% of the full aperture as shown in Fig. 10.6).
    d. Insert the eyepiece in the tube again.

The setting of the condenser diaphragm aperture described in step 10 of this protocol introduces possible inaccuracy in the transmittance measurement. This protocol is now automatized or semiautomatized in most efficient image analysis systems allowing both precision and reproducibility. Figure 10.6 presents the

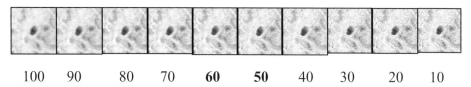

| 100 | 90 | 80 | 70 | **60** | **50** | 40 | 30 | 20 | 10 |

Figure 10.6. Same cell image as seen as a function of the opening of the aperture diaphragm, from (leftmost) 100% of the full area to (rightmost) 10%.

same cell imaged with different aperture diaphragm openings, showing from left to right poor resolution, Koehler optimal settings, and high-resolution noise patterns. The appropriate range according to Koehler illumination appears in bold. When the diaphragm is too wide open, high frequency is lost, whereas noisy high-frequency diffraction patterns appear when the closing of the aperture diaphragm is too strong.

10.4.3. Additive Property of Lambert–Beer Law

The Lambert–Beer law has an additive property such that if the sample comprises several light-absorbing molecular species, for example, s_1 and s_2, having respective concentration C_1 and C_2, the OD of a sample of thickness l (in solution, $l = l_1 = l_2$) can be expressed as:

$$OD = \varepsilon_1 l_1 C_1 + \varepsilon_2 l_2 C_2 \tag{10.4}$$

This situation may occur, for example, in a biological analysis where a "scene" or field of view or portion of the sample has been stained with two dyes consisting of a marker dye for targeting the molecular specie of interest and a counterstain for staining the remainder of the sample (see Fig. 10.7).

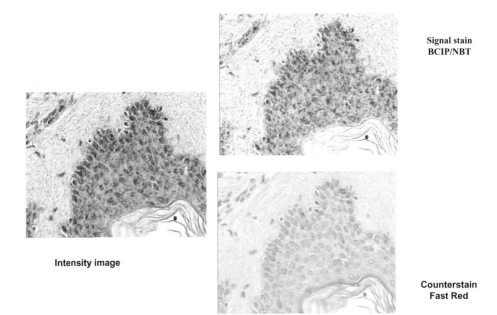

Signal stain
BCIP/NBT

Intensity image

Counterstain
Fast Red

Figure 10.7. Intensity Image of a field of view captured from the microscope, and the representation of the same field showing only the signal stain BCIP/NBT (melastatin marker) or Fast Red counterstain markers after chromogen separation and electronic image synthesis.

10.4.4. Correction of Chromatic Aberration

To accurately measure the concentration of given species imaged under a microscope, one must also make sure that the measurements of the optical densities performed at different wavelengths correspond to the same portion of the sample. In other words, in the world of microscopy, we must make sure that the system is well corrected for chromatic aberration or correct it softwarewise.

The natural dispersion power of glass causes a simple lens to focus blue light at a shorter distance than red light. That is, a simple lens has different focal lengths for light of different wavelength (different colors). Two phenomena occur as a direct consequence: The difference in position along the vertical axis of the focal points for light of different wavelength is called longitudinal chromatic aberration. Thus, when focusing the image for a given color (e.g., green), the images corresponding to other colors tend to be slightly out of focus (blue and red in our example will appear out of focus). And the difference in magnification (focal length) for light of different wavelengths is called lateral chromatic aberration. Thus, the image of a blue (short) wavelength will appear larger than the image of a red (large) wavelength.

In systems with high-quality objectives (apochromatic objectives), most of the obvious chromatic aberration is corrected, but there may be a residual of lateral chromatic aberration resulting from differences in magnification. This aberration may be difficult to observe visually, especially because a human observer tends to look at the center of the field of view where the lateral aberration is absent.

However, when imaging the field of view by means of a CCD camera, a lateral aberration even less that 1% in magnification will result in slight color shifts on the edges of objects located away for the optical center of the objective. Consequently, a pixel located at a given (x,y) position on the image will not exactly depict the same part of the object under investigation depending on the wavelength used to illuminate the object. However, to solve chromogen separation equations, the basic assumption is to investigate the exact same part of the object, therefore requiring to adjust images so that there is a very good matching of the regions where chromatic equations must be solved.

A possible method to solve lateral chromatic aberration is detailed here:

1. Determine the coordinate of the objective center as compared to the camera chip center.
2. Evaluate the observed magnification factor for each wavelength as compared to an arbitrary chosen wavelength (usually the central one, green if RGB).
3. Resample each image according to its relative magnification and the coordinate of the objective center.

To help perform the two first steps, a slide with small dark objects distributed across the slide is required. An image is captured at each wavelength and the center of each object (x,y) is computed. The image taken with the wavelength the closest to the mean of all used wavelength is considered as the reference. For each other wavelength, for each object, the difference in x, δx, and the difference in y, δy, with the same object in the reference image are recorded. The linear equations that minimize the reconstruction error of δx as a function of x and δy as a function of y are then determined. From these two equations the center of the objective (x_0, y_0) within the camera frame is determined with x_0 = solution of the equation in x when $\delta x = 0$ and y_0 = solution of the equation in y when $\delta y = 0$. The linear equation that minimizes the reconstruction error of δd $\left(\delta d = \sqrt{\delta x^2 + \delta y^2}\right)$ as a function of the distance to (x_0, y_0) is then determined and its slope s gives the magnification of the specified wavelength according to the reference wavelength. This image will spatially resample with an origin located in (x_0, y_0) and a magnification of s.

10.5. CHROMOGEN SEPARATION

Once the microscope has been set in Koehler illumination mode for image acquisition and chromatic aberrations have been taken care of, we can make use of the additive property of the Lambert–Beer law to perform chromogen separation using the mathematics of linear algebraic equations (see Figs. 10.7 and 10.8).

10.5.1. Looking at Each Pixel as a Set of Linear Equations

The additive property of the Lambert–Beer law can also be expanded to a situation in which the scene is analyzed in a color image environment, such as, for example, generated by an RGB camera, separated into a red, green, and blue channel. In such an instance, the marker dye (or "dye 1") would exhibit absorption coefficients, ε_{1r}, ε_{1g}, and ε_{1b}, in the red, green, and blue channels, respectively. Note that, in some instances, the analysis of the image in each of the red, green, and blue channels is equivalent to analyzing a red representation of the image across the red spectra, a green representation of the image across the green spectra, and a blue representation of the image across the blue spectra. Accordingly, the counterstain (or "dye 2") would exhibit absorption coefficients, ε_{2r}, ε_{2g}, and ε_{2b}, in the red, green, and blue channels, respectively. Therefore, according to the additive property of the Lambert–Beer law, analysis of the sample in the RGB environment would lead to the system of three equations for the optical density thereof:

$$OD_r = \varepsilon_{1r}l_1C_1 + \varepsilon_{2r}l_2C_2 \tag{10.5}$$

$$OD_g = \varepsilon_{1g}l_1C_1 + \varepsilon_{2g}l_2C_2 \tag{10.6}$$

$$OD_b = \varepsilon_{1b}l_1C_1 + \varepsilon_{2b}l_2C_2 \tag{10.7}$$

where OD_r, OD_g, and OD_b represent the optical densities of the sample measured in the red, green, and blue channels, respectively. Still further, in the case of

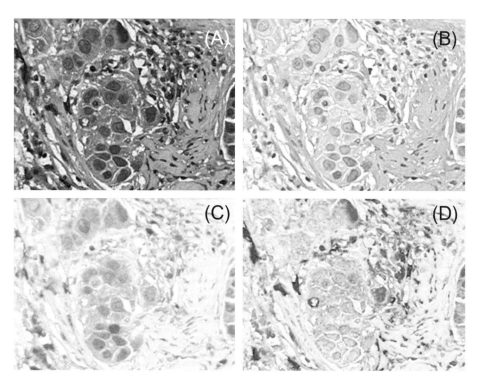

Figure 10.8. RGB image as seen in (A) the microscope field of view, and the color representation of the same field showing only the (B) hematoxylin, (C) DAB, or (D) Fast Red markers, after chromogen separation and electronic image synthesis. See insert for color representation of this figure.

increased sample preparation complexity such as, for example, the treatment of the sample with three different dyes, equations become

$$OD_r = \varepsilon_{1r}l_1C_1 + \varepsilon_{2r}l_2C_2 + \varepsilon_{3r}l_3C_3 \tag{10.8}$$

$$OD_g = \varepsilon_{1g}l_1C_1 + \varepsilon_{2g}l_2C_2 + \varepsilon_{3g}l_3C_3 \tag{10.9}$$

$$OD_b = \varepsilon_{1b}l_1C_1 + \varepsilon_{2b}l_2C_2 + \varepsilon_{3b}l_3C_3 \tag{10.10}$$

In such a situation, the three dyes may comprise, for instance, one marker dye and two counterstains, or two marker dyes and one counterstain, or even three separate marker dyes.

In applying the Lambert–Beer law to a digital microscopy system, it is difficult and complex, inaccurate, or sometimes not possible to measure the thickness of the sample. Consequently, the concentration C of the molecular entity can be extended and examined as the product of l and C (lC), and the results treated accordingly. For example, where the concentration of one dye is being compared to the concentration of another dye in a particular sample, the sample thickness term will be common to both concentrations, and thus it becomes less important to determine the sample thickness as an absolute and accurate value. Determining the thickness of the sample is usually not required but assumed constant and therefore negligible in the equation.

Furthermore, the Lambert–Beer law can also be expressed as:

$$OD_{(x,y)} = \log I_{0(x,y)} - \log I_{(x,y)} \tag{10.11}$$

Within a digital image, according to a Cartesian coordinate system, where (x,y) signifies a particular pixel in the image, $OD_{(x,y)}$ is the optical density of the sample field of view at that pixel, $I_{(x,y)}$ is the measured light intensity or transmittance of the sample at that pixel, and $I_{0(x,y)}$ is the light intensity of the light source as measured without the light-absorbing sample. Accordingly:

$$IOD = \sum\nolimits_{N} \left(\log I_{0(x,y)} - \log I_{(x,y)} \right) \tag{10.12}$$

where IOD is the integrated optical density of the digital image of the sample, and N is the number of pixels of the object under investigation within the image. The logarithmic relationship may be expressed in various bases, base 2, base 10, or natural logarithms, wherein the various bases are related by proportionality constants [e.g., $\ln(x)$ or $\log_e(x) = 2.3026\log_{10}(x)$]. Thus, the proportionality constant may be appropriately considered where relative comparisons are drawn in light intensities. Further, in quantitative microscopy according to the Lambert–Beer law, the proportionality relationship between the optical density OD of the sample and the dye concentrations is conserved. Therefore, for a prepared sample examined by the system, the appropriate relation is expressed as:

$$\ln I_0 - \ln I = \ln \frac{I_0}{I} = OD = \varepsilon l C \tag{10.13}$$

10.5.2. Shading Correction

When an 8-bit per channel RGB camera is used in the system, the light intensity transmitted through the sample will be expressed as $2^8(=256)$ values between 0 and 255. For example, the initial intensity I_0 of the light source, which corresponds to 100% transmittance, will be expressed as values close to 255 (representing the brightest possible value) in each of the red, green, and blue channels. Indeed, the operator adjusts the camera frame grabber/light source so that a pure "white" light in the absence of the sample, corresponding to 100% transmittance, would have an intensity value close to 255 in each of the red, green, and blue channels, whereas in the absence of light, 0% transmittance, the "black image" will have an intensity value close to 0 in each of the red, green, and blue channels. At any pixel (x,y), 100% transmittance, I_0, is therefore expressed as the difference between the value measured by the camera in the presence of the light source when no object is present, minus the value measured by the camera in the absence of the light source, for each of the red, green, and blue channels. Like I_0, I is expressed as the difference between the value measured by the camera in the presence of the light source and object to be evaluated, minus the value measured by the camera in the absence of the light source, for each of the red, green, and blue channels,

For a field of view, the shading correction protocol for each channel is therefore:

$$FOV[x,y] = \frac{\text{amplitude}(FOV[x,y] - \text{Black})}{\text{WhiteRef}[x,y] - \text{Black}} \quad (10.14)$$

where $[x,y]$ refers to the pixel coordinates within the FOV, the amplitude is set to 255 on an 8-bit system, WhiteRef is the image recorded in the absence of tissue material, and Black is the mean value observed when no light illuminates the camera target.

Because the intensity of the light source may vary spatially over the measured field of view, and because the optics may heterogeneously absorb light, 100% transmittance may correspond to a different dynamic range over the measured field of view. The OD of the sample is expressed as the logarithm of the ratio of the corrected transmittance in the absence of the sample (I_0), and transmittance in the presence of the sample (I), and therefore largely spatially independent to the small variations in the real dynamic range measured at 100% transmittance.

Since the light source intensity remains substantially constant over time, or can be easily reevaluated, the reading of the light intensity in any pixel can therefore be translated into a measure of the relative transmittance at the pixel location for each of the red, green, and blue channels. Once I_0 and I are known, the corresponding OD can be computed.

Any location on the field of view where a unique dye is present (the only absorbing material) allows measuring the relative extinction coefficients of the dye for the different RGB channels. Because in the Lambert–Beer law the product lC is de facto equal for each of the RGB channels at a given (x,y) location, both l and C are known at this particular location, the exact extinction coefficient can be computed as being the $OD/(lC)$. The absorption coefficients $\varepsilon_{r,g,b}$ in each of the red, green, and blue channels are consequently extracted as being:

$$\varepsilon_r = \frac{OD_r}{(lC)} = \frac{\ln(I_{0r}/I_r)}{lC} \quad (10.15)$$

$$\varepsilon_g = \frac{OD_g}{lC} = \frac{\ln(I_{0g}/I_g)}{lC} \quad (10.16)$$

$$\varepsilon_b = \frac{OD_b}{lC} = \frac{\ln(I_{0b}/I_b)}{lC} \quad (10.17)$$

Unfortunately, IC is usually unknown and, therefore, the extinction coefficient $\varepsilon_{r,g,b}$ are computed arbitrarily, as being the ratio of the OD measured at the given pixel in the considered channel and the maximum OD measured at this location for any of the RGB channels. The determination of the absorption coefficient ε in each of the red, green, and blue channels in the absence of a priori knowledge concerning IC is a matter of linear equation manipulation in order to achieve a relative solution where I and C are arbitrarily set to 1, wherein

$$\varepsilon_r = \frac{\mathrm{OD}_r}{1} = \mathrm{OD}_r = \ln\left(\frac{I_{0r}}{I_r}\right) \tag{10.18}$$

$$\varepsilon_g = \frac{\mathrm{OD}_g}{1} = \mathrm{OD}_g = \ln\left(\frac{I_{0g}}{I_g}\right) \tag{10.19}$$

$$\varepsilon_b = \frac{\mathrm{OD}_b}{1} = \mathrm{OD}_b = \ln\left(\frac{I_{0b}}{I_b}\right) \tag{10.20}$$

Consequently, if the absolute concentration of the dye will remain unknown, it will remain possible to compute arbitrary concentrations in any pixel, with a known absolute coefficient factor equal to (IC). Because I is unique at a given pixel location and can arbitrarily be set to 1, previous equations may be rewritten as follow where C_1, C_2, and C_3 are I related.

$$\mathrm{OD}_r = \varepsilon_{1r}C_1 + \varepsilon_{2r}C_2 + \varepsilon_{3r}C_3 \tag{10.21}$$

$$\mathrm{OD}_g = \varepsilon_{1g}C_1 + \varepsilon_{2g}C_2 + \varepsilon_{3g}C_3 \tag{10.22}$$

$$\mathrm{OD}_b = \varepsilon_{1b}C_1 + \varepsilon_{2b}C_2 + \varepsilon_{3b}C_3 \tag{10.23}$$

When all the extinction coefficients have been evaluated for the different dyes, and optical densities are known from the reading of the image data, solving these equations to extract C_1, C_2, and C_3 is just a matter of solving a set of linear equations.

10.5.3. Solution of Linear Algebraic Equations—Matrices

A set of linear algebraic equations looks like this:

$$\begin{aligned}
a_{11}x_1 + a_{12}x_2 + a_{13}x_3 + \cdots + a_{1N}x_N &= b_1 \\
a_{21}x_1 + a_{22}x_2 + a_{23}x_3 + \cdots + a_{2N}x_N &= b_2 \\
a_{31}x_1 + a_{32}x_2 + a_{33}x_3 + \cdots + a_{3N}x_N &= b_3 \\
&\vdots \\
a_{M1}x_1 + a_{M2}x_2 + a_{M3}x_3 + \cdots + a_{MN}x_N &= b_M
\end{aligned} \tag{10.24}$$

Here the N unknowns x_j, $j = 1, 2, \dots , N$ are related by M equations. The coefficients a_{ij} with $i = 1, 2, \dots , M$ and $j = 1, 2, \dots , N$ are known numbers, as are the *right-hand side* quantities b_i, $i = 1, 2, \dots , M$.

- If $M < N$, there is effectively fewer equations than unknowns. In this case there can be either no solution or else more than one solution vector **x**.
- If $N = M$, then there are as many equations as unknowns, and there is a good chance of solving for a unique solution set of x_j's.
- If $M > N$ that there are more equations than unknowns, and there is, in general, no solution vector **x** to the equation, the set of equations is said to be *overdetermined*. In such case, the most appropriate solution will be considered in general as the one fitting the best of the equations, that is, the solution minimizing the sum of reconstruction errors.

In case of color image processing, overdetermination issues can easily be bypassed by discarding either the blue channel (usually the weakest in terms of signal-to-noise ratio due to the silicon sensitivity for blue wavelengths) or the channel with less difference between the extinction coefficients of the considered colorimetric markers.

The OD_{rgb} equations written above can be written in matrix form as

$$A \cdot \mathbf{x} = \mathbf{b} \tag{10.25}$$

Here ($\cdot$) denotes matrix multiplication, A is the matrix of coefficients, and **b** is the right-hand side written as a column vector. By convention, the first index on an element a_{ij} denotes its row; the second index its column, a_i, or $a[i]$ denotes a whole row $a[i][j], j = 1, \dots , N$.

Solution of linear algebraic equations: The solution of the matrix equation $A \cdot \mathbf{x} = \mathbf{b}$ for an unknown vector **x**, where A is a square matrix of coefficients, and **b** is a known right-hand side vector usually requires the determination of A^{-1}, which is the matrix inverse of the matrix A:

$$\mathbf{x} = A^{-1} \cdot \mathbf{b} \tag{10.26}$$

where A^{-1} is the matrix inverse of matrix A, that is, $A \cdot A^{-1} = A^{-1} \cdot A = 1$, where 1 is the identity matrix.

Experimental conditions are set up so that there are more (or equal number) equations than unknowns, $M \geq N$. It happens frequently, however, that the best "compromise" solution is the one that comes closest to satisfying all equations simultaneously. If closeness is defined in the least-squares sense, that is, that the sum of the squares of the differences between the left- and right-hand sides of the OD_{rgb} equations be minimized, then the overdetermined linear problem reduces to a (usually) solvable linear problem, called the "linear least-squares" problem. This problem is solved using the mathematics of singular value decomposition (SVD), whose subject is the parametric modeling of data, the method of choice for solving most *linear least-squares* problems (Press et al., 1992).

10.5.4. Absorption Coefficient

The determination of the absorption coefficient ε matrix for different dyes may be performed independently of sample evaluation and stored for further application to samples treated with at least one of the respective dyes. The various absorption coefficient ε vectors for specific dyes, as well as the original light intensity I_0 data for the light source may be stored in, for example, the computer device itself or a server located on the intra- or Internet.

10.5.5. Example

Here is a detailed example of a sample stained with three dyes (see Fig. 10.8A) and measured at a given (x,y) location in the red, green, and blue channel of an 8-bit channel RGB camera after shading correction ($I_0 = 255$ in each of the red, green, and blue channels).

The three dyes being used have the following transmitted light intensity I characteristics in each of the red, green, and blue channels (see Table 10.3).

The corresponding optical density OD matrix [each element being computed as $\ln(I_0/I)$] thus becomes the values shown in Table 10.4.

However, since OD = εlC, the OD values for each dye can be normalized with respect to the channel having the highest OD so as to provide a matrix of relative absorption coefficients for the respective dyes since the lC values will be constant across the channels, as shown in Table 10.5.

At a particular pixel in the image, located in (x,y), the image RGB transmittance is presented in Table 10.6.

Therefore, in order to determine the concentrations of the three dyes at that pixel, this OD matrix is multiplied by the inverse of the previously determined

TABLE 10.3. Example of Transmittance Values Measured in RGB Channels for Each Individual Dye

I	Red	Green	Blue
Dye 1	168	127	94
Dye 2	94	241	247
Dye 3	120	94	155

TABLE 10.4. OD Values Computed from Transmittance Values Measured in RGB Channels for Each Dye in Table 10.3

OD	Red	Green	Blue
Dye 1	0.417	0.697	0.998
Dye 2	0.998	0.056	0.032
Dye 3	0.754	0.998	0.498

TABLE 10.5. Relative Extinction Coefficients as Evaluated from Table 10.4

ε	Red	Green	Blue
Dye 1	0.418	0.698	1.000
Dye 2	1.000	0.057	0.032
Dye 3	0.755	1.000	0.499

TABLE 10.6. Example of Transmittance and OD Values Measured for Given Pixel Showing a Mixture of Dyes in RGB Channels

	Red	Green	Blue
I	89	168	154
I_0	255	255	255
OD	1.053	0.417	0.504

TABLE 10.7. Relative Dye Concentrations in $(x,y;$ Table 10.3) Computed Using Extinction Coefficients from Table 10.5 and Chromogen Separation Technology

	Dye 1	Dye 2	Dye 3
C (relative)	0.455	0.829	0.058

relative absorption coefficient ε matrix. Accordingly, the relative dye concentrations computed for this particular pixel in (x,y) are shown in Table 10.7.

10.5.6. Generating Artificial Marker Images

Reversibly, the gray levels or, in this example, RGB transmittance values of an artificial image built from any combination of the previous dyes can be generated since they are now known. For that particular pixel and dye concentration, the single dye images would correspond to the following black and white (BW) or RGB pixel intensities (see Table 10.8):

$$\text{OD}_{\text{BW}} = C \quad \text{and} \quad I_{\text{BW}} = \exp[\ln(I_0) - \text{OD}_{\text{BW}}] \qquad (10.27)$$

$$\text{OD}_{\text{r}} = \varepsilon_{\text{r}} C \quad \text{and} \quad I_{\text{r}} = \exp[\ln(I_0) - \text{OD}_{\text{r}}] \qquad (10.28)$$

$$\text{OD}_{\text{g}} = \varepsilon_{\text{g}} C \quad \text{and} \quad I_{\text{g}} = \exp[\ln(I_0) - \text{OD}_{\text{g}}] \qquad (10.29)$$

$$\text{OD}_{\text{b}} = \varepsilon_{\text{b}} C \quad \text{and} \quad I_{\text{b}} = \exp[\ln(I_0) - \text{OD}_{\text{b}}] \qquad (10.30)$$

TABLE 10.8. Dye Concentrations in $(x,y;$ Table 10.3) and Corresponding Single Dye RGB Image Values Computed Using Extinction Coefficients from Table 10.5 and Chromogen Separation Technology

Dye	C Evaluated	Intensities BW	Red	Green	Blue
Dye 1	0.455	161	210	185	161
Dye 2	0.829	111	111	243	248
Dye 3	0.058	240	244	240	247

Manipulating these equations therefore allows:

1. Displaying live or still images representing, in RGB (or in gray levels), an artificial image of the field of view, generated by any combination of the markers and counterstain in use (see Fig. 10.8).
2. Detecting automatically a region of interest from its spectral signature. This region can then be manipulated specifically depending upon its identification.
3. Making use of the spatial frequencies found in the counterstain and/or marker-only image to evaluate the focus adequacy of the field of view.
4. Mapping user-defined visual or sonic alarms based on the image processing of the marker images, which draw the user's attention on a specific field of view when the content of marker reaches a given level either in intensity or in field coverage.
5. Extract-marked point processes/contextual analysis/geostatistics features based on the marker spatial distribution analysis.
6. Sort fields of view or objects of interest based on their overall content of a given marker, or ratios of markers, especially useful in the case of rare or worse events detection.
7. Build classifiers specifically based on the image processing resulting from the counterstain and/or marker-only images. Evaluate the presence of certain cell types or the diagnosis of the field of view. Such classifiers usually also encompass other informative features such as feature based on the morphology or the texture of the cells.
8. Data presentation for easy spectral selection of meaningful objects/areas.

10.6. MEASURING INFORMATION

Once the evaluation of a given marker content can be performed pixelwise in any (x,y) pixel location of a digital image, it is still necessary to segment the image. Image segmentation is considered the main difficulty in tissue section analysis.

The "segmentation" procedure is designed to extract from the original image a mask of the objects of interest, for example, the cells and the nuclei, in order to quantify and measure the desired features for each particular object.

10.6.1. Image Segmentation

As already mentioned, once an image is digitized and stored in an image analyzer or a pathology workstation, the pictorial information offers the possibility of extracting quantitative data and can eventually be improved for qualitative human interpretation as well. In computer vision, segmentation refers to the process of partitioning a digital image into multiple regions (sets of pixels). The goal of segmentation is to simplify and/or change the representation of an image into something that is more meaningful and easier to analyze and quantify. Image segmentation is typically used to locate objects and establish their boundaries (tumor region, cells, cytoplasm, nucleus, membranes). The result of image segmentation is a set of regions that collectively cover the entire image, or a set of contours extracted from the image (edge detection) (Pham et al., 2000). Each of the pixels in a region is similar with respect to some characteristic or computed property, such as color, intensity, or texture. Adjacent regions are significantly different with respect to the same characteristic(s) (Shapiro and Stockman, 2001). Usual segmentation approaches are based on the identification of regions within the image, which adhere to a given set of homogeneity criteria or are well separated from each other by transitional contours.

The diagnostic assessment of a histopathology section is indeed based on the microscopic image, but the process relies to a very large extent on information that is not offered by the microscopic image itself. A tissue section analyzer thus requires sophisticated methods, with built in external knowledge or the capability of referring to an external set of a priori laws when facing a specific problem.

10.6.2. Cell Scoring

Based upon the features evaluated for each cell through the segmentations masks, a score is attributed depending on the marker intensity and its signal-to-noise ratio in the targeted compartment. A cell is considered positive when the marker content of that cell in the marker-specific targeted compartment optical density (intensity) is significantly higher than in the neighboring compartments. For instance, if the marker is a nucleus marker, the contrast or signal-to-noise ratio is computed from the marker-specific optical density measured in the nucleus versus the residual optical density measured over the cytoplasm. Figure 10.9 presents different levels of segmentation, making use of the chromogen separation process to result in the scoring of cells on a 0 to 3 scale based upon their marker content and signal-to-noise ratio. Because the background noise is unspecific by definition, the overall background mean optical density will be measured over all the cytoplasm compartment of the cells within the selected region of interest, for example, for a nucleus marker:

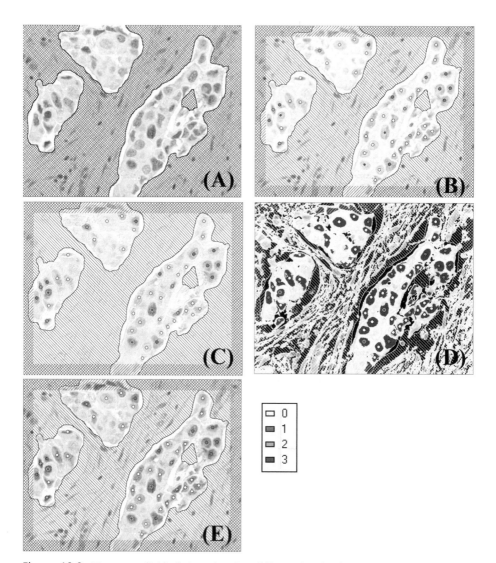

Figure 10.9. 20× tumor field of view showing different levels of segmentation and quantification based on the segmentation masks. (A) Field of view showing the tumor region automatically segmented based upon nucleus size, cell density, and marker content rules. (B, C)
Same field of view showing the chromogen-separated images of the scene. (D) Nuclei masks
segmented within the tumor regions. (E) Marker intensity labeling of cells based upon their
marker intensity observed within the nucleus mask (0, negative; 1, weak; 2, mild; and 3, strong
positive). See insert for color representation of this figure.

$$\text{Nucleus signal} = \text{Nucleus marker IOD} - \text{Nucleus area} \times \\ \text{Cytoplasm marker MOD} \qquad (10.31)$$

$$\text{Cell signal–noise ratio} = \frac{\text{Nucleus marker MOD}}{\text{Cytoplasm marker MOD}} \qquad (10.32)$$

where IOD and MOD refer, respectively, to the integrated and the mean optical densities measured in the chromogen-separated image of the targeted marker.

To best match the pathologist know-how, the contrast required to call a cell as positive can be adapted from strong to weak, as some pathologists will consider only very intense nuclei as positive, when for others any faint positive staining will be consider as appropriate. If required, by choosing different contrast values, it is possible to define cells as negative, weak positive, mild positive, and strong positives (0, 1, 2, and 3, respectively) and therefore mimic a pathologist's appreciation.

10.6.3. Multiplexing and Tissue Microarrays

As an increasing number of genes are being suspected to play a role in cancer biology, it is usually required to examine a high number of well-characterized primary tumors in order to evaluate the clinical significance of newly detected potential cancer genes. Traditional methods of molecular pathology are time consuming, and a new tissue microarray (TMA) technology has to be developed that can rapidly evaluate those samples (Kononen et al., 1998). The TMAs allow an entire cohort to be analyzed in one batch on a single slide. Thus reagent concentrations are identical for each case, as are incubation times and temperatures, wash conditions, and antigen retrieval.

Tissue microarrays are a method of relocating tissue from conventional histologic paraffin blocks in order to see tissues from multiple patients or blocks on the same slide. Hundreds of tiny cylindrical tissue cores (typically 0.6 mm in diameter) are densely and precisely arrayed into a single histologic paraffin block (see Fig. 10.10). The block may be divided into serial sections, 4 to 8 μm thick, which we refer to as tissue array slides. Typically, cores contain small histologic sections from unique tissues or tumors. These tissue array slides serve as targets for immunohistochemical staining reactions. Several biomarkers can be embedded in TMAs. TMA blocks can then be utilized for the simultaneous analysis of all different tumors at the DNA, RNA, or protein level. Each TMA slide yields information about protein staining pattern, distribution, intensity, background, and target tissue. In many cases, each spot/core on a TMA is scored by a skilled pathologist and recorded manually. See Figures 10.11 and 10.12 for a detailed process of the image segmentation steps required to extract marker intensities leading to cell scoring within the targeted subcellular compartment of each cell of the tumor regions defined within each core of a given TMA.

High-resolution digital images are automatically assembled into montage images. These digital images are used for analysis of both anatomical features

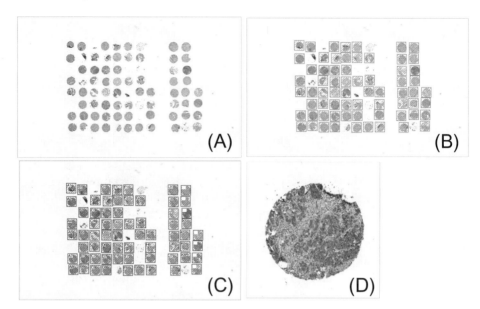

Figure 10.10. Tissue microarray showing a breast cancer tumor cohort showing HER2 expression. (A) Image of the glass slide, (B) identification of the cores, (C) cores registration, and (D) low-resolution image of a given core.

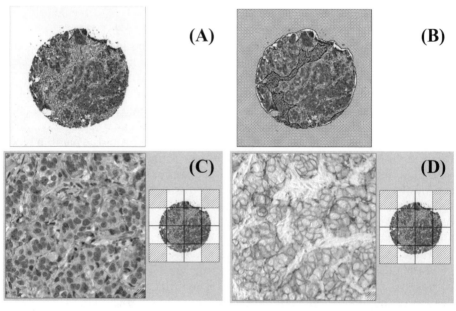

Figure 10.11. Processing of a given core within a TMA, (A) image of the core, (B) automatic identification of the region of interest, (C, D) high-resolution acquisition of the fields of view covering the core and chromogen separation of the same field of view with (C) hematoxylin and (D) HER2-positive signal.

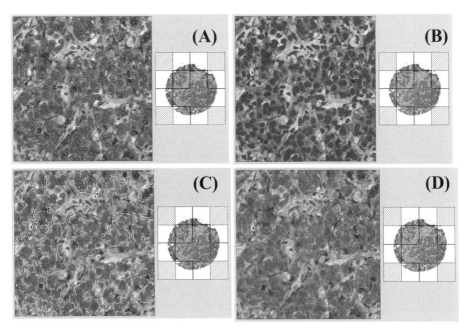

Figure 10.12. Cell segmentation of a given field of view extracted from the high-resolution image of a core within a TMA and processed using the chromogen separation engine: (A) image of the field of view and identification of each automatically found cell with their respective masks, (B) nucleus, and (C) positive HER2 membrane stain; (D) estimation of cytoplasmic boundaries based upon found membranes and iso-distance maps between nuclei of adjacent cells. See insert for color representation of this figure.

and fine tissue structures. Machine learning algorithms combined with data mining allow the extraction of essential features that classify particular tissue elements: geometric features such as the locations of cells, area, perimeter, compactness, elongation, and transmittance. These parameters may describe the shape and orientation of cells, nuclei, cytoplasms, and membranes. The optical densities of pixels within each cell are recorded as well, linked to the respective marker contents (from chromogen separation evaluation), and summarized using standard statistics (mean, median, standard deviation, quartiles) (Emily et al., 2005).

Multimarker Study Paradigm. The common underlying paradigm used for marker selection is that marker overexpression should capture a subpopulation of patients, specific for their bad diagnostic or prognostic value and show a very high specificity. If a study aims at the prognostic value of a set of markers, for instance, a given marker should show (1) in the good outcome patients, little or no marker expression level and (2) in the bad outcome patients, an expression level either similar to the good outcome patients or should be significantly

TABLE 10.9. List of Minimum Specificity Required per Marker When an Overall Specificity of 0.8 Targeted for Given Combination of up to 5 Markers

Marker Number in Combination	Required Specificity per Marker
1	0.800000
2	0.894427
3	0.928318
4	0.945742
5	0.956352

overexpressed for a fraction of those. Hence, combining markers would potentially allow reaching high sensitivity and high specificity (e.g., 80 and 80% target).

In a study aimed to reach the best sensitivity at a given specificity (e.g., 80% specificity), the specificity target for each marker is by definition mathematically dependent on the number of markers to combine. As an example, a combination of 3 markers will reach 80% specificity if each individual marker, independent of each other, shows specificity of at least $0.8^{\frac{1}{3}} = 93\%$. Table 10.9 gives the list of required specificity according to the number of markers in the combination, from 1 to 5 markers.

A good approach to the evaluation of a new marker with established markers is to compare the predictive ability of the multivariable model that contains the marker to the predictive ability of the model that lacks the marker (Kattan, 2004). Hence, an attractive solution is to show the improvement in predictive accuracy that is obtained when the new marker is added to a model containing the established markers. This means that the predictive ability should be representative of what would be expected when the model is applied to new patients. This can be done by comparing cross-validated predicted probabilities (i.e., probabilities produced for patients not used to derive the prediction model). Similarly, bootstrapping can be used to provide 95% confidence intervals and p values.

It is also possible from the sensitivity and specificity of each marker within the targeted population to build a model determining the probability of occurrence of each possible marker sequence, that is, the marker positive/negative status for all studied markers for a given patient. This model takes into account the prevalence of the pathology into the test population. This model is based on the assumption that markers are independent from one another and can therefore be used to test marker independence by comparing observed sequence prevalence to expected prevalence. Figure 10.13 shows probability computation for a single marker analysis, and Figure 10.14 details the formulas used to compute the conditional probabilities model when multiple markers are tested (e.g., two markers).

A simulated example is shown where three independent markers show a slight increase in marker intensity when looking at the bad outcome population versus the good outcome population. Figure 10.15 shows the marker intensity

- **Good outcome 0**
- **Bad outcome 1**
- $P(0|Bad) = 1-Sens$
- $P(1|Bad) = Sens$
- $P(0|Good) = Spec$
- $P(1|Good) = 1-Spec$
- $P(0) = P(0| Good) \times Prev_{Good} + P(0|Bad) \times Prev_{Bad}$
- $P(1) = P(1| Good) \times Prev_{Good} + P(1|Bad) \times Prev_{Bad}$
- $P(0) = Spec \times Prev_{Good} + (1-Sens) \times Prev_{Bad}$
- $P(1) = (1-Spec) \times Prev_{Good} + Sens \times Prev_{Bad}$
- $P(Good|0) = P(0| Good) \times Prev_{Good} / P(0)$
- $P(Good|1) = P(1| Good) \times Prev_{Good} / P(1)$
- $P(Bad|0) = P(0| Bad) \times Prev_{Bad} / P(0) = 1 - P(Good|0)$
- $P(Bad|1) = P(1| Bad) \times Prev_{Bad} / P(1) = 1 - P(Good|1)$

Figure 10.13. Probability formulas used during a single marker analysis. Conditional probabilities are read as follows: for example, P(0|Bad): probability of a bad outcome patient to be evaluated as being negative in regard to the marker, that is, to be considered as a false negative.

- $P(00|Good) = SpecM_1 \times SpecM_2$
- $P(01|Good) = SpecM_1 \times (1-SpecM_2)$
- $P(10|Good) = (1-SpecM_1) \times SpecM_2$
- $P(11|Good) = (1-SpecM_1) \times (1-SpecM_2)$
- $P(00|Bad) = (1-SensM_1) \times (1-SensM_2)$
- $P(01|Bad) = (1-SensM_1) \times SensM_2$
- $P(10|Bad) = SensM_1 \times (1-SensM_2)$
- $P(11|Bad) = SensM_1 \times SensM_2$
- $P(00) = P(00|Good) \times Prev_{Good} + P(00|Bad) \times Prev_{Bad}$
- $P(01) = P(01|Good) \times Prev_{Good} + P(01|Bad) \times Prev_{Bad}$
- $P(10) = P(10|Good) \times Prev_{Good} + P(10|Bad) \times Prev_{Bad}$
- $P(11) = P(11|Good) \times Prev_{Good} + P(11|Bad) \times Prev_{Bad}$
- $P(00) = SpecM_1 \times SpecM_2 \times Prev_{Good} + (1-SensM_1) \times (1-SensM_2) \times Prev_{Bad}$
- $P(01) = SpecM_1 \times (1- SpecM_2) \times Prev_{Good} + (1- SensM_1) \times SensM_2 \times Prev_{Bad}$
- $P(10) = (1- SpecM_1) \times SpecM_2 \times Prev_{Good} + SensM_1 \times (1- SensM_2) \times Prev_{Bad}$
- $P(11) = (1- SpecM_1) \times (1- SpecM_2) \times Prev_{Good} + SensM_1 \times SensM_2 \times Prev_{Bad}$
- $P(Good|00) = [P(00|Good) / P(00)] \times Prev_{Good}$
- $P(Bad|00) = [P(00|Bad) / P(00)] \times Prev_{Bad}$
- $P(Good|01) = [P(01|Good) / P(01)] \times Prev_{Good}$
- $P(Bad|01) = [P(01|Bad) / P(01)] \times Prev_{Bad}$
- $P(Good|10) = [P(10|Good) / P(10)] \times Prev_{Good}$
- $P(Bad|10) = [P(10|Bad) / P(10)] \times Prev_{Bad}$
- $P(Good|11) = [P(11|Good) / P(11)] \times Prev_{Good}$
- $P(Bad|11) = [P(11|Bad) / P(11)] \times Prev_{Bad}$

Figure 10.14. Probability formulas used during a two-marker analysis. Conditional probabilities are read as follows: for example, P(01|Bad): probability of a bad outcome patient to be evaluated as being negative for the marker M_1 and positive for the marker M_2. This algorithm can easily be extended to N markers.

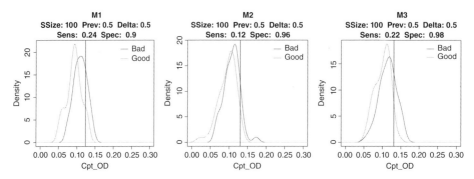

Figure 10.15. Density distributions of three simulated markers showing a shift in marker intensity equal to +0.5 standard deviation when looking at the bad outcome population versus the good outcome population (delta = 0.5). The sensitivity of these three markers (M_1, M_2, and M_3) is measured for marker intensity threshold defining marker positive/negative status with specificities in the range of $0.8^{\frac{1}{3}} = 93\%$.

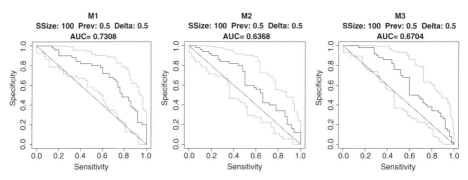

Figure 10.16. ROC curves of the three markers (M_1, M_2, and M_3) and their surrounding 95% confidence intervals. The area under the curve (AUC) is a good measure of the ability of the marker to help distinguish between good and bad outcomes. AUC = 0.5 if the marker presents no interest, AUC ≫ 0.5 if the marker is of high interest.

density distributions for good and bad outcome subpopulations, while Figure 10.16 shows their respective ROC curves with 95% confidence intervals, and Figure 10.17 shows the benefit of combining the three markers as the area under the curve (AUC) shows a significant increase from left to right, as the power of each individual marker is merged in the multiplexed assay to help differentiating the good outcome population from the bad outcome population. The threshold defining marker positive/negative status for each of these three markers (M_1, M_2, and M_3) is chosen in order to measure specificities in the range of $0.8^{\frac{1}{3}} = 93\%$ in order to obtain the best possible sensitivity for an 80% specificity target in the multiplexed assay.

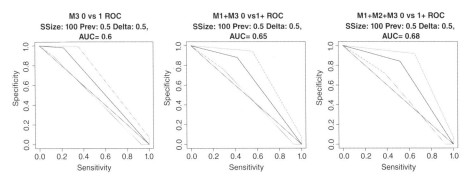

Figure 10.17. ROC curves of the three markers (M_1, M_2, and M_3) combinations and their surrounding 95% confidence intervals, from one maker only (leftmost) to three markers combination (rightmost). The area under the curve (AUC) shows a significant increase from left to right as the power of each marker is merged in the multiplexed assay.

10.7. CONCLUSION

Colorimetric immunohistochemistry, or C-IHC, detection methods and subcellular imaging algorithms based upon multispectral analysis are now available to optimize and standardize the reading of colorimetric markers. This technology is ready to turn molecular pathology into quantitative molecular pathology. Molecular markers may be used to detect and/or quantify gene amplification, gene deletion, gene mutations, and abnormal protein expression that may be visible upon analyzing a tissue section slide treated with an appropriate marker chosen to highlight the abnormal cellular activity that may aid in the diagnosis and/or determination of prognosis for a disease such as cancer. Such methods are useful for obtaining a valuable quantitative measurement of a target molecular species within a given tissue sample. Additional molecular species can be highlighted within the same tissue sample or on consecutive tissue sections by additional biomarkers, leading to a multiplexed assay, in order to more systematically analyze a tissue sample so as to allow a clinician to provide a more accurate diagnosis or prognosis. This will aid patients suffering from complex diseases such as cancer or will help to evaluate the impact of a new drug on a key cellular function in the targeted cellular population and its side effects in other organic tissues. Altogether, developing solutions that redefine the early detection and clinical management of cancer and developing cancer therapy can benefit at an early stage from advanced quantitative colorimetric IHC. Such techniques and analyses can be used in marker and drug assay development to identify the best candidates. In the case of marker assay development it can help to refine the staining protocol to best accommodate and optimize the assay to the microscopic imaging quantification constraints leading to a significant reduction in development costs and maximized detection performances.

REFERENCES

Brugal, G. (1984). Image analysis of microscopic preparations. *Meth. Achiev. Exp. Pathol.* 11:1–33.

Emily, M., Morel, D., Marcelpoil, R., and Francois, O. (2005). Spatial correlation of gene expression measures in tissue microarray core analysis. *J. Theor. Med.* 6(1):33–39.

Geusebroek, J. M. (2000). *Color and Geometrical Structure in Images, Applications in Microscopy.* Univ. of Amsterdam, Faculty of Sciences.

Hedley, D. W., Friedlander, M. L., Taylor, I. W., Rugg, C. A., and Musgrave, E. A. (1983). Method for analysis of cellular DNA content in paraffin-embedded pathological material using flow cytometry. *J. Histochem. Cytochem.* 31:1333–1335.

Kattan, M. W. (2004). Evaluating a new marker's predictive contribution. *Clin. Cancer Res.* 10:822–824.

Kononen, J., Bubendorf, L., Kallioniemi, A., et al. (1998). Tissue microarrays for high-throughput molecular profiling of tumor specimens. *Nat. Med.* 4:844–847.

Krupinski, E. A., Weinstein, R. S., Bloom, K. J., and Rozek, L. S. (1993). *Progress in Telepathology: System Implementation and Testing. Advances in Pathology and Laboratory Medicine,* Vol. 6, Mosby-Year Book, St. Louis.

Mairinger, T., and Gschwendtner, A. (1996). Comparison of different mathematical algorithms to correct DNA-histograms obtained by measurements on thin liver tissue sections. *Anal. Cell. Pathol.* 11:159–171.

Pham, D. L., Xu, C.-Y., and Prince, J. L. (2000). Current methods in medical image segmentation. *Ann. Rev. Biomed. Eng.* 2:315–337.

Press, W. H., Teukolsky, S. A. (1992). *Numerical Recipes in C: The Art of Scientific Computing.* Cambridge University Press, New York.

Russ, J. C. (2006). *The Image Processing Handbook,* 5th edition, CRC Press. Boca Raton, FL.

Shapiro, L. G., and Stockman, G. C. (2001). *Computer Vision,* Prentice-Hall, Upper Saddle River, NJ, pp. 279–325.

Westphal, V., and Hell, S. W. (2005). Nanoscale resolution in the focal plane of an optical microscope. *Phys. Rev. Lett.* 94:143903.1–4.

Williams, T. M., Burns, F., Domnita, C., Dumler, S., Fink, L. M., Frank, T., Greiner, T., Kant, J. A., Matthias-Hagen, V., and Sabatini, L. (1999). Special report, goals and objectives for molecular pathology. Education in residency programs. *J. Mol. Diagn.* 1(1): November. American Society for Investigative Pathology, Association for Molecular Pathology.

Zobel, R. (2005). European Research Consortium for Informatics and Mathematics. *ERCIM News* 60:January; available at: www.ercim.org.

11

AQUA® TECHNOLOGY AND MOLECULAR PATHOLOGY

Mark Gustavson, Marisa Dolled-Filhart, Jason Christiansen, Robert Pinard, and David Rimm

11.1. INTRODUCTION

In the advent of personalized medicine and targeted molecular therapeutics, translational diagnostics that enable selection of patients for specific therapies or treatment regimens have become ever more critical. A classic example is the immunohistochemistry (IHC)-based HER2 companion diagnostic (HercepTest, DAKO, Carpenteria, CA), which is used to determine eligibility for trastuzumab (Herceptin, Genentech Inc., San Francisco, CA), a targeted antibody-based therapeutic shown to have efficacy in the treatment of breast cancer (Cobleigh et al., 1999; Slamon et al., 2001; Vogel et al., 2002). IHC has the advantage of allowing for the assessment of protein expression while preserving tissue architecture and cellular morphology, thus allowing for localization of protein expression [for review see Taylor and Levenson (2006) and Walker (2006)]. It also has the advantage that only a small amount of tissue (typically one 5-μm section) is needed for testing, in contrast to other gene expression methodologies [enzyme-linked immunosorbent assay (ELISA), real-time quantitative polymerase chain reaction (RTQ-PCR), or genechip technology), which require a larger amount of tissue and are destructive techniques that eliminate any morphological information from the analysis.

Molecular Pathology in Drug Discovery and Development, Edited by J. Suso Platero
Copyright © 2009 John Wiley & Sons, Inc.

However, traditional IHC has disadvantages. In addition to those sources of variation that plague all tissue-based methods including time-to-fixation, scoring traditional IHC is subjective and qualitative (nonquantitative) in nature. A pathologist, or observer, assesses how much protein is there by qualitative, "by eye," determination of the level of "brown stain" present in the tissue. Typically, scoring is categorical with four categories: IHC 0 (negative), IHC +1 (low), IHC +2 (medium), and IHC +3 (high). Although there are variations on this theme which take into consideration percentage of positive staining [i.e., Allred scoring (Harvey et al., 1999) or H-score (McCarty et al., 1985)], protein expression determination remains subjective. Second, scoring reproducibility and thus standardization, pathologist to pathologist, is poor because, again, protein expression determination is subjective and qualitative. This is best highlighted by recent studies showing poor concordance between local and central laboratories for the HER2 companion diagnostic (Dowsett et al., 2007; Hofmann et al., 2008; Paik et al., 2002; Perez et al., 2006; Roche et al., 2002). Third, traditional chromagen-based IHC lacks the dynamic range that, for instance, immunofluorescence provides (Rimm, 2006). Despite these disadvantages, traditional IHC remains the "standard-of-care" for tissue-based diagnostics in the clinical pathology laboratory.

One solution is AQUA® technology (AQUA analysis,[1] HistoRx, Inc., New Haven, CT). The AQUA technology was invented to address the disadvantages in IHC-based testing outlined above (Camp et al., 2002). AQUA technology is a fluorescence-based method that provides objective and continuous protein expression scores in tissue using automated fluorescence microscopy and advanced image analysis algorithms. It uses molecular identification of compartments to quantify biomarker expression as a function of pixel intensity in specific tissues or subcellular compartments. It has been demonstrated that AQUA scores are directly proportional to molecules per unit area or protein concentration (McCabe et al., 2005) and that this methodology is broadly applicable to biomarker assessment and clinical characterization (Berger et al., 2004, 2005; Camp et al., 2003; Chung et al., 2004; Divito et al., 2004a; Dolled-Filhart et al., 2006a, 2006b; Giltnane et al., 2007; Pozner-Moulis et al., 2006; Psyrri et al., 2005a, 2005b; Zerkowski et al., 2007).

AQUA has distinct advantages over traditional IHC and other immune-based assays: *standardization, quantification, and localization* (Fig. 11.1). While some immunoassays that are nontissue based or extraction based (i.e., ELISA and flow cytometry) can provide strict quantification of protein expression, spatial information (cellular and subcellular localization) is lost by virtue of the assay. In contrast, tissue or cell-based assays (i.e., IHC or fluorescence in situ hybridization (FISH)] preserve tissue architecture and hence protein localization

---

[1] AQUA®, PM2000, and AQUAsition are registered trademarks or trademarks of HistoRx, Inc. (New Haven, CT). The PM2000 and/or AQUA analysis software may be covered by one or more patent applications issued or pending in the United States and worldwide.

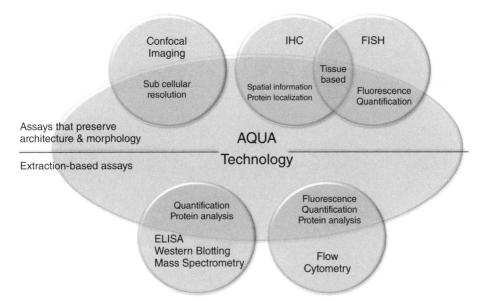

Figure 11.1. AQUA technology landscape. Venn diagram outlining the AQUA technology landscape and the features AQUA technology has in common with other protein/gene expression technologies. The top circles represent technologies that preserve tissue architecture and morphology but lack true quantification. The bottom circles represent technologies that are quantitative (extraction-based assays) but that do not preserve tissue architecture and hence cellular and subcellular localization. As depicted, the AQUA technology encompasses aspects of all these technologies by not only being quantitative but also tissue architecture and localization is preserved.

but lack the ability to be truly quantitative. AQUA technology encompasses features of all these technologies by not only being strictly quantitative but also preserving tissue architecture and protein localization (Fig. 11.1).

The function and application of AQUA technology as it relates to drug discovery as well as diagnostic development is the primary subject of this chapter. We will first describe in detail how the AQUA technology works from immunostaining to image validation and analysis. We will then describe the ability of the AQUA platform to standardize protein expression scores across instruments (sites), operators, and even staining days. This is a key feature of any technology that is geared toward the development of diagnostics to advance drug discovery and personalized medicine. Next, examples will be provided that illustrate how AQUA quantifies and localizes protein expression and how this relates to biomarker discovery. Finally, we will discuss how AQUA technology can be employed for diagnostic assay development in drug discovery and companion diagnostics.

11.2. AQUA TECHNOLOGY—HOW IT WORKS

The AQUA protocol is defined by three main components: (1) tissue staining, (2) image acquisition, and (3) image analysis (compartmentalization and AQUA scoring). The foundation of the AQUA technology is the PLACE image analysis algorithm (pixel-based locale assignment for compartmentalization of expression) (Camp et al., 2002). Tissue is a complex mixture of various components (i.e., epithelium, stroma, and blood vessels) and subcellular components (i.e., cytoplasm, nuclei, and membrane). PLACE enables differential localization of image pixel intensities associated with target gene expression within these different components or *masks*. In the traditional AQUA software, masks are defined through a series of pixel intensity thresholding steps producing binary images followed by image exclusion steps (see Fig. 11.4). In the next generation of software, compartmentalization is performed in a completely unsupervised fashion using mathematical algorithms. Both compartmentalization methodologies are described in detail below.

Once localized, pixel intensities, defined as 256 (8-bit) or 4096 (12-bit) shades of gray, can be summed and then normalized for compartment (mask) area producing the generalized AQUA score:

$$\text{AQUA score} = \sum \text{target pixel intensity/compartment area}$$

By normalizing for area, an AQUA score is effectively equivalent to protein concentration or molecules per unit area. This has been demonstrated using cell lines comparing AQUA scores and protein concentration by ELISA (McCabe et al., 2005).

11.2.1. Staining Methodology

In the typical AQUA experiment looking at target gene expression in an epithelial cancer, 4′-6-diamidino-2-phenylindole (DAPI) is used for the nuclear mask [ultraviolet (UV) channel], anticytokeratin antibodies are used to identify and differentiate epithelium from stroma (tumor mask) as well as to establish the cytoplasmic mask (Cy2 and/or Cy3 channel), and an antibody directed against the target is used to visualize the target gene of interest (Cy5 and/or Cy7 channel). However, an AQUA experiment is not limited to these parameters in that, depending on the tissue/compartment mask desired, the experiment can employ a number of different masking (i.e., GFAP to identify neuronal cells for glioblastoma or S100 to identify differentiate melanoma) and/or target antibodies.

Although AQUA technology employs multiple fluorescent stains, its staining methodology is similar to that of traditional IHC and is easily adapted to the typical pathology laboratory work flow. The AQUA staining methodology and its comparison to traditional IHC is outlined in Figure 11.2 (Camp et al., 2002). The primary difference is that AQUA technology employs multiple primary antibodies as a cocktail in order to not only identify target(s) of interest for quantification

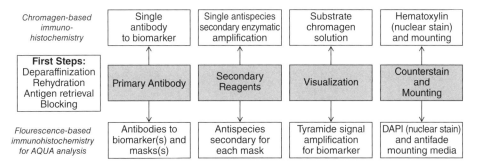

Figure 11.2. Comparison of AQUA IHC assay with traditional IHC. Schematic representation of the assay process for both traditional chromagen-based immunohistochemistry (top) and fluorescence-based immunohistochemistry for AQUA analysis (bottom). Both assays employ the same basic principles (middle boxes) with differences outlined as indicated.

(typically using Cy5 and/or Cy7 to minimize tissue autofluorescence), but to also to identify targets for molecular identification of tissues (i.e., cytokeratin to differentiate epithelium from stroma) and/or subcellular compartments (i.e., pan-cadherin to identify membrane; cytokeratin to identify cytoplasm). These compartment-specific antibodies are typically visualized using secondary antibodies directly conjugated to fluors (i.e., Cy2 or Cy3), while secondary antibodies to target gene antibodies are typically conjugated to horseradish peroxidase (HRP) for visualization using Cy5-tyramide, which is the fluorescence equivalent to chromagen-based solution or DAB (3,3′-diaminobenzidine).

An example indirect immunofluorescent staining protocol used for AQUA analysis of HER2 is provided next:

Precut paraffin-coated tissue microarray slides were deparaffinized and antigen retrieved by heat-induced epitope retrieval in 10 mM Tris (pH 9.0). Using an autostainer (LabVision, Fremont, CA), slides were preincubated with Background Sniper (BioCare Medical, Concord, CA). Slides were then incubated with primary antibodies against HER2 (Dako, Carpinteria, CA, rabbit polyclonal, 1:8000 dilution) and pan-cytokeratin (rabbit polyclonal, 1:200 dilution, Dako, Carpinteria, CA) diluted in DaVinci Green (BioCare Medical, Concord, CA) for 1 hour at room temperature. Slides were washed 3 × 5 minutes with 1X Tris-buffered saline (TBS) containing 0.05% Tween-20. Corresponding secondary antibodies were diluted in Da Vinci Green and incubated for 30 minutes at room temperature. These included either antibodies directly conjugated to a fluorophore for anticytokeratin (Alexa 555-conjugated goat antirabbit; 1:100, Molecular Probes, Eugene, OR), and/or conjugated to an HRP via, antimouse or rabbit Envision (Dako, Carpinteria, CA). Slides were again washed 3 × 5 minutes with TBS containing 0.05% Tween-20. Slides were incubated with a fluorescent chromagen amplification system (Cy5-tyramide, NEN Life Science Products, Boston, MA), which, like DAB, is activated by HRP and results in the deposition of numerous covalently associated Cy-5 dyes immediately adjacent to the

DAPI/nuclei   Cy3/tumor mask   Cy5/biomarker

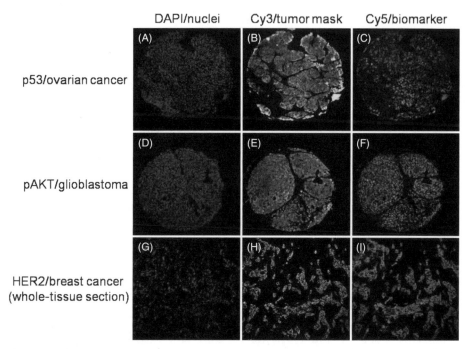

Figure 11.3. AQUA images. Representative 20× images of typical AQUA experiments to determine expression of p53 in an ovarian cancer TMA (A–C), pAKT expression in a glioblastoma TMA (D–F), and HER2 expression in breast cancer whole-tissue sections (G–I). Indicated are DAPI images for identification of nuclei, Cy3 images for identification of tumor masks, and Cy5 images for identification and quantification of biomarkers of interest. The use of these images in AQUA analysis is outlined in Figure 11.4.

HRP-conjugated secondary antibody. Cy-5 (red) was used because its emission peak is well outside the green-orange spectrum of tissue autofluorescence. Slides for automated analysis were cover slipped with an antifade DAPI-containing mounting medium (ProLong Gold, Molecular Probes, Eugene, OR).

Some example images are given in Figure 11.3. Staining for AQUA analysis has been performed successfully in a multitude of tissue types, including breast, colon, lung, prostate, ovarian, melanoma, glioblastoma, pancreas, lymphoma, multiple myeloma, adrenal carcinoma, thyroid, and others (Bamias et al., 2006; Berger et al., 2004; Camp et al., 2003; Chung et al., 2006; Divito et al., 2004a; Giltnane et al., 2006; Harigopal et al., 2005; Psyrri et al., 2005a; Yu et al., 2005a, 2005b; Zheng et al., 2007).

Careful consideration needs to be given to antibody selection with respect to host species so as to avoid antibody cross-reactivity. For example, when using a mouse primary antibody to identify target/biomarker expression, a rabbit (or other species) must be used for the mask (i.e., cytokeratin). As controls for antibody cross-reactivity, no primary controls should be employed. In the future, other visualization techniques could theoretically be employed, including fluorescent dendrimers, rolling circle amplification, and/or aptamer technology. This would free the experiment from the constraints of antibody species considerations and enable direct labeling of primary antibodies.

11.2.2. Tissue Microarray Technology

Tissue microarrays (TMAs), with their value in screening large populations of tissues, have become valuable tools for biomarker discover [for review see Rimm et al. (2001)]. TMAs make it practical to screen antibodies or markers on the basis of patient outcome. This method of tissue analysis has numerous advantages: (1) Instead of staining hundreds of slides, an entire cohort of cases can be analyzed by staining just one or two master blocks; (2) each specimen is treated with identical antibody concentration for identical times in identical buffer at identical temperatures along with appropriate controls; (3) antigen retrieval is identical for each specimen; and (4) only a very small (a few microliters) amount of antibody is required to analyze an entire cohort. A potential disadvantage of this technique is tissue and/or tumor heterogeneity. This laboratory and others have completed validation studies of tissue microarrays (Bova et al., 2001; Camp et al., 2000; Hoos et al., 2001). This work showed that, in breast cancer, equivalent results can be obtained in 95% of the cases by simply scoring two spots, suggesting a twofold redundant array is approximately representative of outcomes achieved using conventional histological methods. Similar redundancy appears to be appropriate for lung and colon cancer (unpublished data from our lab).

AQUA technology, in part, was developed to address the issue of imaging TMAs in an efficient and automated fashion. The front end of AQUA technology, as described below, is an automated fluorescence microscopy imaging platform, the PM2000, which is ideally suited for capturing TMA images. With minimal operator setup, the PM2000 can be programmed, through an automated stage (Prior Scientific, Rockland, MA), to move to each TMA spot and take the requisite high-resolution images. In addition to TMAs, the latest version of image acquisition software allows for streamlined image acquisition of whole tissue sections and provides overlay capabilities enabling identification of specific regions of interest based on hematoxylin and eosin (H&E) (or other) stains.

11.2.3. Automated Fluorescence Microscopy and Image Acquisition

Once tissues have been stained appropriately, image acquisition can proceed using the PM2000 system. The PM2000 platform, which is an automated epi-fluorescence microscopy system with accompanied image acquisition software (AQUAsition), is designed for high-resolution automated image acquisition for both TMA and whole-tissue sections (WTS). The PM2000 system, commercialized by HistoRx, Inc. (New Haven, CT), is based on a system described previously

(Camp et al., 2002). In brief, it is comprised of the Olympus BX51 epi-fluorescence microscope (Olympus America, Inc., Center Valley, PA), which is equipped with a motorized nosepiece to control selection of objectives (i.e., 4×, 10×, 20×, 40×, and 60×), a motorized filter turret to control selection of different filter cubes (i.e., DAPI, Cy2, Cy3, Cy5, and Cy7 or equivalent wavelengths), a motorized stage to control stage movements (Prior Scientific Inc., Rockland, MA), an X-Cite 120 mercury/metal halide light source (EXFO Life Sciences & Industrial Division, Ontario, Candada), and a QUANTFIRE monochromatic digital camera (Optronics, Inc., Goleta, CA).

Automated image capture is then performed using the AQUAsition software package. For the typical experiment as outlined above, high-resolution, 8-bit (resulting in 256 discrete intensity values per pixel of an acquired image) digital images of the cytokeratin staining visualized with Cy3, DAPI for visualization of nuclei, and target staining with Cy5 can be captured and saved for every histospot on the array or field of view (FOV) for whole-tissue sections.

Importantly, exposure time setting is done automatically for each histospot or FOV. This eliminates operator variability in setting exposure times. Auto-exposure also functions to maximize pixel dynamic range and reduce image over- and undersaturation. This is critical in providing the most pixel information (resolution) for each image. This is also critical for providing the maximal dynamic range of AQUA scores across a population of patients.

Once exposure times are set, pixels are written to image files as a function of power:

$$\text{Power}(P) = \frac{\text{Pixel intensity}/256}{\text{exposure time}}$$

Recording pixel information in terms of power helps to compensate for experimental variations in staining intensity and to normalize for exposure times; thus, for two spots with equal intensity but far varying exposure times, different AQUA scores will be appropriately calculated.

11.2.4. Automated Image Validation

Although the operator and/or the pathologist are the ultimate arbiters of image quality, automated image validation software algorithms have been developed that expedite this process. Three key algorithms are employed that detect image oversaturation, out-of-focus, and split-spot images (TMAs only). In fluorescence imaging, oversaturation is a key concern. If an image is oversaturated, pixel-based information/resolution (which translates into biomarker expression information) is lost by virtue of a percentage of pixels that cannot be discerned from one another (see autoexposure description above). An image is considered over-saturated if greater than 1% of pixels (41,943 pixels in 2048 × 2048 pixel image) are at maximal intensity. Although autoexposure algorithms function to ensure that no image has greater than 0.02% saturated pixels, this serves as control for this process. Furthermore, regardless of autoexposure, regions of image capture that have debris or dust often show increased fluorescence saturation and can be identified using this metric. Automated image validation software also can detect out-of-focus images through a series of pixel kurtosis-based algorithms. Finally, automated image validation is designed to detect split-spot images for TMA-based analysis by examining the borders of each image for increased fluorescence intensity. This is a key component in that inclusion of images that represent two spots is prevented.

11.2.5. AQUA (Image) Analysis—Producing an AQUA Score

Molecular-Based Compartmentalization of Biomarker Expression. AQUA analysis is outlined in Figure 11.4. It takes you through a step-by-step illustration of how AQUA image analysis is accomplished given a typical experiment with an epithelial tumor using the target estrogen receptor (ER) as an example. Again, this AQUA analysis is easily applicable to any number of different permutations depending on the outcome desired. AQUA analysis begins (Figs. 11.4A and 11.4C; step 1) with generation of a tumor mask through pixel intensity thresholding (binary gating) and spatial image analysis procedures (i.e., fill holes). Using identified tumor mask pixels as a template, we use the same type of pixel intensity thresholding to identify nuclear and/or cytoplasmic pixels (resulting in Figs. 11.4D and 11.4E; steps 2a and 2b). Then, through a process of 100% mutual exclusion, these images are combined to provide pixel assignments for compartmentalization (Fig. 11.4F; step 3). Then, for purposes of visualization only, Figure 11.4 (step 4) shows overlay of the target image (colorized in red) with the compartment image demonstrating co-localization of ER with nuclei (magenta pixels from the overlay of the target in red with nuclei in blue; Fig. 11.4H). AQUA scoring proceeds as described below.

AQUA Scoring. Once compartment pixels have been assigned, the AQUA score is generated according to following calculation:

$$AQ = \left(\frac{1}{\sum C_i}\right)\left(\sum T_i C_i\right)$$

In this equation, target pixel power (T_i) is multiplied by its congruent compartment pixel value (C_i), and then all pixel products are summed ($\sum T_i C_i$). Since compartment pixel values are either 0 or 1 (binary gating), target pixels not in the compartment (compartment pixel value = 0) are valued at 0, while target pixels in the compartment (compartment pixel value = 1) are given their raw target pixel value. Thus this represents the sum of target pixel values (power) in a designated compartment. Then, this sum is divided by the total number of pixels in the compartment to normalize for compartment area, yielding the AQUA score. Because pixel power ranges from 0 to 0.3 (see power equation), in the

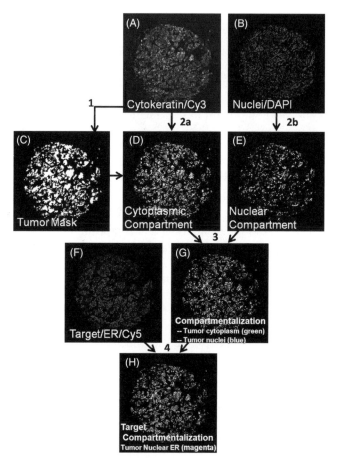

Figure 11.4. AQUA image analysis. Schematic representation of the AQUA analysis process for a typical experiment looking at biomarker expression in an epithelial cancer. (1) Tumor mask generation through pixel intensity thresholding (binary gating) and spatial image analysis procedures. (2a and 2b) Generation of cytoplasmic and nuclear-specific pixel mask through binary gating. (3) Combining cytoplasmic and nuclear-specific pixel masks in by 100% mutual exclusion. (4) Identification of coincidental target pixels with compartment pixels (for visualization only). See insert for color representation of this figure.

latest version of software, the AQUA score is multiplied by a constant of 100,000 to yield AQUA scores ranging from 0 to 33,000.

Next Version of AQUA Analysis. When performing an AQUA experiment on a TMA or even whole-tissue section, the same thresholding for compartmentalization or image segmentation, as described above, is applied across every histospot or FOV. This has the limitation that the set threshold value may not be optimal for each spot. Furthermore, threshold setting is a subjective deter-

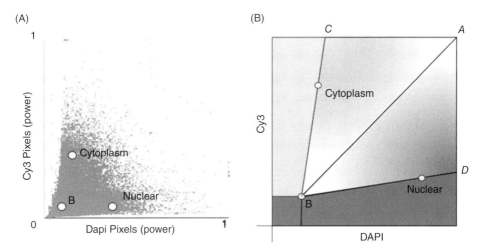

Figure 11.5. Clustering AQUA analysis. (A) 2 × 2 scatter plot showing Cy3 (Y) and DAPI (X) pixel intensities graphed against one another with indicated centroids (B, background; C, cytoplasm; N, nuclear). (B) Model description of C-AQUA method showing specific pixel assignment: background (gray box), 100% cytoplasm/Cy3 (light gray box; Y-axis; 0% nuclear/DAPI), 0–100% cytoplasm/Cy3 (triangle *ABC*; 0% nuclear/DAPI), 0–100% nuclear/DAPI (triangle *ABD*, 0% cytoplasm/Cy3), and 100% nuclear/DAPI (dark gray box; X-axis; 0% cytoplasm/Cy3). (Adapted from Gustavson et al., 2009a.)

mination made by the operator. In order to remove this subjectivity and provide optimal, objective image segmentation on an image-by-image basis, in development is a new version of AQUA analysis. This version, outlined in Figure 11.5, employs unsupervised clustering algorithms to objectively determine compartment membership (Gustavson et al., 2009a).

Image segmentation by clustering is accomplished using unsupervised k-means clustering based on Euclidean distances (Miller et al., 2008). First, all pixels were assigned characteristics based on power (see image acquisition) reported for subcellular images and can be represented as coordinates (P_{DAPI}, P_{Cy3}). As a result of this, pixels could be presented in a two-dimensional scatter plot of compartment intensities (see Fig. 11.5A). The model used to perform the image segmentation asserts that pixels will fall into two classifications: (1) those that have low signal in all compartments tested (i.e., background), and (2) pixels with the property that one compartment marker is showing higher staining than the others (i.e., higher Cy3 intensity than DAPI). For the data presented here, for two subcellular compartments, this would result in the need to identify three data centroids (Figs. 11.5A and 11.5B). For the model described here, the background cluster is initialized to the origin while the cytoplasmic and nuclear centers are initialized to their respective maximum values and zero (i.e., for the DAPI marker, the initial value is ($P_{DAPI(max)}$, 0). Pixels are then assigned to each cluster based on Euclidean distance. Cluster centroid values are then calculated and cluster pixel membership is reassessed. The method runs iteratively and terminates after there is convergence (no membership changes) or 30 iterations.

From examination of the scatter plots in Figure 11.5A, it can be seen that there will generally be pixels that have intensities higher than background but have similar intensity contribution for each channel. Thus, once convergence is reached, a geometric method is then used in order to further define the certainty of a pixel as being a member of either cluster. Each pixel is characterized based upon its location in the cluster and proximity to other clusters. If both the Cy3 and DAPI pixels value are less than B, then there is zero certainty in both compartments and the pixel value is set to zero in both compartments (Fig. 11.5B, medium gray box). This represents background in the image. If Cy3 is greater than B and DAPI is less than B, then there is 100% probability for cytoplasm and 0% probability for nuclear (Fig. 11.5B, light gray box). Conversely, if DAPI is greater than B and Cy3 is less than B, then there is 100% probability for nuclear and 0% probability for cytoplasm (Fig. 11.5B, dark gray box). For values in the center region of the scatter plot that are not definitively assigned to either compartment, a probability function region is defined by the triangles ABC and ABD. In these regions, pixels are assigned to either Cy3 (triangle ABC) or DAPI (triangle ABD) exclusively. However, their contribution to the overall calculation is modified by their location within the triangles. Pixels in triangle ABC are assigned a probability based on their proximity to the vertices. As a pixel approaches C, the value approaches 100%; as a pixel approaches the vertices A or B (or the line segment connected A and B), the value approaches zero. Triangle ABD follows the same logic, with values approaching 100% as pixels approach the vertex D.

As a proof of concept and to demonstrate the precision of this new AQUA analysis (C-AQUA), two highly trained operators set up a traditional AQUA and a C-AQUA experiment on the same data set. Setup for the traditional AQUA experiment took an average of 20 minutes, whereas average set up time for C-AQUA was less than 2 minutes and does not require subjective operator intervention. Linear regression analysis between two operators for the two methods is shown in Figure 11.6. Although highly correlative [Fig. 11.6A; linear regression coefficient = 0.97 ($P < 0.001$); $R^2 = 0.984$], resultant AQUA scores from AQUA analysis were nonetheless different between operators, whereas AQUA scores generated with C-AQUA were identical [Fig. 11.6B; linear regression coefficient = 1.00 ($P = 0$); $R^2 = 1.00$]. This next generation of AQUA analysis will thus minimize operator time and subjective input as well as enhance compartmentalization. This level of efficiency and objectivity, in conjunction with standardization capabilities as described below, will be important in moving forward in the development of robust clinical diagnostic tests.

As a more objective and relevant metric, compartmentalization was compared with a known clinical feature, histological grade. It has been demonstrated that histological grade correlates with percent nuclear volume in breast (Khan et al., 2003) and ovarian cancers (Hsu et al., 2005). Percent nuclear volume [(nuclear pixels/(nuclear pixels + cytoplasmic pixels)*100] was calculated in three serial sections of the invasive breast cancer cohort and then categorized these

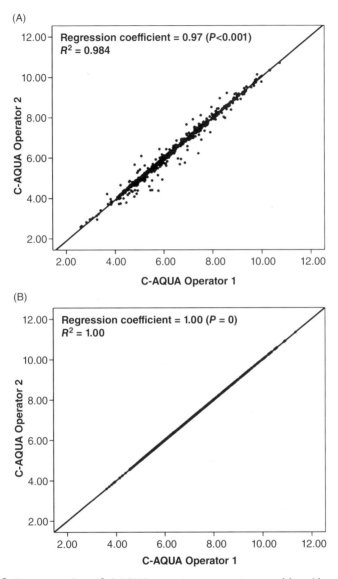

Figure 11.6. Demonstration of C-AQUA operator-to-operator precision. Linear regression analysis with indicated linear regression coefficients and R^2 values between AQUA scores generated by (A) two highly trained operators using traditional AQUA analysis algorithms and (B) two highly trained operators using C-AQUA algorithms on the same data set as in (A). (Adapted from Gustavson et al., 2009a.)

results by histological grade. As shown in Figure 11.7, there was a statistically significant [$P = 0.002, 0.006$, and 0.08 for section 1 (11.7A), section 2 (11.7B), and section 3 (11.7C), respectively] difference in mean percent nuclear volume, as calculated with compartmentalization values using C-AQUA, between low- and

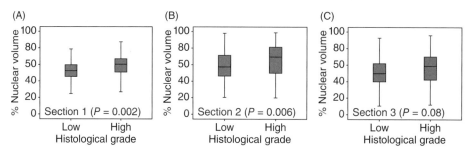

Figure 11.7. Correlation of percent nuclear volume with histological grade for demonstration of C-AQUA accuracy. Box plots of percent nuclear volume [(nuclear pixels/(nuclear pixels + cytoplasmic pixes))*100] (*y* axis) categorized by histological grade (low and high) for three independent serial sections of the same breast tissue microarray cohort (indicated; A–C). One-way ANOVA analysis for comparison of means across categories was significant at least at the 10% level as indicated. (Adapted from Gustavson et al., 2009a.)

high-grade tumors for three independent experiments. Furthermore, percent nuclear volume significantly correlated (all $P \leq 0.001$) with histological grade by rank-order analysis.

11.3. STANDARDIZATION

The ability to standardize IHC results across laboratories is becoming increasingly more demanded, especially in the advent of personalized medicine and targeted molecular therapeutics that ultimately will require reliable biomarker diagnostics to ensure their success. Due to the subjective and qualitative nature of traditional IHC, standardization across laboratories and observers is quite problematic. Because AQUA technology is objective and strictly quantitative, it has the ability to be standardized across instruments (i.e., laboratories) and operators (i.e., observers). Instrument calibration methodologies have been developed by HistoRx, which enable captured signal to be normalized across multiple instruments. This is accomplished through a combination of light source and intrinsic machine calibration methodologies (Fig. 11.8). Software algorithmic methodologies have also been developed that predominantly remove operator decisions from the image acquisition (i.e., autoexposure) and scoring process (i.e., unsupervised pixel-based clustering). These methodologies can be applied to any target of interest to achieve % coefficients of variations (CVs) of less than 5%, which rival other quantitative immunoassays (i.e., ELISA and flow cytometry). These standardization methodologies have been applied to numerous markers including HER2 (Fig. 11.10), mTOR (as further described in Fig. 11.9), EGFR, and ER, and is described in detail (Gustavson et al., 2009b).

For machine and AQUA score normalization, three calibration factors are employed: calibration cube (CC) factor, light source (LS) factor, and Cy5 optical path (OP) factor. Calculation of these factors is based on pixel intensity

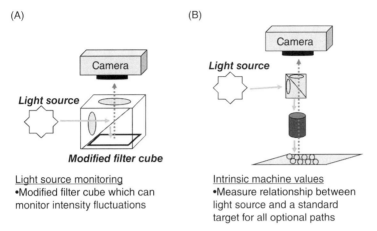

Figure 11.8. Schematic representation of machine calibration techniques. (A) Light source monitoring using modified cube. (B) Intrinsic machine values are monitored using a specialized calibration slide. This enables normalization of optical path and filter cube differences.

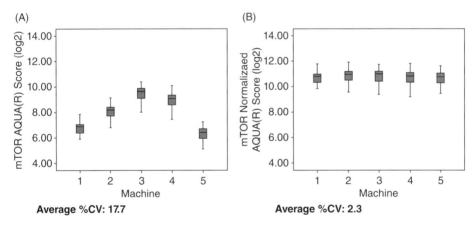

Figure 11.9. Standardization of AQUA scores across five independent instruments. mTOR AQUA scores were generated for a 30-spot TMA and represented as box plots for each machine for (A) before and (B) after standardization with indicated %CVs.

measurements given by images acquired under described conditions. All factors rely on a specialized filter cube (calibration cube) designed whereby light is reflected directly from the light source to the camera via white filter paper attached to the objective end of the filter cube. To account for variations in the different cube constructions, calibration cubes for each machine were standardized by calculating the percentage of the average total light intensity compared to average total light intensity of a "gold standard" calibration cube (producing the CC factor). This is a constant factor that is calculated and maintained for each cube, and thus each microscope system with that cube installed. The light source factor is calculated for each histospot acquired and is the total light intensity as measured by the calibration cube divided into a constant (100,000). The OP factor accounts for the amount of light passed through a specific microscope objective/ filter combination relative to the measured incoming light intensity. For these measurements, a standard sample is required that can be transferred between different machines and maintain reproducibility in its construction. A commercially available blue fluorescent standard slide was selected for this purpose (Omega Optical Inc., Brattleboro, VT). To produce this measurement, a ratio is taken between the incident light intensity and the measured intensity of the standard sample. The Cy5 OP factor is the quotient of the average total light intensity of 16 images taken for each cube/sample combination. The CC and OP factors are intrinsic to the specific hardware system being studied and need only be calculated once or at an interval where one would suspect some type of modification in the optics has occurred. The normalized AQUA score is thus

Normalized AQUA score =
Raw AQUA score × CC factor × LS factor × OP factor

where the CC and OP factors are defined upon system setup/construction and the LS factor is measured simultaneously. Thus, the system standardization results described here do not add significant extra time to the data acquisition from the current methods.

Two examples of these standardization methods are provided in Figures 11.9 and 11.10. First, using mTOR on a TMA of 30 histospots of invasive colorectal carcinoma, raw AQUA scores ($\log_2$ transformed) are compared in a box plot across 5 different PM2000 instruments with an average %CV of 17.7 (Fig. 11.9A). After normalization, %CV is reduced to 2.3 (Fig. 11.9B). Second, examination of HER2 on a large TMA of 669 invasive breast cancer cases across 3 instruments, 3 operators, and 3 independent staining days shows average %CV of 9.3 ± 2.6 before normalization (Fig. 11.10B), and this is reduced to 3.9 ± 2.1 after normalization (Fig. 11.10B).

Of importance for drug discovery and the development of robust clinical diagnostics is the ability to reproducibly classify patients or, in other words, reproduce a cutoff within data across independent patients and patient populations. Current American Society of Clinical Oncalogy/Callege of American Pathologists (ASCO-CAP) guidelines are suggesting laboratories achieve 95% positive/negative concordance for current HER2 assay methodologies (Wolff et al., 2007). A recent study shows that for HER2 IHC-based scoring, concordance between observers ranges from 54 to 85%, falling short of these guidelines (Hameed et al. 2008). We examined positive/negative concordance for AQUA scoring across instruments, operators, and staining days using optimal cut points established using X-tile (Camp et al., 2004). As shown in Figure 11.11, overall concordance ranged from 94.5% (instrument 1 to instrument 3; Fig.

(A)

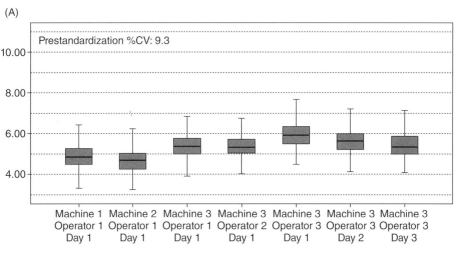

(B)

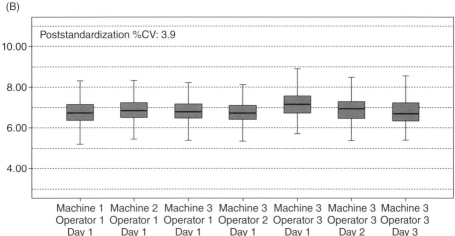

Figure 11.10. Standardization of AQUA scores across three operators, three instruments (machines), and three independent staining days. HER2 AQUA scores were generated for a 669-spot TMA and represented as box plots for each parameter for (A) before and (B) after standardization with indicated %CVs. (Adapted from Gustavson et al., 2009b.)

11.11B) to 99.3% (operator 1 to operator 2; Fig. 11.11C). It is important to note that these analyses include all cases, even those that would be considered equivocal.

Of those cases that are differentially classified, the question arises where along the distribution of AQUA scores these cases occur. To address that question, we generated paneled frequency histograms to examine where differentially classified cases were occurring. As shown in Figure 11.12, for instrument to instrument, operator to operator, and run to run, differentially classified cases occur at

(A)

Instrument 2	Instrument 1 (Reference)		
	POS	NEG	TOT
POS	87	9	96
NEG	4	483	487
TOT	91	482	583

Overall Concordance: 97.8% (95CI:96.3–98.6)
Positive Agreement: 95.6% (95CI:90.9–98.1)
Negative Agreement: 98.2% (95CI:97.3–98.6)

(B)

Instrument 3	Instrument 1 (Reference)		
	POS	NEG	TOT
POS	71	12	83
NEG	20	480	400
TOT	91	482	583

Overall Concordance: 94.5% (95CI:92.5–96.0)
Positive Agreement: 78.0% (95CI:71.6–92.7)
Negative Agreement: 97.6% (95CI:96.4–98.4)

(C)

Operator 2	Operator 1 (Reference)		
	POS	NEG	TOT
POS	71	1	72
NEG	3	508	511
TOT	74	509	583

Overall Concordance: 99.3% (95CI:98.3–99.6)
Positive Agreement: 95.9% (95CI:91.9–97.0)
Negative Agreement: 99.8% (95CI:99.2–100)

(D)

Operator 3	Operator 1 (Reference)		
	POS	NEG	TOT
POS	73	10	83
NEG	1	499	500
TOT	74	509	583

Overall Concordance: 98.1% (95CI:96.9–98.4)
Positive Agreement: 98.6% (95CI:93.9–99.8)
Negative Agreement: 90.0% (95CI:97.3–98.2)

(E)

Run 2	Run 1 (Reference)		
	POS	NEG	TOT
POS	52	1	53
NEG	20	510	530
TOT	72	511	583

Overall Concordance: 96.4% (95CI:95.1–96.7)
Positive Agreement: 72.2% (95CI:67.0–73.4)
Negative Agreement: 99.8% (95CI:99.1–100)

(F)

Run 3	Run 1 (Reference)		
	POS	NEG	TOT
POS	60	18	78
NEG	12	493	505
TOT	72	511	583

Overall Concordance: 94.9% (95CI:92.9–96.3)
Positive Agreement: 83.3% (95CI:75.5–89.2)
Negative Agreement: 96.5% (95CI:95.4–97.3)

Figure 11.11. Percent agreement for positive/negative population classification. 2 × 2 contingency tables comparing positive (POS) vs. negative (NEG) population segregation based on X-tile cut points generated for the reference (i.e., instrument 1) for each indicated instrument set (A, B), operator set (C, D), and run set (E, F). Also shown are overall concordance, positive agreement, and negative agreement rates with 95% confidence intervals. (Adapted from Gustavson et al., 2009b.)

the cut point and not over the entire distribution. These data suggest that the classification error concerns cut-point selection not generation and reproducibility of the HER2 AQUA score. Taken together, these data suggest that, although there is an equivocal region in the vicinity of the cut point, classification of patients for interinstrument, interoperator, and interrun assessment of HER2 expression using AQUA scoring is highly reproducible with concordance rates approaching, if not exceeding, that suggested by ASCO/CAP (Wolff et al., 2007).

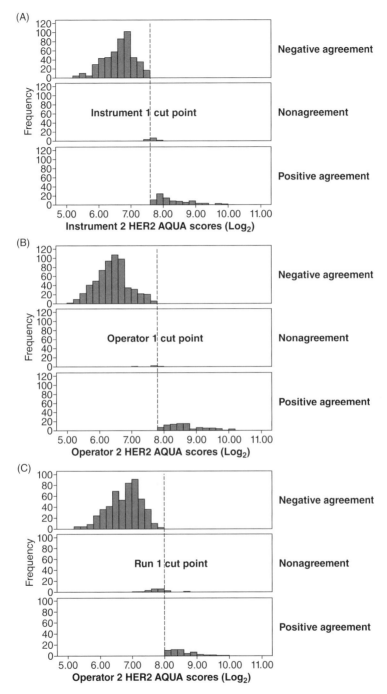

Figure 11.12. Distribution analysis of cases based on agreement. Frequency distributions separated into negative agreement, positive agreement, and nonagreement cases for (A) instrument 2 (AQUA scores) to instrument 1 (cut point); (B) operator 2 (AQUA scores) to operator 1 (cut point); and (C) run 2 (AQUA scores) to run 1 (cut point) to demonstrate where disagreement occurs within the population of breast cancer cases. Cases that disagree reside in and around the indicated cut points and do not span over the entire distribution. (Adapted from Gustavson et al., 2009b.)

11.4. QUANTIFICATION

The AQUA score represents average intensity of a biomarker per unit area. As such, an AQUA is equivalent to concentration of protein in a tissue section. This has been demonstrated by using cell line controls whereby matched cell lysates and cell pellets (see www.tissuearray.org for protocols to make cell line TMAs) are created for assessment of protein expression by ELISA and AQUA score assessment, respectively. As shown in Figure 11.13, AQUA scores are directly proportional to pictogram/microgram protein concentration as determined for HER2 [Fig. 11.13A (McCabe et al., 2005)] and EGFR (Fig. 11.13B).

Although AQUA scores do correlate with traditional IHC categorical scoring, significant overlap is observed as seen with HER2 [Fig. 11.14, right top panel (Camp et al., 2003)]. This is most likely due to the quantitative abilities of AQUA analysis over traditional IHC, but it is also potentially due to the way scoring is accomplished. With traditional IHC, specifically for HER2, only a small percentage of the tissue (10% for HER2) must appear positive (i.e., IHC +3) in order to be scored positive (Paik et al., 2002). However, an AQUA score represents average expression over the entire tissue section. This actually translates into enhanced resolution of patient survival, compared to traditional IHC, where low-level expression is differentiated from mid- and high level (Fig. 11.14, bottom panels).

Because AQUA technology is objective and quantitative on a continuous scale, it is ideally suited for population-based studies. Complimentary to this is the ability of the AQUA platform for automated image acquisition of TMAs (Camp et al., 2002) as well as whole-tissue sections (Chung et al., 2007). Figure 11.15 shows a typical AQUA score output in the form of a frequency distribution of AQUA scores across a population-based study. As delineated by the various circles, AQUA analysis can not only differentiate high from low (on from off) but offers increased resolution to delineate within low-level expressing patients and even very low level expressing patients. There are now over 40 peer-reviewed publications using the AQUA platform, mostly for population-based studies examining biomarker expression as a function of outcome in either survival or treatment for cancer patients (Bamias et al., 2006; Berger et al., 2004, 2005; Chung et al., 2007; DiVito et al., 2004b; Dolled-Filhart et al., 2006a, 2006b; Giltnane et al., 2006, 2007; Harigopal et al., 2005, 2008; McCabe et al., 2005; McCarthy et al., 2008, 2005; Pick et al., 2007; Pozner-Moulis et al., 2006; Psyrri et al., 2005b; Rothberg et al., 2008). Here, we will discuss three examples of AQUA analysis utility in population-based studies for biomarker discovery.

The first example is a study by Giltnane et al. (2007) looking at epidermal growth factor receptor (EGFR) expression by AQUA analysis to determine response to tamoxifen in ER-positive early-stage breast cancer patients (Giltnane et al., 2007). Treatment with antiestrogen therapies such as tamoxifen has substantially decreased the risk of recurrence and mortality in women with hormone receptor–positive disease (Early Breast Cancer Trials Collaborative Group, 1998). Unfortunately, both de novo and acquired resistance remain a major

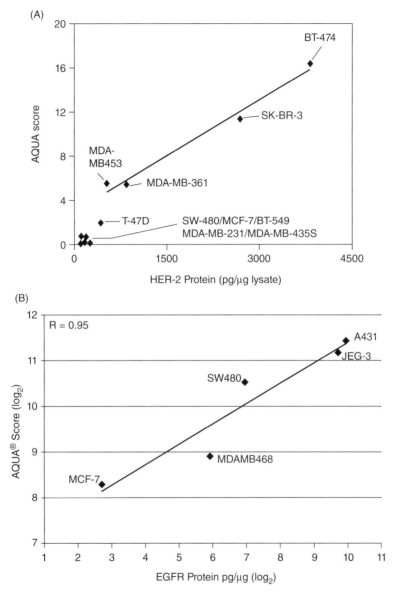

Figure 11.13. AQUA analysis compared to ELISA. Linear regression analysis showing direct linear relationship between AQUA scores and protein concentration as determined by ELISA for indicated cell lines for (A) HER2 and (B) EGFR. (Fig. 11.13A adapted from McCabe et al., 2005.)

clinical problem and the mechanisms for resistance are under active investigation (Arpino et al., 2004, 2005; Dowsett et al., 2006; Osborne, 1998). One possible mechanism of resistance is cross-talk with growth factor receptor (i.e., EGFR) signaling pathways (Osborne, 1998). EGFR is a receptor tyrosine kinase involved

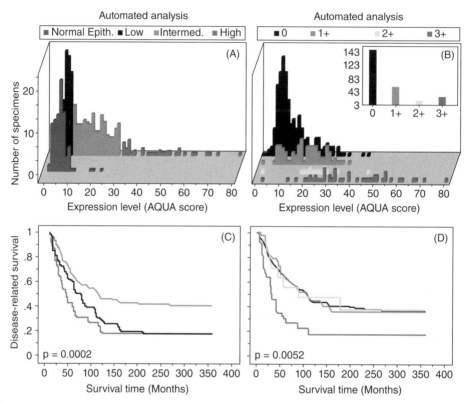

Figure 11.14. Comparison of traditional IHC and AQUA scoring for HER2 in breast cancer. Frequency histograms (top) and associated Kaplan–Meier (KM) survival curves as function of AQUA analysis (left) or manual scoring (right). AQUA analysis is able to resolve patients that manual scoring cannot (see black curve in KM analysis for automated analysis). (Adapted from Camp et al., 2003.)

in a number of cellular processes including growth and proliferation and is critically involved in tumorigenesis for many cancers (Hynes and Lane, 2005).

In this study, AQUA analysis was used to quantitatively measure EGFR. Although traditional IHC was unable to differentiate patient populations with respect to response to tamoxifen in ER-positive patients, AQUA analysis of EGFR expression demonstrated low-level EGFR expression associates with response to tamoxifen (Fig. 11.16). Furthermore, a cell line model system was described whereby a biological cut point (on or off) for EGFR expression could be reproducibly determined. Development of cell line control models for not only quantitative control but reproducible assessment of cut points is potentially a key aspect to the success of AQUA-based clinical diagnostics. Taken together, these data demonstrate the potential utility of quantitative assessment of EGFR positivity by AQUA analysis as a clinical diagnostic that would be used to make

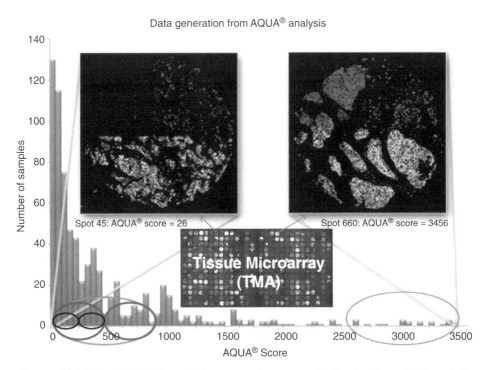

Figure 11.15. Typical AQUA analysis output. Frequency distribution from TMA analysis showing a low-resolution TMA image (inset) with example fluorescence images (inset). Different shaded circles in frequency histogram delineated resolving capacity of AQUA scoring. See insert for color representation of this figure.

treatment decisions in ER-positive women with invasive breast cancer. Further studies are required and are currently underway to validate these findings as well as apply them to additional indications.

The second example is looking at PTEN expression in glioblastoma (GBM). PTEN is a tumor suppressor protein whose expression is frequently lost in numerous cancers (Sansal and Sellers, 2004). GBM is a particularly aggressive form of brain cancer with median survival times ranging only from 11 to 13 months (Miller and Perry, 2007). At this time there are no clinical diagnostics available to assess prognosis of these patients, let alone response to treatment. Although mutations in *PTEN* have been shown to predict outcome in GBM (Kato et al., 2004; Kraus et al., 2000; Smith et al., 2001), assessment of PTEN protein expression has not been demonstrated with respect to prognosis. The difficulty in measuring PTEN protein expression with respect to survival is related to the fact that PTEN expression is inherently low in GBM relative to normal brain tissue (Fig. 11.17A), thus differentiating very low level expression versus low-level expression for outcome differentiation is problematic using traditional IHC.

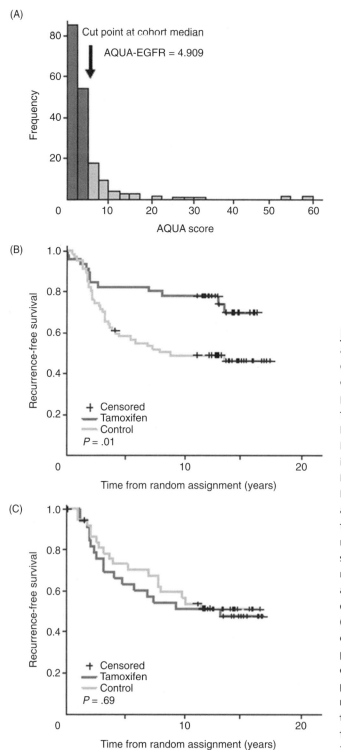

Figure 11.16. AQUA analysis of EGFR expression in breast cancer can determine patients that respond to tamoxifen. (A) Frequency histogram of EGFR AQUA scores with indicated cut point. (B) KM survival analysis of EGFR negative patients as a function of treatment; EGFR negative patients show significant ($p = 0.01$) response to tamoxifen as a function of 5-year disease-specific survival. (C) KM survival analysis of EGFR positive patients as a function of treatment; EGFR positive patients show no significant response to tamoxifen. (Adapted from Giltname et al., 2007.)

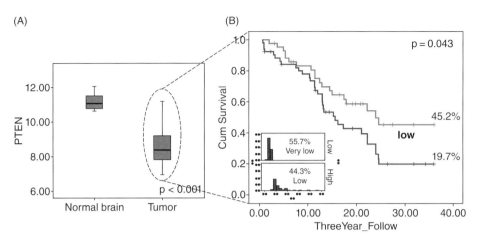

Figure 11.17. Ability of AQUA analysis to assess and differentiate low-level PTEN expressing glioblastoma tumors. (A) Box plot of AQUA scores comparing normal brain to tumor tissue; significant difference in expression by one-way ANOVA ($p < 0.001$). (B) KM survival analysis of low-level expressing tumors with indicated cut points [frequency histograms (inset)] showing a significant ($p = 0.043$) increase in 3-year disease-specific survival for patients expressing higher levels of PTEN.

Measurement of PTEN by AQUA analysis, much like that described for EGFR in the example above, offers potential prognostic utility.

In this study, comparing normal level expression to tumor expression for PTEN by AQUA analysis, tumor expression is significantly lower as compared to normal (Fig. 11.17A). Nonetheless, differences in low-level expression are resolved with respect to patient survival where patients that have relatively higher level PTEN expression have increased survival compared to lower level expressing patients (25.5% decrease from 45.2 to 19.7% three-year disease-specific survival; $p = 0.043$; Fig. 11.17B). Patients with higher PTEN levels had an 8.3-month improvement in median survival, which is quite substantial for GBM. Although these findings need to be validated, these data demonstrate the quantitative ability of AQUA analysis to differentiate low-level PTEN expression and could lead to a prognostic clinical assay for management of patients with GBM.

The third example is looking at two independent biomarkers, ERCC1 and RRM1, to predict prognosis in stage I non-small-cell lung cancer (NSCLC) in a study by Zheng et al. (2007). ERCC1 and RRM1 are enzymes involved in DNA repair and metabolism, respectively, and have both been shown to contribute to tumorigenesis when abnormally regulated (Bepler et al., 2006, 2004; Gautam et al., 2003; Pitterle et al., 1999; Simon et al., 2005). Assessment of prognosis of stage I NSCLC is a critical clinical question in that there is considerable debate as to the utility of chemotherapy in stage I patients (Calhoun et al., 2008). A

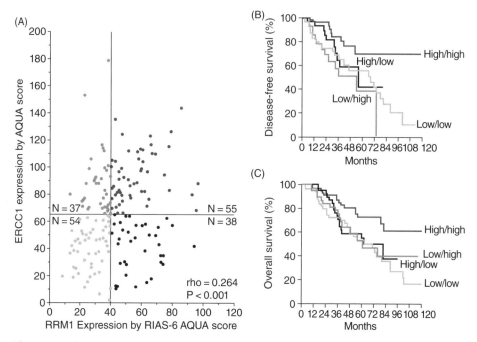

Figure 11.18. Ability of AQUA analysis to multiplex two independent biomarkers. (A) Scatter plot of AQUA scores for ERCC1 and RRM1 in stage I NSCLC with indicated cut points (groupings). KM analysis for (B) overall survival and (C) time to recurrence using groups established in (A) demonstrated increased overall survival and time to recurrence for patients with both high ERCC1 and high RRM1 expression as determined by AQUA analysis. (Adapted from Zheng et al., 2006.) See insert for color representation of this figure.

prognostic biomarker(s) for stage I NSCLC would provide clinicians with additional information for making this decision.

Taking advantage of the quantitative and multiplexing capabilities of AQUA analysis, Zheng et al. (2007) regressed continuous AQUA scores from ERCC1 and RRM1 (Fig. 11.18A). Then, based on median cut points from each biomarker, they divided their patient cohort into four quantitative groups as shown in Figure 11.18A. By Kaplan–Meier survival analysis, they were able to show a significant association between both recurrence-free and overall survival and these groupings (Fig. 11.18B), specifically the high/high group showed improved survival compared to the other groups (Zheng et al., 2007).

Although this study demonstrates the prognostic value for AQUA analysis of ERCC1 and RRM1 and, as discussed above, is a key clinical question, ERCC1 and RRM1 by other gene expression assays have been shown to predict response to cisplatinum-based and anti-metabolite-based therapies in advanced stage NSCLC. Thus, AQUA analysis of ERCC1 and RRM1 may lead to a predictive diagnostic assay whereby treatment decisions could be made based on a patient's ERCC1 or RRM1 AQUA score. In fact, these studies are currently underway (personal communication with G. Bepler). Furthermore, this is an example of how AQUA technology can be used in a multivariate setting to predict outcome. This topic will be discussed in more detail later in this chapter.

11.5. LOCALIZATION

Another aspect of the AQUA technology is the ability to localize or compartmentalize protein expression and thus quantify protein expression in different subcellular compartments. Many proteins reside in different cellular compartments depending on their specific function or activation state. For example, thymidylate synthase (TS) resides in both cytoplasm for its DNA synthesis role and nucleus for its translational inhibition function (Liu et al., 2002). Another example is cellular signaling molecules such as AKT, STAT, and ERK that move from cytoplasm to nucleus upon their activation. Although activation of these proteins is typically mediated by phosphorylation, detection of phosphorylated proteins is problematic in tissue, thus the ability to assess activation by localization is valuable (Baker et al., 2005).

The Rimm laboratory has published several studies that specifically take advantage of the localization capabilities of AQUA analysis by using expression ratios (i.e., nuclear-to-cytoplasmic) to assess differential compartment expression and/or to normalize expression (Berger et al., 2003; Dolled-Filhart et al., 2006a; Psyrri et al., 2005a). One study examined TS expression in two large cohorts of colorectal carcinoma, using one cohort as a training set to establish expression cut points and the other as a validation set for these cut points (Gustavson et al., 2008). Figure 11.19 shows the principle result where neither nuclear (Figs. 11.19A and 11.19B) nor cytoplasmic expression (Figs. 11.19C and 11.19D) could reproducibly predict survival, whereas a nuclear-to-cytoplasmic ratio reproducibly predicted survival in both the training and validation set. It was also demonstrated that the expression ratio did not correlate with total expression suggesting that the expression ratio predicts outcome regardless of total expression.

Overall, these studies demonstrate that a nuclear-to-cytoplasmic expression ratio is a more powerful predictor of overall survival and disease-free survival in colorectal cancer patients than nuclear and/or cytoplasmic expression alone. As supported by multivariate analysis (data not shown), this biomarker could be used with other common clinical-pathological criteria to better assess prognosis of patients in the clinic for determination of treatment course. With further study, this biomarker may also prove to be a potent, independent predictor for response to 5'FU treatment and thus lead to the development of a clinical diagnostic using AQUA technology, based on the ability of AQUA analysis to quantitatively localize expression.

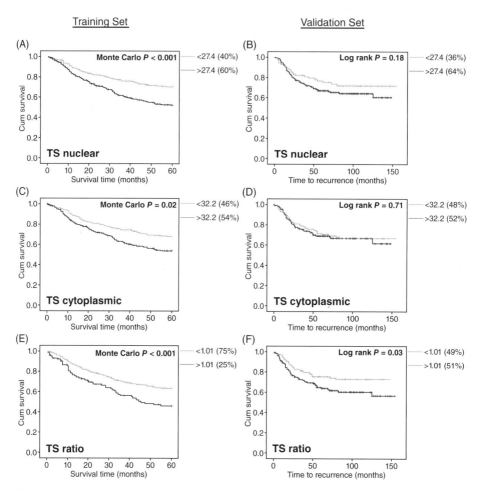

Figure 11.19. Kaplan–Meier survival analysis for differential compartmentalization of thymidylate synthase in two independent (training and validation sets) colorectal cancer cohorts. Figure shows results of optimal cut point determination for the training set (left) and application of cut point to the validation set (right) for indicated compartments and compartment ratios. Only nuclear-to-cytoplasmic ratio resulted in significant validation on the second cohort (E, F). (Adapted from Gustavson et al., 2008.)

11.6. MULTIPARAMETRIC ANALYSIS

Multiparametric-type analyses, or the ability to assess multiple genes and/or proteins at once, have tremendous power in research as well as clinical diagnostics. These types of analyses have been seen for over a decade in gene microarray technology [i.e., messenger ribonucleic acid (mRNA) profiling] where thousands of genes can be assessed concurrently for mRNA expression and then patterns within these gene expression profiles examined by statistical analyses such as hierarchical clustering. Because AQUA analysis produces continuous expression scores, these types of analyses can now be extended to protein expression in tissue. An example is given in Figures 11.20A and 11.20B where 35 ER-related proteins were assessed by AQUA analysis on a breast cancer cohort ($n = 161$) and analyzed by unsupervised hierarchical clustering (Dolled-Filhart et al., 2006b). Four predominant patient clusters can be observed (Fig. 11.20A), and these patient clusters have differential survival characteristics (Fig. 11.20B).

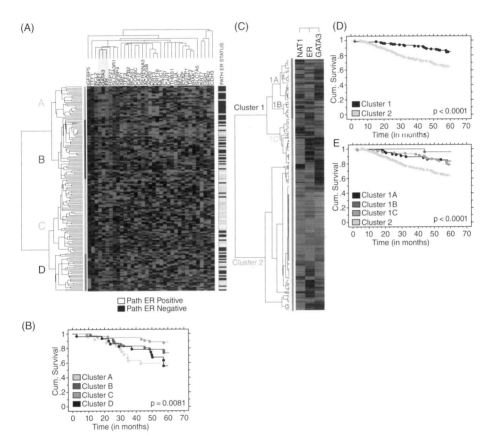

Figure 11.20. Hierarchical clustering analysis using AQUA analysis in breast cancer. (A) Unsupervised hierarchical clustering of 35 ER-related genes on 161 tumor samples with indicated cluster groupings. (B) KM survival analysis indicating a significant differentiation ($p = 0.0083$) of cluster groupings with respect to 5-year disease-specific survival. (C) Unsupervised hierarchical clustering analysis of ER and two most closely related genes from (A) and indicated cluster groupings (indicated: two main clusters, 1 and 2; and subsequent subcluster 1 groupings). (D, E) KM survival analysis of main clusters and cluster 1 subclusters indicate a significant association with 5-year disease-specific survival. (Adapted from Dolled-Filhart et al., 2006b.) See insert for color representation of this figure.

Another example of multiparametric analysis is given in Figure 11.21. In this analysis, four proteins in the AKT pathway (PTEN, mTOR, phosphor-mTOR, and phospho-AKT) were assessed by AQUA analysis in a cohort of glioblastoma tumors ($n = 110$); then their interaction as continuous variables with survival and each other was assesses by Cox proportional hazards modeling. The overall model with all four proteins was significant; however, only two proteins (PTEN and pAKT) contributed significantly to the model (Fig. 11.21; top table). The optimal model with only these two proteins is highly significant ($p = 0.009$). Using the optimal model, a Cox proportional hazards model can be used to calculate overall risk of future patients on a continuum (Fig. 11.21, bottom right panel) much like the model established by Genomic Health with its OncotypeDx diagnostic for early-stage breast cancer patients (Paik, 2007). The power of this type of analysis also comes from the use of AQUA data as a continuous variable in the actual survival analysis, rather than determining a cut point.

Model	Marker	HR	95 CI	Marker p	Model p
All	PTEN	0.44	0.24–0.80	0.007	
	mTOR	0.84	0.43–1.64	0.604	0.013
	pmTOR	0.70	0.45–1.10	0.122	
	pAKT	7.41	2.30–23.90	0.001	
Optimal	PTEN	0.47	0.26–0.86	0.015	0.009
	pAKT	4.38	1.62–11.85	0.004	

Cox Proportional Hazards Model
Risk = (1.48 * pAKT) – (0.75 * PTEN)

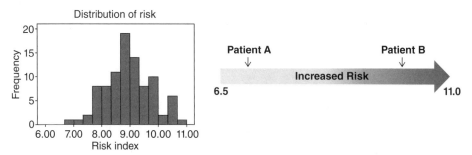

Figure 11.21. Results of Cox proportional hazards model using continuous AQUA scores. Four markers (PTEN, pAKT, mTOR, and pmTOR) were analyzed in a TMA cohort of glioblastoma ($n = 110$). Table indicates two models (all and optimal) with described hazard ratios and associated *p* values for each marker and overall model. A Cox proportional hazards model equation to calculate overall risk was formulated using the optimal model coefficients. (B) Distribution of risk based on indicated model. (C) Schematic representation of possible model diagnostic for determining patient risk based on AQUA scoring of a PTEN/pAKT diagnostic test.

11.6.1. Pathway Diagnostics

Targeted molecular therapeutics are typically looking to shut down specific cellular pathways within the tumor cell. If these therapies are to be successful, patients must be identified that will have the greatest chance to respond to the therapy. Response to therapy will predominantly be determined by whether a patient has that specific pathway activated within his or her tumor (Weinstein and Joe, 2008, 2006). Therefore, assessment of pathway activation will be critical for determining what patients will respond to a given treatment. Because assessment of pathway activation will most likely involve quantification and association of multiple protein biomarkers as well as measurements of protein translocations, as has been demonstrated in this chapter, AQUA analysis is well suited for this task. An example of such a diagnostic would be assessment of EGFR pathway activation for prediction of response to EGFR-targeted therapeutics by not only quantification of EGFR protein expression but also expression and localization, as well as quantitative association thereof, of downstream effector molecules such as ERK, STAT, and/or AKT.

11.7. APPLICATION OF AQUA TECHNOLOGY TO DRUG DISCOVERY AND COMPANION DIAGNOSTICS

The promise of personalized medicine lies in the further discovery of targeted molecular therapeutics. Targeted molecular therapeutics, however, will not be of benefit for every patient with a given indication, thus the requirement for robust clinical diagnostics that enable patient selection. Two classic examples of this are that for ER and HER2. Roughly 60% of breast cancer cases are ER positive (Harvey et al., 1999) and 15 to 20% of cases are HER2 positive (Natali et al., 1990). In the case of HER2, only 10% of all-comers will respond to HER2, but with the development of a companion diagnostic (HercepTest, DAKO, Carpinteria, CA) to identify patients that express the receptor, that response rate jumped to 50%, thus ensuring the success of the drug (Paik et al., 2002). Therefore it is quite apparent that the development of diagnostics that can differentiate patients that will respond to a given therapeutic is paramount for the ongoing success of drug discovery. This concept is outlined in Figure 11.22 using AQUA technology as an example of how to bring about success.

As has been demonstrated to this point, the AQUA platform is a powerful technology whereby robust clinical diagnostics, both companion and standard of care, could be developed. Although development of single biomarker diagnostics has potential in the short term, it is the ability of the AQUA platform to provide multiparametric analysis of biomarker expression that, we feel, promises the greatest potential. As discussed above, most molecular therapeutics in development are targeting specific cellular pathways and only tumors that rely, or are addicted to this pathway for their growth and survival, will most likely respond to the drug. The ability of the AQUA platform to not only quantify but localize

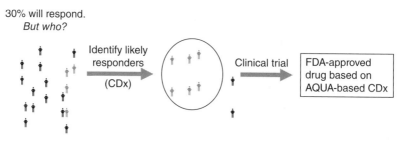

Figure 11.22. Role of companion diagnostics in drug development and approval. In a given population of patients, only a certain percentage of those will respond to a given drug. One of the critical steps today in drug development is the identification of likely responders through the use of companion diagnostics. Identification of likely responders before a clinical trial increases the chances of success and FDA approval.

expression of multiple biomarkers and return meaningful expression data that can be analyzed in a truly multiparametric fashion provides the greatest opportunity to assess pathway activation (or inactivation) in tumor tissue.

With respect to drug discovery, we believe AQUA technology can be employed on two major fronts. First, AQUA technology can be employed to examine drug efficacy and/or potentially drug toxicity. This could be accomplished in both animal and human trials. An example of its use in animal models is given in Figure 11.23 where AQUA scores for a given biomarker were assessed with respect to drug plasma levels in mice. As plasma levels of the drug increase (black line), AQUA scores for the chosen biomarker concomitantly decrease. These data not only demonstrate that the drug is working but also give a sense of effective dosage. This same paradigm could be employed in human trials in the presurgical and/or neoadjuvant setting whereby biomarker expression can be assessed in biopsy tissue. Then, followed by a treatment period, biomarker expression can be assessed in resected tissue or a second biopsy to determine whether the drug is showing efficacy based on AQUA measurements of a given biomarker(s). Because AQUA technology is strictly quantitative, small changes in biomarker expression can be quantified that lead to highly resolved determination of drug efficacy. This could be of particular importance in the determination of the minimal effective dose, thus maximizing efficacy and minimizing toxicity.

Second is the development of companion diagnostics. As discussed above, the success of targeted molecular therapeutics relies on the accurate and precise identification of patients that are most likely going to respond to a given drug. The development of companion diagnostics using AQUA technology would come in two phases. First, experiments examining quantitative expression of a multitude of biomarkers (i.e., multiple pathway activation/inactivation assessment in the case of an EGFR-targeted therapeutic) in retrospective clinical trial cohorts and/or historical cohorts where the outcome and response data have already been collected will be performed looking for quantitative association of

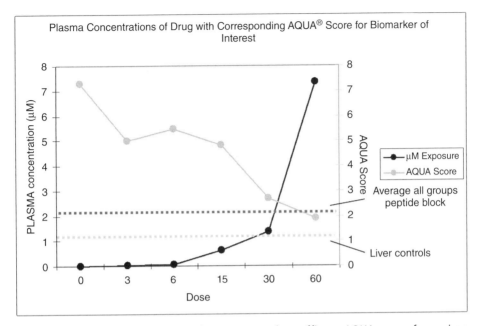

Figure 11.23. Use of AQUA technology to assess drug efficacy. AQUA scores for a given biomarker (gray line) are shown to inversely correlated with plasma levels of a given drug (black line). This demonstrates the ability of AQUA analysis to potentially measure drug efficacy.

biomarkers with response and/or outcome. Once a potential biomarker or set of biomarkers has been identified, prospective clinical trials can be designed incorporating the use of these biomarkers to segregate patients and enrich the population of likely responders. And as with the case with HER2, the ability to identify patients that will most likely respond going into a clinical trial can ensure the success and, ultimately, Food and Drug Administration approval of the drug.

11.8. SUMMARY AND CONCLUSIONS

In summary, we have demonstrated that AQUA technology is a powerful tool for molecular pathology and ultimately a tool that can enhance drug discovery and development. We demonstrated the function of the AQUA technology as an objective and standardized platform whereby robust clinical diagnostics could be developed. It is important to note that because AQUA technology employs routine immunostaining techniques on formalin-fixed paraffin-embedded tissue sections, its adoption into current pathology laboratory infrastructure is simplified. We also summarized the ability of AQUA analysis as a tool for strict quantification and to localization of protein expression in tissue allowing for discovery of biomarkers that cannot be discerned using traditional technologies. Furthermore, because of the continuous nature of AQUA data, enhanced statistical and multiparametric type of analyses can be performed leading to more robust diagnostics. For the advent of personalized medicine and targeted molecular therapeutics, the development of robust clinical diagnostics will be essential. In conclusion, the AQUA platform has significant potential for the development of companion diagnostics that can facilitate drug discovery and adoption in the clinic leading to greater success in the treatment of disease.

REFERENCES

Arpino, G., Green, S. J., Allred, D. C., Lew, D., Martino, S., Osborne, C. K., and Elledge, R. M. (2004). HER-2 amplification, HER-1 expression, and tamoxifen response in estrogen receptor-positive metastatic breast cancer: A southwest oncology group study. *Clin. Cancer Res.* 10:5670–5676.

Arpino, G., Weiss, H., Lee, A. V., Schiff, R., De Placido, S., Osborne, C. K., and Elledge, R. M. (2005). Estrogen receptor-positive, progesterone receptor-negative breast cancer: Association with growth factor receptor expression and tamoxifen resistance. *J. Natl. Cancer Inst.* 97:1254–1261.

Baker, A. F., Dragovich, T., Ihle, N. T., Williams, R., Fenoglio-Preiser, C., and Powis, G. (2005). Stability of phosphoprotein as a biological marker of tumor signaling 1. *Clin. Cancer Res.* 11:4338–4340.

Bamias, A., Yu, Z., Weinberger, P. M., Markakis, S., Kowalski, D., Camp, R. L., Rimm, D. L., Dimopoulos, M. A., and Psyrri, A. (2006). Automated quantitative analysis of DCC tumor suppressor protein in ovarian cancer tissue microarray shows association with beta-catenin levels and outcome in patients with epithelial ovarian cancer. *Ann. Oncol.* 17:1797–1802.

Bepler, G., Sharma, S., Cantor, A., Gautam, A., Haura, E., Simon, G., Sharma, A., Sommers, E., and Robinson, L. (2004). RRM1 and PTEN as prognostic parameters for overall and disease-free survival in patients with non-small-cell lung cancer. *J. Clin. Oncol.* 22:1878–1885.

Bepler, G., Kusmartseva, I., Sharma, S., Gautam, A., Cantor, A., Sharma, A., and Simon, G. (2006). RRM1 modulated in vitro and in vivo efficacy of gemcitabine and platinum in non-small-cell lung cancer. *J. Clin. Oncol.* 24:4731–4737.

Berger, A. J., Kluger, H. M., Li, N., Kielhorn, E., Halaban, R., Ronai, Z., and Rimm, D. L. (2003). Subcellular localization of activating transcription factor 2 in melanoma specimens predicts patient survival 25. *Cancer Res.* 63:8103–8107.

Berger, A. J., Camp, R. L., DiVito, K. A., Kluger, H. M., Halaban, R., and Rimm, D. L. (2004). Automated quantitative analysis of HDM2 expression in malignant melanoma shows association with early-stage disease and improved outcome 11. *Cancer Res.* 64:8767–8772.

Berger, A. J., Davis, D. W., Tellez, C., Prieto, V. G., Gershenwald, J. E., Johnson, M. M., Rimm, D. L., and Bar-Eli, M. (2005). Automated quantitative analysis of activator protein-2alpha subcellular expression in melanoma tissue microarrays correlates with survival prediction. *Cancer Res.* 65:11185–11192.

Bova, G. S., Parmigiani, G., Epstein, J. I., Wheeler, T., Mucci, N. R., and Rubin, M. A. (2001). Web-based tissue microarray image data analysis: Initial validation testing through prostate cancer Gleason grading 1. *Hum. Pathol.* 32:417–427.

Calhoun, R., Jablons, D., Lau, D., and Gandara, D. R. (2008). Adjuvant treatment of stage IB NSCLC: The problem of stage subset heterogeneity. *Oncology (Williston Park)* 22:511–516; discussion 516, 521–513.

Camp, R. L., Charette, L. A., and Rimm, D. L. (2000). Validation of tissue microarray technology in breast carcinoma. *Lab. Invest.* 80:1943–1949.

Camp, R. L., Chung, G. G., and Rimm, D. L. (2002). Automated subcellular localization and quantification of protein expression in tissue microarrays. *Nat. Med.* 8:1323–1327.

Camp, R. L., Dolled-Filhart, M., King, B. L., and Rimm, D. L. (2003). Quantitative analysis of breast cancer tissue microarrays shows that both high and normal levels of HER2 expression are associated with poor outcome. *Cancer Res.* 63:1445–1448.

Camp, R. L., Dolled-Filhart, M., and Rimm, D. L. (2004). X-tile: A new bio-informatics tool for biomarker assessment and outcome-based cut-point optimization. *Clin. Cancer Res.* 10:7252–7259.

Chung, G. G., Zerkowski, M. P., Ocal, I. T., Dolled-Filhart, M., Kang, J. Y., Psyrri, A., Camp, R. L., and Rimm, D. L. (2004). Beta-Catenin and p53 analyses of a breast carcinoma tissue microarray. *Cancer* 100:2084–2092.

Chung, G. G., Yoon, H. H., Zerkowski, M. P., Ghosh, S., Thomas, L., Harigopal, M., Charette, L. A., Salem, R. R., Camp, R. L., Rimm, D. L., Burtness, B. A. (2006). Vascular endothelial growth factor, FLT-1, and FLK-1 analysis in a pancreatic cancer tissue microarray. *Cancer* 106:1677–1684.

Chung, G. G., Zerkowski, M. P., Ghosh, S., Camp, R. L., and Rimm, D. L. (2007). Quantitative analysis of estrogen receptor heterogeneity in breast cancer. *Lab. Invest.* 87:662–669.

Cobleigh, M. A., Vogel, C. L., Tripathy, D., Robert, N. J., Scholl, S., Fehrenbacher, L., Wolter, J. M., Paton, V., Shak, S., Lieberman, G., Slamon, D. J. (1999). Multinational study of the efficacy and safety of humanized anti-HER2 monoclonal antibody in women who have HER2-overexpressing metastatic breast cancer that has progressed after chemotherapy for metastatic disease. *J. Clin. Oncol.* 17:2639–2648.

Divito, K. A., Berger, A. J., Camp, R. L., Dolled-Filhart, M., Rimm, D. L., and Kluger, H. M. (2004a). Automated quantitative analysis of tissue microarrays reveals an association between high Bcl-2 expression and improved outcome in melanoma. *Cancer Res.* 64:8773–8777.

DiVito, K. A., Berger, A. J., Camp, R. L., Dolled-Filhart, M., Rimm, D. L., and Kluger, H. M. (2004b). Automated quantitative analysis of tissue microarrays reveals an association between high Bcl-2 expression and improved outcome in melanoma. *Cancer Res.* 64:8773–8777.

Dolled-Filhart, M., McCabe, A., Giltnane, J., Cregger, M., Camp, R. L., and Rimm, D. L. (2006a). Quantitative in situ analysis of beta-catenin expression in breast cancer shows decreased expression is associated with poor outcome. *Cancer Res.* 66:5487–5494.

Dolled-Filhart, M., Ryden, L., Cregger, M., Jirstrom, K., Harigopal, M., Camp, R. L., and Rimm, D. L. (2006b). Classification of breast cancer using genetic algorithms and tissue microarrays. *Clin. Cancer Res.* 12:6459–6468.

Dowsett, M., Houghton, J., Iden, C., Salter, J., Farndon, J., A'Hern, R., Sainsbury, R., and Baum, M. (2006). Benefit from adjuvant tamoxifen therapy in primary breast cancer patients according oestrogen receptor, progesterone receptor, EGF receptor and HER2 status. *Ann. Oncol.* 17:818–826.

Dowsett, M., Hanna, W. M., Kockx, M., Penault-Llorca, F., Ruschoff, J., Gutjahr, T., Habben, K., and van de Vijver, M. J. (2007). Standardization of HER2 testing: Results of an international proficiency-testing ring study. *Mod. Pathol.* 20:584–591.

Early Breast Cancer Trialists' Collaborative Group (1998). Tamoxifen for early breast cancer: An overview of the randomised trials. *Lancet* 351:1451–1467.

Gautam, A., Li, Z. R., and Bepler, G. (2003). RRM1-induced metastasis suppression through PTEN-regulated pathways. *Oncogene* 22:2135–2142.

Giltnane, J. M., Murren, J. R., Rimm, D. L., and King, B. L. (2006). AQUA and FISH analysis of HER-2/neu expression and amplification in a small cell lung carcinoma tissue microarray. *Histopathology* 49:161–169.

Giltnane, J. M., Ryden, L., Cregger, M., Bendahl, P. O., Jirstrom, K., and Rimm, D. L. (2007). Quantitative measurement of epidermal growth factor receptor is a negative predictive factor for tamoxifen response in hormone receptor positive premenopausal breast cancer. *J. Clin. Oncol.* 25:3007–3014.

Gustavson, M. D., Bourke-Martin, B., Reilly, D. M., Cregger, M., Williams, C., Tedeschi, G., Pinard, R., and Christiansen, J. (2009a). Development of an Unsupervised Pixel-based Clustering Algorithm for Compartmentalization of Immunohistochemical Expression Using Automated Quantitative Analysis. *Appl Immunohistochem Mol Morphol.* (in press)

Gustavson, M. D., Bourke-Martin, B., Reilly, D. M., Cregger, M., Williams, C., Mayotte, J., Zerkowski, M., Tedeschi, G., Pinard, R., and Christiansen, J. (2009b). Standardization of HER2 testing: using AQUA to provide a standardized and quantitative HER2 immunohistochemical result. *Arch Pathol Lab Med.* (in press).

Gustavson, M. D., Molinaro, A. M., Tedeschi, G., Camp, R. L., and Rimm, D. L. (2008). AQUA analysis of thymidylate synthase reveals localization to be a key prognostic biomarker in 2 large cohorts of colorectal carcinoma. *Arch Pathol Lab Med* 132:1746–1752.

Hameed, O., Adams, A. L., Baker, A. C., Balmer, N. E., Bell, W. C., Burford, H. N., Chhieng, D. C., Jhala, N. C., Klein, M. J., and Winokur, T. (2008). Using a higher cutoff for the percentage of HER2+ cells decreases interobserver variability in the interpretation of HER2 immunohistochemical analysis. *Am J Clin Pathol* 130:425–427.

Harigopal, M., Berger, A. J., Camp, R. L., Rimm, D. L., and Kluger, H. M. (2005). Automated quantitative analysis of E-cadherin expression in lymph node metastases is predictive of survival in invasive ductal breast cancer. *Clin. Cancer Res.* 11:4083–4089.

Harigopal, M., Heymann, J., Ghosh, S., Anagnostou, V., Camp, R. L., and Rimm, D. L. (2008). Estrogen receptor co-activator (AIB1) protein expression by automated quantitative analysis (AQUA) in a breast cancer tissue microarray and association with patient outcome. *Breast Cancer Res Treat* 115:77–85.

Harvey, J. M., Clark, G. M., Osborne, C. K., and Allred, D. C. (1999). Estrogen receptor status by immunohistochemistry is superior to the ligand-binding assay for predicting response to adjuvant endocrine therapy in breast cancer. *J. Clin. Oncol.* 17:1474–1481.

Hofmann, M., Stoss, O., Gaiser, T., Kneitz, H., Heinmoller, P., Gutjahr, T., Kaufmann, M., Henkel, T., and Ruschoff, J. (2008). Central HER2 IHC and FISH analysis in a trastuzumab (Herceptin) phase II monotherapy study: Assessment of test sensitivity and impact of chromosome 17 polysomy. *J. Clin. Pathol.* 61:89–94.

Hoos, A., Urist, M. J., Stojadinovic, A., Mastorides, S., Dudas, M. E., Leung, D. H., Kuo, D., Brennan, M. F., Lewis, J. J., and Cordon-Cardo, C. (2001). Validation of tissue microarrays for immunohistochemical profiling of cancer specimens using the example of human fibroblastic tumors. *Am. J. Pathol.* 158:1245–1251.

Hsu, C. Y., Kurman, R. J., Vang, R., Wang, T. L., Baak, J., and Shih Ie, M. (2005). Nuclear size distinguishes low- from high-grade ovarian serous carcinoma and predicts outcome. *Hum. Pathol.* 36:1049–1054.

Hynes, N. E., and Lane, H. A. (2005). ERBB receptors and cancer: The complexity of targeted inhibitors. *Nat. Rev. Cancer* 5:341–354.

Kato, H., Fujimura, M., Kumabe, T., Ishioka, C., Kanamaru, R., and Yoshimoto, T. (2004). PTEN gene mutation and high MIB-1 labeling index may contribute to dissemination in patients with glioblastoma. *J. Clin. Neurosci.* 11:37–41.

Khan, M. Z., Haleem, A., Al Hassani, H., and Kfoury, H. (2003). Cytopathological grading, as a predictor of histopathological grade, in ductal carcinoma (NOS) of breast, on air-dried Diff-Quik smears. *Diagn. Cytopathol.* 29:185–193.

Kraus, J. A., Glesmann, N., Beck, M., Krex, D., Klockgether, T., Schackert, G., and Schlegel, U. (2000). Molecular analysis of the PTEN, TP53 and CDKN2A tumor suppressor genes in long-term survivors of glioblastoma multiforme. *J. Neurooncol.* 48:89–94.

Liu, J., Schmitz, J. C., Lin, X., Tai, N., Yan, W., Farrell, M., Bailly, M., Chen, T., and Chu, E. (2002). Thymidylate synthase as a translational regulator of cellular gene expression. *Biochim. Biophys. Acta* 1587:174–182.

McCabe, A., Dolled-Filhart, M., Camp, R. L., and Rimm, D. L. (2005). Automated quantitative analysis (AQUA) of in situ protein expression, antibody concentration, and prognosis. *J. Natl. Cancer Inst.* 97:1808–1815.

McCarty, K. S., Jr., Miller, L. S., Cox, E. B., Konrath, J., and McCarty, K. S., Sr. (1985). Estrogen receptor analyses. Correlation of biochemical and immunohistochemical methods using monoclonal antireceptor antibodies. *Arch. Pathol. Lab. Med.* 109:716–721.

McCarthy, M. M., Sznol, M., DiVito, K. A., Camp, R. L., Rimm, D. L., and Kluger, H. M. (2005). Evaluating the expression and prognostic value of TRAIL-R1 and TRAIL-R2 in breast cancer. *Clin. Cancer Res.* 11:5188–5194.

McCarthy, M. M., Pick, E., Kluger, Y., Gould-Rothberg, B., Lazova, R., Camp, R. L., Rimm, D. L., and Kluger, H. M. (2008). HSP90 as a marker of progression in melanoma. *Ann. Oncol.* 19:590–594.

Miller, C. R., and Perry, A. (2007). Glioblastoma. *Arch. Pathol. Lab. Med.* 131: 397–406.

Miller, D. J., Wang, Y., and Kesidis, G. (2008). Emergent unsupervised clustering paradigms with potential application to bioinformatics. *Front. Biosci.* 13:677–690.

Natali, P. G., Nicotra, M. R., Bigotti, A., Venturo, I., Slamon, D. J., Fendly, B. M., and Ullrich, A. (1990). Expression of the p185 encoded by HER2 oncogene in normal and transformed human tissues. *Int. J. Cancer* 45:457–461.

Osborne, C. K. (1998). Tamoxifen in the treatment of breast cancer. *N. Engl. J. Med.* 339:1609–1618.

Paik, S. (2007). Development and clinical utility of a 21-gene recurrence score prognostic assay in patients with early breast cancer treated with tamoxifen. *Oncologist* 12:631–635.

Paik, S., Bryant, J., Tan-Chiu, E., Romond, E., Hiller, W., Park, K., Brown, A., Yothers, G., Anderson, S., Smith, R., Wickerham, D. L., and Wolmark, N. (2002). Real-world performance of HER2 testing—National Surgical Adjuvant Breast and Bowel Project experience. *J. Natl. Cancer Inst.* 94:852–854.

Perez, E. A., Suman, V. J., Davidson, N. E., Martino, S., Kaufman, P. A., Lingle, W. L., Flynn, P. J., Ingle, J. N., Visscher, D., and Jenkins, R. B. (2006). HER2 testing by local, central, and reference laboratories in specimens from the North Central Cancer Treatment Group N9831 intergroup adjuvant trial. *J. Clin. Oncol.* 24:3032–3038.

Pick, E., Kluger, Y., Giltnane, J. M., Moeder, C., Camp, R. L., Rimm, D. L., and Kluger, H. M. (2007). High HSP90 expression is associated with decreased survival in breast cancer. *Cancer Res.* 67:2932–2937.

Pitterle, D. M., Kim, Y. C., Jolicoeur, E. M., Cao, Y., O'Briant, K. C., and Bepler, G. (1999). Lung cancer and the human gene for ribonucleotide reductase subunit M1 (RRM1). *Mamm. Genome* 10:916–922.

Pozner-Moulis, S., Pappas, D. J., and Rimm, D. L. (2006). Met, the hepatocyte growth factor receptor, localizes to the nucleus in cells at low density. *Cancer Res.* 66:7976–7982.

Psyrri, A., Bamias, A., Yu, Z., Weinberger, P. M., Kassar, M., Markakis, S., Kowalski, D., Efstathiou, E., Camp, R. L., Rimm, D. L., and Dimopoulos, M. A. (2005a). Subcellular localization and protein levels of cyclin-dependent kinase inhibitor p27 independently predict for survival in epithelial ovarian cancer. *Clin. Cancer Res.* 11:8384–8390.

Psyrri, A., Kassar, M., Yu, Z., Bamias, A., Weinberger, P. M., Markakis, S., Kowalski, D., Camp, R. L., Rimm, D. L., and Dimopoulos, M. A. (2005b). Effect of epidermal growth factor receptor expression level on survival in patients with epithelial ovarian cancer. *Clin. Cancer Res.* 11:8637–8643.

Rimm, D. L. (2006). What brown cannot do for you. *Nat. Biotechnol.* 24:914–916.

Rimm, D. L., Camp, R. L., Charette, L. A., Costa, J., Olsen, D. A., and Reiss, M. (2001). Tissue microarray: A new technology for amplification of tissue resources. *Cancer J.* 7:24–31.

Roche, P. C., Suman, V. J., Jenkins, R. B., Davidson, N. E., Martino, S., Kaufman, P. A., Addo, F. K., Murphy, B., Ingle, J. N., and Perez, E. A. (2002). Concordance between local and central laboratory HER2 testing in the breast intergroup trial N9831. *J. Natl. Cancer Inst.* 94:855–857.

Rothberg, B. E., Moeder, C. B., Kluger, H., Halaban, R., Elder, D. E., Murphy, G. F., Lazar, A., Prieto, V., Duncan, L. M., and Rimm, D. L. (2008). Nuclear to nonnuclear Pmel17/gp100 expression (HMB45 staining) as a discriminator between benign and malignant melanocytic lesions. *Mod. Pathol.* 21:1121–1129.

Sansal, I., and Sellers, W. R. (2004). The biology and clinical relevance of the PTEN tumor suppressor pathway. *J. Clin. Oncol.* 22:2954–2963.

Simon, G. R., Sharma, S., Cantor, A., Smith, P., and Bepler, G. (2005). ERCC1 expression is a predictor of survival in resected patients with non-small cell lung cancer. *Chest* 127:978–983.

Slamon, D. J., Leyland-Jones, B., Shak, S., Fuchs, H., Paton, V., Bajamonde, A., Fleming, T., Eiermann, W., Wolter, J., Pegram, M., Baselga, J., Norton, L. (2001). Use of chemotherapy plus a monoclonal antibody against HER2 for metastatic breast cancer that overexpresses HER2. *N. Engl. J. Med.* 344:783–792.

Smith, J. S., Tachibana, I., Passe, S. M., Huntley, B. K., Borell, T. J., Iturria, N., O'Fallon, J. R., Schaefer, P. L., Scheithauer, B. W., James, C. D., Buckner, J. C., Jenkins, R. B. (2001). PTEN mutation, EGFR amplification, and outcome in patients with anaplastic astrocytoma and glioblastoma multiforme. *J. Natl. Cancer Inst.* 93:1246–1256.

Taylor, C. R., and Levenson, R. M. (2006). Quantification of immunohistochemistry— issues concerning methods, utility and semiquantitative assessment II. *Histopathology* 49:411–424.

Vogel, C. L., Cobleigh, M. A., Tripathy, D., Gutheil, J. C., Harris, L. N., Fehrenbacher, L., Slamon, D. J., Murphy, M., Novotny, W. F., Burchmore, M., Shak, S., Stewart, S. J., Press, M. (2002). Efficacy and safety of trastuzumab as a single agent in first-line treatment of HER2-overexpressing metastatic breast cancer. *J. Clin. Oncol.* 20:719–726.

Walker, R. A. (2006). Quantification of immunohistochemistry—issues concerning methods, utility and semiquantitative assessment I. *Histopathology* 49:406–410.

Weinstein, I. B., and Joe, A. K. (2006). Mechanisms of disease: Oncogene addiction— a rationale for molecular targeting in cancer therapy. *Nat. Clin. Pract. Oncol.* 3:448–457.

Weinstein, I. B., and Joe, A. (2008). Oncogene addiction. *Cancer Res.* 68:3077–3080; discussion 3080.

Wolff, A. C., Hammond, M. E., Schwartz, J. N., Hagerty, K. L., Allred, D. C., Cote, R. J., Dowsett, M., Fitzgibbons, P. L., Hanna, W. M., Langer, A., McShane, L. M., Paik, S., Pegram, M. D., Perez, E. A., Press, M. F., Rhodes, A., Sturgeon, C., Taube, S. E., Tubbs, R., Vance, G. H., van de Vijver, M., Wheeler, J. M., Hayes, D. F. (2007). American Society of Clinical Oncology/College of American Pathologists Guideline Recommendations for Human Epidermal Growth Factor Receptor 2 Testing in Breast Cancer. *Arch. Pathol. Lab. Med.* 131:18.

Yu, Z., Weinberger, P. M., Haffty, B. G., Sasaki, C., Zerillo, C., Joe, J., Kowalski, D., Dziura, J., Camp, R. L., Rimm, D. L., Psyrri, A. (2005a). Cyclin d1 is a valuable prognostic marker in oropharyngeal squamous cell carcinoma. *Clin. Cancer Res.* 11:1160–1166.

Yu, Z., Weinberger, P. M., Provost, E., Haffty, B. G., Sasaki, C., Joe, J., Camp, R. L., Rimm, D. L., and Psyrri, A. (2005b). Beta-Catenin functions mainly as an adhesion molecule in patients with squamous cell cancer of the head and neck. *Clin. Cancer Res.* 11:2471–2477.

Zerkowski, M. P., Camp, R. L., Burtness, B. A., Rimm, D. L., and Chung, G. G. (2007). Quantitative analysis of breast cancer tissue microarrays shows high cox-2 expression is associated with poor outcome. *Cancer Invest.* 25:19–26.

Zheng, Z., Chen, T., Li, X., Haura, E., Sharma, A., and Bepler, G. (2007). DNA synthesis and repair genes RRM1 and ERCC1 in lung cancer. *N. Engl. J. Med.* 356:800–808.

INDEX